Mandell, Douglas, and Bennett's
Infectious Disease
ESSENTIALS

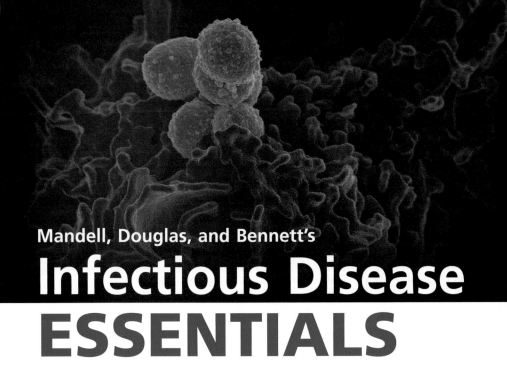

Mandell, Douglas, and Bennett's
Infectious Disease
ESSENTIALS

JOHN E. BENNETT, MD, MACP
Adjunct Professor of Medicine
Uniformed Services University of the Health Sciences
F. Edward Hebert School of Medicine
Bethesda, Maryland

RAPHAEL DOLIN, MD
Maxwell Finland Professor of Medicine (Microbiology and Molecular Genetics)
Harvard Medical School;
Attending Physician
Beth Israel Deaconess Medical Center;
Brigham and Women's Hospital
Boston, Massachusetts

MARTIN J. BLASER, MD
Muriel G. and George W. Singer Professor of Translational Medicine
Professor of Microbiology
Director, Human Microbiome Program
Departments of Medicine and Microbiology
New York University School of Medicine
Langone Medical Center
New York, New York

ELSEVIER

ELSEVIER

1600 John F. Kennedy Blvd.
Ste 1800
Philadelphia, PA 19103-2899

Notices

Knowledge and best practice in this field are constantly changing. As new research and experience broaden our understanding, changes in research methods, professional practices, or medical treatment may become necessary.

Practitioners and researchers must always rely on their own experience and knowledge in evaluating and using any information, methods, compounds, or experiments described herein. In using such information or methods they should be mindful of their own safety and the safety of others, including parties for whom they have a professional responsibility.

With respect to any drug or pharmaceutical products identified, readers are advised to check the most current information provided (i) on procedures featured or (ii) by the manufacturer of each product to be administered, to verify the recommended dose or formula, the method and duration of administration, and contraindications. It is the responsibility of practitioners, relying on their own experience and knowledge of their patients, to make diagnoses, to determine dosages and the best treatment for each individual patient, and to take all appropriate safety precautions.

To the fullest extent of the law, neither the Publisher nor the authors, contributors, or editors, assume any liability for any injury and/or damage to persons or property as a matter of products liability, negligence or otherwise, or from any use or operation of any methods, products, instructions, or ideas contained in the material herein.

Library of Congress Cataloging-in-Publication Data
Names: Bennett, John E. (John Eugene), 1933- , editor. | Dolin, Raphael, editor. | Blaser, Martin J., editor.
Title: Mandell, Douglas, and Bennett's infectious disease essentials / [edited by] John E. Bennett, Raphael Dolin, Martin J. Blaser.
Other titles: Infectious disease essentials
Description: Philadelphia, PA : Elsevier, [2017]
Identifiers: LCCN 2015048664 | ISBN 9780323431019 (paperback : alk. paper)
Subjects: | MESH: Communicable Diseases | Handbooks
Classification: LCC RA643 | NLM WC 39 | DDC 616.9–dc23 LC record available at http://lccn.loc.gov/2015048664

Senior Content Strategist: Suzanne Toppy
Senior Content Development Manager: Taylor Ball
Publishing Services Manager: Catherine Jackson
Book Production Specialist: Kristine Feeherty
Design Direction: Renee Duenow

Printed in the United States of America

Last digit is the print number: 9 8 7 6 5 4 3

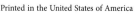

Working together
to grow libraries in
developing countries

www.elsevier.com • www.bookaid.org

Contributors

Fredrick M. Abrahamian, DO
Professor of Medicine, David Geffen School of
Medicine at UCLA, Los Angeles, California;
Director of Education, Department of Emergency
Medicine, Olive View–UCLA Medical Center,
Sylmar, California
Bites

Ban Mishu Allos, MD
Associate Professor, Departments of Medicine
and Preventive Medicine, Division of Infectious
Diseases, Vanderbilt University School of
Medicine, Nashville, Tennessee
Campylobacter jejuni and Related Species

Michael A. Apicella, MD
Professor and Head, Department of Microbiology,
University of Iowa Carver College of Medicine,
Iowa City, Iowa
Neisseria meningitidis; Neisseria gonorrhoeae
(Gonorrhea)

Kevin L. Ard, MD, MPH
Instructor in Medicine, Harvard Medical School;
Associate Physician, Department of Medicine,
Brigham and Women's Hospital, Boston,
Massachusetts
Pulmonary Manifestations of Human
Immunodeficiency Virus Infection

Cesar A. Arias, MD, MSc, PhD
Associate Professor of Medicine, Department of
Internal Medicine, Division of Infectious Diseases
and Department of Microbiology and Molecular
Genetics, University of Texas Medical School at
Houston, Houston, Texas; Director, Molecular
Genetics and Antimicrobial Resistance Unit,
Universidad El Bosque, Bogota, Colombia
Enterococcus Species, Streptococcus gallolyticus
Group, and Leuconostoc Species

Michael H. Augenbraun, MD
Professor of Medicine, Chief, Division of
Infectious Diseases, Department of Medicine,
SUNY Downstate Medical Center, Brooklyn,
New York
Genital Skin and Mucous Membrane Lesions;
Urethritis; Vulvovaginitis and Cervicitis

Francisco Averhoff, MD, MPH
Division of Viral Hepatitis, National Center for
HIV/AIDS, Viral Hepatitis, STD, and TB
Prevention, Centers for Disease Control and
Prevention, Atlanta, Georgia
Hepatitis A Virus

Dimitri T. Azar, MD, MBA
Dean and B.A. Field Chair of Ophthalmologic
Research, Distinguished Professor of
Ophthalmology, Pharmacology, and
Bioengineering, College of Medicine, University
of Illinois at Chicago, Chicago, Illinois
Microbial Conjunctivitis; Microbial Keratitis

Larry M. Baddour, MD
Professor of Medicine, Mayo Clinic College of
Medicine; Consultant, Infectious Diseases, Mayo
Clinic, Rochester, Minnesota
Prosthetic Valve Endocarditis

Carol J. Baker, MD
Professor of Pediatrics, Molecular Virology, and
Microbiology, Department of Pediatrics,
Infectious Diseases Section, Baylor College of
Medicine; Attending Physician, Texas Children's
Hospital, Houston, Texas
Streptococcus agalactiae (Group B Streptococcus)

Ronald C. Ballard, MSB, PhD
Associate Director for Laboratory Science, Center
for Global Health, Centers for Disease Control
and Prevention, Atlanta, Georgia
Klebsiella granulomatis (Donovanosis, Granuloma
Inguinale)

Scott D. Barnes, MD
Chief, Warfighter Refractive Eye Surgery Clinic,
Womack Army Medical Center, Fort Bragg,
North Carolina
Microbial Conjunctivitis; Microbial Keratitis

Dan H. Barouch, MD, PhD
Professor of Medicine, Harvard Medical School;
Director, Center for Virology and Vaccine
Research, Staff Physician, Beth Israel Deaconess
Medical Center; Associate Physician, Brigham
and Women's Hospital, Boston, Massachusetts
Adenoviruses

Alan D. Barrett, PhD
Director, Sealy Center for Vaccine Development,
Professor, Departments of Pathology and
Microbiology & Immunology, University of Texas
Medical Branch, Galveston, Texas
Flaviviruses (Dengue, Yellow Fever, Japanese
Encephalitis, West Nile Encephalitis, St. Louis
Encephalitis, Tick-Borne Encephalitis, Kyasanur
Forest Disease, Alkhurma Hemorrhagic Fever,
Zika)

Miriam Baron Barshak, MD
Assistant Professor of Medicine, Harvard Medical
School; Associate Physician, Department of
Medicine, Massachusetts General Hospital,
Boston, Massachusetts
Pancreatic Infection

Sridhar V. Basavaraju, MD
Centers for Disease Control and Prevention,
Atlanta, Georgia
Transfusion- and Transplantation-Transmitted
Infections

Byron E. Batteiger, MD
Professor of Medicine, Microbiology, and
Immunology, Division of Infectious Diseases,
Indiana University School of Medicine,
Indianapolis, Indiana
Chlamydia trachomatis (Trachoma, Genital
Infections, Perinatal Infections, and
Lymphogranuloma Venereum)

Stephen G. Baum, MD
Professor of Medicine, Microbiology, and
Immunology, Albert Einstein College of
Medicine, Bronx, New York
Mumps Virus

Arnold S. Bayer, MD
Professor of Medicine, Department of Internal
Medicine, David Geffen School of Medicine at
UCLA, Los Angeles, California; Associate Chief,
Adult Infectious Diseases, Department of Internal
Medicine, Harbor-UCLA Medical Center; Senior
Investigator, St. John's Cardiovascular Research
Center, Los Angeles Biomedical Research
Institute, Torrance, California
Endocarditis and Intravascular Infections

J. David Beckham, MD
Assistant Professor, Departments of Medicine,
Neurology, and Microbiology, Division of
Infectious Diseases, Director, Infectious Disease
Fellowship Training Program, Medical Director,
Occupational Health, University of Colorado
Anschutz Medical Campus, Aurora, Colorado
Encephalitis

Susan E. Beekmann, RN, MPH
University of Iowa Carver College of Medicine,
Iowa City, Iowa
Infections Caused by Percutaneous Intravascular
Devices

Beth P. Bell, MD, MPH
Director, National Center for Emerging and
Zoonotic Infectious Diseases, Centers for Disease
Control and Prevention, Atlanta, Georgia
Hepatitis A Virus

John E. Bennett, MD, MACP
Adjunct Professor of Medicine, Uniformed
Services University of the Health Sciences, F.
Edward Hebert School of Medicine, Bethesda,
Maryland
Chronic Meningitis

Dennis A. Bente, DVM, PhD
Assistant Professor, Department of Microbiology
and Immunology, University of Texas Medical
Branch, Galveston, Texas
California Encephalitis, Hantavirus Pulmonary
Syndrome, and Bunyavirus Hemorrhagic Fevers

Elie F. Berbari, MD
Professor of Medicine, Division of Infectious
Diseases, Mayo Clinic, Rochester, Minnesota
Osteomyelitis

Adarsh Bhimraj, MD
Head, Section of Neurologic Infectious Diseases,
Associate Program Director, Internal Medicine
Residency Program, Cleveland Clinic, Cleveland,
Ohio
Cerebrospinal Fluid Shunt and Drain Infections

Alan L. Bisno, MD
Professor Emeritus, Department of Medicine,
University of Miami Miller School of Medicine;
Staff Physician, Miami Veterans Affairs Medical
Center, Miami, Florida
Nonsuppurative Poststreptococcal Sequelae:
Rheumatic Fever and Glomerulonephritis

Brian G. Blackburn, MD
Clinical Associate Professor, Division of
Infectious Diseases and Geographic Medicine,
Stanford University School of Medicine;
Attending Physician, Department of Internal
Medicine, Division of Infectious Diseases and
Geographic Medicine, Stanford Hospital and
Clinics, Stanford, California
Free-Living Amebae

Lucas S. Blanton, MD
Assistant Professor, Department of Internal
Medicine, Division of Infectious Diseases,
University of Texas Medical Branch, Galveston,
Texas
Rickettsia rickettsii and Other Spotted Fever
Group Rickettsiae (Rocky Mountain Spotted Fever
and Other Spotted Fevers); Rickettsia prowazekii
(Epidemic or Louse-Borne Typhus); Rickettsia typhi
(Murine Typhus)

Martin J. Blaser, MD
Muriel G. and George W. Singer Professor of
Translational Medicine, Professor of
Microbiology, Director, Human Microbiome
Program, Departments of Medicine and
Microbiology, New York University School of
Medicine, Langone Medical Center, New York,
New York
Campylobacter jejuni and Related Species;
Helicobacter pylori and Other Gastric Helicobacter
Species

Thomas P. Bleck, MD
Professor of Neurological Sciences, Neurosurgery,
Medicine, and Anesthesiology, Rush Medical
College; Associate Chief Medical Officer (Critical
Care), Associate Vice President, Director,
Laboratory of Electroencephalography and
Evoked Potentials, Rush University Medical
Center, Chicago, Illinois
Rabies (Rhabdoviruses); Tetanus (Clostridium
tetani); Botulism (Clostridium botulinum)

David A. Bobak, MD
Associate Professor of Medicine, Associate Chair
for Clinical Affairs, Division of Infectious
Diseases and HIV Medicine, Case Western
Reserve University School of Medicine; Director,
Traveler's Healthcare Center, Chair, Health System
Medication Safety and Therapeutics Committee,
Staff Physician, Transplant Infectious Diseases
Clinic, University Hospitals Case Medical Center,
Cleveland, Ohio
Nausea, Vomiting, and Noninflammatory Diarrhea

William Bonnez, MD
Professor of Medicine, Department of Medicine,
Division of Infectious Diseases, University of
Rochester School of Medicine and Dentistry,
Rochester, New York
Papillomaviruses

John C. Boothroyd, MD
Professor of Microbiology and Immunology,
Stanford University School of Medicine, Stanford,
California
Toxoplasma gondii

Patrick J. Bosque, MD
Associate Professor, Department of Neurology,
University of Colorado Denver School of
Medicine; Neurologist, Department of Medicine,
Denver Health Medical Center, Denver, Colorado
Prions and Prion Diseases of the Central Nervous
System (Transmissible Neurodegenerative
Diseases)

John Bower, MD
Associate Professor of Pediatrics, Northeast Ohio
Medical University, Rootstown, Ohio
Croup in Children (Acute
Laryngotracheobronchitis); Bronchiolitis

Robert W. Bradsher, Jr., MD
Ebert Professor of Medicine, Department of
Medicine, Division of Infectious Diseases,
University of Arkansas for Medical Sciences,
Central Arkansas Veterans Healthcare System,
Little Rock, Arkansas
Blastomycosis

Kevin E. Brown, MD, MRCP
Consultant Medical Virologist, Virus Reference
Department, Public Health England,
Microbiology Services, London, United Kingdom
Human Parvoviruses, Including Parvovirus B19V
and Human Bocaparvoviruses

Patricia D. Brown, MD
Professor of Medicine, Department of Internal
Medicine, Division of Infectious Diseases, Wayne
State University School of Medicine; Corporate
Vice President of Quality and Patient Safety,
Detroit Medical Center, Detroit, Michigan
Infections in Injection Drug Users

**Barbara A. Brown-Elliott, MS,
MT(ASCP)SM**
Research Assistant Professor, Microbiology,
Supervisor, Mycobacteria/Nocardia Laboratory,
University of Texas Health Science Center, Tyler,
Texas
Infections Caused by Nontuberculous
Mycobacteria Other than Mycobacterium avium
Complex

Roberta L. Bruhn, MS, PhD
Staff Scientist, Department of Epidemiology,
Blood Systems Research Institute, San Francisco,
California
Human T-Lymphotropic Virus (HTLV)

Amy E. Bryant, PhD
Research Career Scientist, Infectious Diseases
Section, Veterans Affairs Medical Center, Boise,
Idaho
Streptococcus pyogenes

Eileen M. Burd, PhD
Associate Professor, Department of Pathology and
Laboratory Medicine, Emory University School of
Medicine; Director, Clinical Microbiology, Emory
University Hospital, Atlanta, Georgia
Other Gram-Negative and Gram-Variable Bacilli

Jane C. Burns, MD
Professor of Pediatrics, University of California
San Diego School of Medicine, La Jolla, California
Kawasaki Disease

Larry M. Bush, MD
Affiliated Associate Professor of Medicine,
University of Miami Miller School of Medicine,
JFK Medical Center, Palm Beach County, Florida;
Affiliated Professor of Medicine, Charles E.
Schmidt School of Medicine, Florida Atlantic
University, Boca Raton, Florida
Peritonitis and Intraperitoneal Abscesses

Luz Elena Cano, PhD
Head of Medical and Experimental Mycology
Group, Corporación para Investigaciones
Biológicas; Titular Professor, Microbiology
School, Universidad de Antioquia, Medellín,
Colombia
Paracoccidioidomycosis

Charles C. J. Carpenter, MD
Professor of Medicine, Warren Alpert Medical
School of Brown University; Attending Physician,
Division of Infectious Diseases, Miriam Hospital,
Providence, Rhode Island
Other Pathogenic Vibrios

Mary T. Caserta, MD
Professor of Pediatrics, University of Rochester
School of Medicine and Dentistry, Rochester,
New York
Pharyngitis; Acute Laryngitis

Elio Castagnola, MD
Infectious Diseases Unit, Istituto Giannina
Gaslini, Genova, Italy
Prophylaxis and Empirical Therapy of Infection in
Cancer Patients

Richard E. Chaisson, MD
Professor of Medicine, Epidemiology, and
International Health, Johns Hopkins University
School of Medicine, Baltimore, Maryland
General Clinical Manifestations of Human
Immunodeficiency Virus Infection (Including Acute
Retroviral Syndrome and Oral, Cutaneous, Renal,
Ocular, Metabolic, and Cardiac Diseases)

Sharon C-A. Chen, MBBS, PhD
Clinical Associate Professor, University of Sydney
Faculty of Medicine, Sydney, New South Wales,
Australia; Senior Staff Specialist, Centre for
Infectious Diseases and Microbiology, Westmead
Hospital, Westmead, New South Wales, Australia
Nocardia Species

Anthony W. Chow, MD
Professor Emeritus, Department of Internal
Medicine, Division of Infectious Diseases,
University of British Columbia; Honorary
Consultant, Department of Internal Medicine,
Division of Infectious Diseases, Vancouver
Hospital, Vancouver, British Columbia, Canada
Infections of the Oral Cavity, Neck, and Head

Jeffrey I. Cohen, MD
Chief, Laboratory of Infectious Diseases, National
Institute of Allergy and Infectious Diseases,
National Institutes of Health, Bethesda, Maryland
Introduction to Herpesviridae; Human
Herpesvirus Types 6 and 7 (Exanthem Subitum);
Herpes B Virus

Myron S. Cohen, MD
Yergin-Bates Eminent Professor of Medicine,
Microbiology, and Epidemiology, Director,
Institute of Global Health and Infectious Diseases,
University of North Carolina at Chapel Hill,
Chapel Hill, North Carolina
The Acutely Ill Patient with Fever and Rash

Lawrence Corey, MD
Professor of Medicine and Laboratory Medicine,
University of Washington School of Medicine;
President and Director, Fred Hutchinson Cancer
Research Center, Seattle, Washington
Herpes Simplex Virus

Timothy L. Cover, MD
Professor of Medicine, Professor of Pathology,
Microbiology and Immunology, Vanderbilt
University Medical Center; Veterans Affairs
Tennessee Valley Healthcare System, Nashville,
Tennessee
Helicobacter pylori and Other Gastric Helicobacter
Species

Kent B. Crossley, MD, MHA
Professor, Department of Medicine, University of
Minnesota Medical School; Chief of Staff,
Minneapolis Veterans Administration Healthcare
System, Minneapolis, Minnesota
Infections in the Elderly

Clyde S. Crumpacker II, MD
Professor of Medicine, Harvard Medical School;
Attending Physician, Division of Infectious
Diseases, Beth Israel Deaconess Medical Center,
Boston, Massachusetts
Cytomegalovirus (CMV)

Bart J. Currie, MBBS, DTM&H
Professor in Medicine, Department of Infectious
Diseases, Royal Darwin Hospital; Global and
Tropical Health Division, Menzies School of
Health Research, Darwin, Australia
Burkholderia pseudomallei and *Burkholderia
mallei:* Melioidosis and Glanders

Erika D'Agata, MD, MPH
Associate Professor of Medicine, Brown
University; Department of Medicine, Division of
Infectious Diseases, Rhode Island Hospital,
Providence, Rhode Island
Pseudomonas aeruginosa and Other
Pseudomonas Species

Inger K. Damon, MD, PhD
Adjunct Clinical Faculty, Department of
Medicine, Emory University School of Medicine;
Director, Division of High-Consequence
Pathogens and Pathology, Centers for Disease
Control and Prevention, Atlanta, Georgia
Orthopoxviruses: Vaccinia (Smallpox Vaccine),
Variola (Smallpox), Monkeypox, and Cowpox;
Other Poxviruses That Infect Humans:
Parapoxviruses (Including Orf Virus), Molluscum
Contagiosum, and Yatapoxviruses

Rabih O. Darouiche, MD
VA Distinguished Service Professor, Departments
of Medicine, Surgery, and Physical Medicine and
Rehabilitation, Michael E. DeBakey VA Medical
Center and Baylor College of Medicine, Houston,
Texas
Infections in Patients with Spinal Cord Injury

Roberta L. DeBiasi, MD
Acting Chief, Division of Pediatric Infectious
Diseases, Children's National Medical Center;
Professor of Pediatrics and Microbiology,
Immunology and Tropical Medicine, George
Washington University School of Medicine;
Principal Investigator, Center for Clinical and
Translational Science, Children's Research
Institute, Washington, DC
Orthoreoviruses and Orbiviruses; Coltiviruses and
Seadornaviruses

George S. Deepe, Jr., MD
Professor, Department of Internal Medicine,
Division of Infectious Diseases, University of
Cincinnati College of Medicine, Cincinnati, Ohio
Histoplasma capsulatum (Histoplasmosis)

Andrew S. Delemos, MD
Transplant Hepatologist, Carolinas Healthcare
System, Charlotte, North Carolina
Viral Hepatitis

Gregory P. DeMuri, MD
Associate Professor, University of Wisconsin
School of Medicine and Public Health; Attending
Physician, American Family Children's Hospital,
Madison, Wisconsin
Sinusitis

Robin Dewar, PhD
Principal Scientist, Leidos Biomedical Research—
Frederick, National Cancer Institute—Frederick,
Frederick, Maryland
Diagnosis of Human Immunodeficiency Virus
Infection

James H. Diaz, MD, MPHTM, DrPH
Professor of Public Health and Preventive
Medicine, School of Public Health, Louisiana
State University Health Sciences Center, New
Orleans, Louisiana
Introduction to Ectoparasitic Diseases; Lice
(Pediculosis); Scabies; Myiasis and Tungiasis;
Mites, Including Chiggers; Ticks, Including Tick
Paralysis

Jules L. Dienstag, MD
Dean for Medical Education, Carl W. Walter
Professor of Medicine, Harvard Medical School;
Physician, Massachusetts General Hospital,
Boston, Massachusetts
Viral Hepatitis

Raphael Dolin, MD
Maxwell Finland Professor of Medicine
(Microbiology and Molecular Genetics), Harvard
Medical School; Attending Physician, Beth Israel
Deaconess Medical Center; Brigham and
Women's Hospital, Boston, Massachusetts
Zoonotic Paramyxoviruses: Nipah, Hendra, and
Menangle; Noroviruses and Sapoviruses
(Caliciviruses); Astroviruses and Picobirnaviruses

Michael S. Donnenberg, MD
Professor of Medicine, Microbiology, and
Immunology, University of Maryland School of
Medicine, Baltimore, Maryland
Enterobacteriaceae

Gerald R. Donowitz, MD
Professor of Medicine and Infectious Diseases/
International Health, Department of Medicine,
University of Virginia, Charlottesville, Virginia
Acute Pneumonia

Philip R. Dormitzer, MD, PhD
Head of U.S. Research, Global Head of Virology,
Vice President, Novartis Vaccines, Cambridge,
Massachusetts
Rotaviruses

James M. Drake, MB BCh, MSc
Professor of Surgery, University of Toronto
Faculty of Medicine; Neurosurgeon-in-Chief and
Harold Hoffman Shopper's Drug Mart Chair in
Pediatric Neurosurgery, Division of Neurosurgery,
Hospital for Sick Children, Toronto, Ontario,
Canada
Cerebrospinal Fluid Shunt and Drain Infections

J. Stephen Dumler, MD
Professor, Departments of Pathology and
Microbiology and Immunology, University of
Maryland School of Medicine, Baltimore,
Maryland
Rickettsia typhi (Murine Typhus)

Herbert L. DuPont, MD
Professor and Director, Center for Infectious
Diseases, University of Texas School of Public
Health; Chief, Internal Medicine Service, Baylor
St. Luke's Medical Center; Professor and Vice
Chairman, Department of Medicine, Baylor
College of Medicine, Houston, Texas
Bacillary Dysentery: Shigella and Enteroinvasive
Escherichia coli

David T. Durack, MB, DPhil
Consulting Professor of Medicine, Duke
University School of Medicine, Durham, North
Carolina
Prophylaxis of Infective Endocarditis

Marlene L. Durand, MD
Associate Professor of Medicine, Harvard Medical
School; Physician, Infectious Disease Unit,
Massachusetts General Hospital; Director,
Infectious Disease Service, Massachusetts Eye and
Ear Infirmary, Boston, Massachusetts
Endophthalmitis; Infectious Causes of Uveitis;
Periocular Infections

Paul H. Edelstein, MD
Professor of Pathology and Laboratory Medicine,
University of Pennsylvania Perelman School of
Medicine; Director of Clinical Microbiology,
Pathology and Laboratory Medicine, Hospital of
the University of Pennsylvania, Philadelphia,
Pennsylvania
Legionnaires' Disease and Pontiac Fever

Morven S. Edwards, MD
Professor of Pediatrics, Baylor College of
Medicine; Attending Physician, Department of
Pediatrics, Infectious Diseases Section, Texas
Children's Hospital, Houston, Texas
Streptococcus agalactiae (Group B Streptococcus)

Richard T. Ellison III, MD
Professor, Departments of Medicine and
Microbiology & Physiological Systems, Division
of Infectious Diseases, University of
Massachusetts Medical School, Worcester,
Massachusetts
Acute Pneumonia

Timothy P. Endy, MD, MPH
Professor of Medicine, Division Chief of
Infectious Diseases, Upstate Medical University,
State University of New York, Syracuse, New York
Flaviviruses (Dengue, Yellow Fever, Japanese
Encephalitis, West Nile Encephalitis, St. Louis
Encephalitis, Tick-Borne Encephalitis, Kyasanur
Forest Disease, Alkhurma Hemorrhagic Fever,
Zika)

N. Cary Engleberg, MD
Professor, Departments of Infectious Diseases and
Microbiology and Immunology, University of
Michigan Medical School, Ann Arbor, Michigan
Chronic Fatigue Syndrome

Hakan Erdem, MD
Department of Infectious Diseases and Clinical
Microbiology, GATA Haydarpasa Training
Hospital, Istanbul, Turkey
Brucellosis (Brucella Species)

Joel D. Ernst, MD
Professor, Departments of Medicine, Pathology,
and Microbiology, New York University School of
Medicine, New York, New York
Mycobacterium leprae (Leprosy)

Rick M. Fairhurst, MD, PhD
Chief, Malaria Pathogenesis and Human
Immunity Unit, Laboratory of Malaria and Vector
Research, National Institute of Allergy and
Infectious Diseases, Rockville, Maryland
Malaria (Plasmodium Species)

Jessica K. Fairley, MD
Assistant Professor of Medicine, Emory
University School of Medicine, The Emory Clinic,
Atlanta, Georgia
Tapeworms (Cestodes)

Ann R. Falsey, MD
Professor of Medicine, Infectious Diseases Unit,
University of Rochester School of Medicine,
Rochester, New York
Human Metapneumovirus

Thomas Fekete, MD
Professor of Medicine and Chief, Section of
Infectious Diseases, Temple University School of
Medicine, Philadelphia, Pennsylvania
Bacillus Species and Related Genera Other Than
Bacillus anthracis

Paul D. Fey, PhD
Professor, Department of Pathology and
Microbiology, University of Nebraska Medical
Center, Omaha, Nebraska
Staphylococcus epidermidis and Other Coagulase-
Negative Staphylococci

Steven M. Fine, MD, PhD
Associate Professor of Medicine, Division of
Infectious Diseases, University of Rochester
Medical Center, Rochester, New York
Vesicular Stomatitis Virus and Related
Vesiculoviruses

Daniel W. Fitzgerald, MD
Associate Professor of Medicine, Microbiology,
and Immunology, Weill Cornell Medical College,
New York, New York
Mycobacterium tuberculosis

Anthony R. Flores, MD, MPH, PhD
Assistant Professor, Department of Pediatrics,
Section of Infectious Diseases, Baylor College of
Medicine, Houston, Texas
Pharyngitis

Derek Forster, MD
Section on Infectious Diseases, Wake Forest
School of Medicine, Winston-Salem, North
Carolina
Infectious Arthritis of Native Joints

Vance G. Fowler, Jr., MD, MHS
Professor of Medicine, Division of Infectious
Diseases, Duke University School of Medicine,
Durham, North Carolina
Endocarditis and Intravascular Infections

David O. Freedman, MD
Professor of Medicine and Epidemiology, Gorgas
Center for Geographic Medicine, Division of
Infectious Diseases, University of Alabama at
Birmingham School of Medicine; Director,
University of Alabama at Birmingham Travelers
Health Clinic, University of Alabama at
Birmingham Health System, Birmingham,
Alabama
Protection of Travelers; Infections in Returning
Travelers

Arthur M. Friedlander, MD
Adjunct Professor of Medicine, School of
Medicine, Uniformed Services University of the
Health Sciences, Bethesda, Maryland; Senior
Scientist, U.S. Army Medical Research Institute of
Infectious Diseases, Frederick, Maryland
Bacillus anthracis (Anthrax)

John N. Galgiani, MD
Professor of Internal Medicine, Director, Valley
Fever Center for Excellence, University of
Arizona College of Medicine; Chief Medical
Officer, Valley Fever Solutions, Tucson, Arizona
Coccidioidomycosis (*Coccidioides* Species)

Robert C. Gallo, MD
Director, Institute of Human Virology, Professor,
Department of Medicine, University of Maryland
School of Medicine, Baltimore, Maryland
Human Immunodeficiency Viruses

Tejal N. Gandhi, MD
Clinical Assistant Professor of Medicine,
Department of Internal Medicine, Division of
Infectious Diseases, University of Michigan, Ann
Arbor, Michigan
Bartonella, Including Cat-Scratch Disease

Wendy S. Garrett, MD, PhD
Assistant Professor, Immunology & Infectious
Diseases and Genetic & Complex Diseases,
Department of Medicine, Harvard School of
Public Health; Department of Medical Oncology,
Dana-Farber Cancer Institute, Boston,
Massachusetts
Gas Gangrene and Other *Clostridium*-Associated
Diseases; *Bacteroides, Prevotella, Porphyromonas,*
and *Fusobacterium* Species (and Other Medically
Important Anaerobic Gram-Negative Bacilli)

Charlotte A. Gaydos, DrPH, MPH, MS
Professor of Medicine, Division of Infectious
Diseases, Johns Hopkins University School of
Medicine; Emergency Medicine Department and
Epidemiology, Population, Family and
Reproductive Health, Bloomberg Johns Hopkins
School of Public Health; Director, International
Sexually Transmitted Diseases Research
Laboratory, Baltimore, Maryland
Chlamydia pneumoniae

Thomas W. Geisbert, PhD
Professor, Department of Microbiology and
Immunology, University of Texas Medical Branch,
Galveston, Texas
Marburg and Ebola Hemorrhagic Fevers
(Filoviruses)

Jeffrey A. Gelfand, MD
Clinical Professor of Medicine, Harvard Medical
School; Attending Physician, Infectious Diseases
Division, Massachusetts General Hospital, Boston,
Massachusetts
Babesia Species

Dale N. Gerding, MD
Professor of Medicine, Loyola University Chicago
Stritch School of Medicine, Maywood, Illinois;
Research Physician, Department of Medicine,
Edward Hines, Jr., Veterans Affairs Hospital,
Hines, Illinois
Clostridium difficile Infection

Anne A. Gershon, MD
Professor of Pediatrics, Columbia University
College of Physicians and Surgeons, New York,
New York
Rubella Virus (German Measles); Measles Virus
(Rubeola)

Janet R. Gilsdorf, MD
Robert P. Kelch Research Professor of Pediatrics
and Communicable Diseases, University of
Michigan Medical School and C.S. Mott
Children's Hospital, Ann Arbor, Michigan
Infections in Asplenic Patients

Ellie J. C. Goldstein, MD
Clinical Professor of Medicine, David Geffen
School of Medicine at University of California,
Los Angeles, California; Director, R.M. Alden
Research Laboratory, Santa Monica, California
Bites

Fred M. Gordin, MD
Professor of Medicine, George Washington
University School of Medicine; Chief, Infectious
Diseases, Veterans Affairs Medical Center,
Washington, DC
Mycobacterium avium Complex

Paul S. Graman, MD
Professor of Medicine, University of Rochester
School of Medicine and Dentistry; Attending
Physician and Clinical Director, Infectious
Diseases Division, Strong Memorial Hospital,
Rochester, New York
Esophagitis

Patricia M. Griffin, MD
Chief, Enteric Diseases Epidemiology Branch,
Division of Foodborne, Waterborne, and
Environmental Diseases, National Center for
Emerging and Zoonotic Infectious Diseases,
Centers for Disease Control and Prevention,
Atlanta, Georgia
Foodborne Disease

Richard L. Guerrant, MD
Professor of Medicine, Infectious Diseases, and
International Health, University of Virginia
School of Medicine, Charlottesville, Virginia
Nausea, Vomiting, and Noninflammatory
Diarrhea; Bacterial Inflammatory Enteritides

H. Cem Gul, MD
Department of Infectious Diseases and
Microbiology, Gulhane Military Medical
Academy, Ankara, Turkey
Brucellosis (*Brucella* Species)

David A. Haake, MD
Professor, Departments of Medicine, Urology, and
Microbiology, Immunology, & Molecular
Genetics, The David Geffen School of Medicine at
UCLA; Staff Physician, Department of Medicine,
Division of Infectious Diseases, The Veterans
Affairs Greater Los Angeles Healthcare System,
Los Angeles, California
Leptospira Species (Leptospirosis)

David W. Haas, MD
Professor of Medicine, Pharmacology, Pathology,
Microbiology, and Immunology, Vanderbilt
University School of Medicine, Nashville,
Tennessee
Mycobacterium tuberculosis

Charles Haines, MD, PhD
Division of Infectious Diseases, Johns Hopkins
University School of Medicine, Baltimore,
Maryland
Gastrointestinal, Hepatobiliary, and Pancreatic
Manifestations of Human Immunodeficiency Virus
Infection

Caroline Breese Hall, MD†
Professor of Pediatrics and Medicine, University
of Rochester School of Medicine and Dentistry,
Rochester, New York
Respiratory Syncytial Virus (RSV)

Joelle Hallak, BS, MS
Research Assistant, Department of
Ophthalmology and Visual Science, University
of Illinois at Chicago, Chicago, Illinois
Microbial Keratitis

Scott A. Halperin, MD
Professor, Departments of Pediatrics and
Microbiology & Immunology, Director, Canadian
Center for Vaccinology, Dalhousie University;
Head, Pediatric Infectious Diseases, IWK Health
Centre, Halifax, Nova Scotia, Canada
Bordetella pertussis

Margaret R. Hammerschlag, MD
Professor of Pediatrics and Medicine, State
University of New York Downstate College of
Medicine; Director, Division of Pediatric
Infectious Diseases, State University of New York
Downstate Medical Center, Brooklyn, New York
Chlamydia pneumoniae

†Deceased.

Rashidul Haque, MD
Scientist and Head of Parasitology Laboratory,
Laboratory Sciences Division, International
Centre for Diarrhoeal Disease Research,
Bangladesh, Dhaka, Bangladesh
Entamoeba Species, Including Amebic Colitis and Liver Abscess

Jason B. Harris, MD, MPH
Assistant Professor of Pediatrics, Harvard Medical
School; Division of Infectious Diseases,
MassGeneral Hospital for Children, Boston,
Massachusetts
Enteric Fever and Other Causes of Fever and Abdominal Symptoms

Claudia Hawkins, MD, MPH
Assistant Professor, Department of Medicine,
Division of Infectious Diseases, Northwestern
University Feinberg School of Medicine, Chicago,
Illinois
Hepatitis B Virus and Hepatitis Delta Virus

Roderick J. Hay, DM
Professor of Cutaneous Infection, Department of
Dermatology (KCH Campus), Kings College
London, London, United Kingdom
Dermatophytosis (Ringworm) and Other Superficial Mycoses

David K. Henderson, MD
Deputy Director for Clinical Care, Clinical
Center, National Institutes of Health, Bethesda,
Maryland
Infections Caused by Percutaneous Intravascular Devices; Human Immunodeficiency Virus in Health Care Settings; Nosocomial Herpesvirus Infections

David R. Hill, MD, DTM&H
Professor, Department of Medical Sciences,
Director, Global Public Health, Frank H. Netter
MD School of Medicine, Quinnipiac University,
Hamden, Connecticut
Giardia lamblia

Martin S. Hirsch, MD
Professor of Medicine, Harvard Medical School;
Professor of Infectious Diseases and Immunology,
Harvard School of Public Health; Senior
Physician, Infectious Diseases Service,
Massachusetts General Hospital, Boston,
Massachusetts
Antiretroviral Therapy for Human Immunodeficiency Virus Infection

Aimee Hodowanec, MD
Assistant Professor, Department of Medicine,
Division of Infectious Diseases, Rush University
Medical Center, Chicago, Illinois
Tetanus (Clostridium tetani); Botulism (Clostridium botulinum)

Robert S. Holzman, MD
Professor Emeritus of Medicine, Department of
Medicine, Division of Infectious Diseases and
Immunology, New York University School of
Medicine, New York, New York
Mycoplasma pneumoniae and Atypical Pneumonia

Edward W. Hook III, MD
Professor and Director, Division of Infectious
Diseases, University of Alabama at Birmingham,
Birmingham, Alabama
Endemic Treponematoses

Thomas M. Hooton, MD
Professor of Clinical Medicine, Department of
Medicine, Clinical Director, Division of Infectious
Diseases, University of Miami Miller School of
Medicine; Chief of Medicine, Miami Veterans
Affairs Healthcare System, Miami, Florida
Nosocomial Urinary Tract Infections

Harold W. Horowitz, MD
Professor of Medicine, Infectious Diseases and
Immunology, Department of Medicine, New York
University School of Medicine; Chief of Service
Infectious Diseases, Bellevue Hospital Center,
New York, New York
Acute Exacerbations of Chronic Obstructive Pulmonary Disease

C. Robert Horsburgh, Jr., MD, MUS
Professor of Epidemiology, Biostatistics, and
Medicine, Boston University Schools of Public
Health and Medicine, Boston, Massachusetts
Mycobacterium avium Complex

James M. Horton, MD
Chief, Division of Infectious Diseases,
Department of Internal Medicine, Carolinas
Medical Center, Charlotte, North Carolina
Relapsing Fever Caused by Borrelia Species

Duane R. Hospenthal, MD, PhD
Adjunct Professor of Medicine, Department of
Medicine, Infectious Disease Division, University
of Texas Health Science Center at San Antonio,
San Antonio, Texas
Agents of Chromoblastomycosis; Agents of Mycetoma; Uncommon Fungi and Related Species

Nicole M. Iovine, MD, PhD
Assistant Professor of Medicine, Director,
Antimicrobial Stewardship Program, Department
of Medicine, Division of Infectious Diseases and
Global Medicine, University of Florida School of
Medicine, Gainesville, Florida
Campylobacter jejuni and Related Species

Jonathan R. Iredell, MBBS, PhD
Associate Professor, University of Sydney Faculty of Medicine, Sydney, New South Wales, Australia; Director, Department of Infectious Diseases, Centre for Infectious Diseases and Microbiology, Westmead Hospital, Westmead, New South Wales, Australia
Nocardia Species

Michael G. Ison, MD, MS
Associate Professor, Divisions of Infectious Diseases and Organ Transplantation, Northwestern University Feinberg School of Medicine, Chicago, Illinois
Parainfluenza Viruses

J. Michael Janda, PhD, D(ABMM)
Laboratory Director, Public Health Laboratory, Department of Public Health, County of Los Angeles, Downey, California
Capnocytophaga

Edward N. Janoff, MD
Professor of Medicine, Microbiology, and Immunology, Departments of Medicine and Infectious Diseases, University of Colorado Denver, Aurora, Colorado; Director, Mucosal and Vaccine Research Center, Denver Veterans Affairs Medical Center, Denver, Colorado
Streptococcus pneumoniae

Eric C. Johannsen, MD
Assistant Professor of Medicine, University of Wisconsin School of Medicine and Public Health; Physician, Division of Infectious Diseases, University of Wisconsin Hospitals and Clinics, Madison, Wisconsin
Epstein-Barr Virus (Infectious Mononucleosis, Epstein-Barr Virus–Associated Malignant Diseases, and Other Diseases)

Donald Kaye, MD
Professor of Medicine, Drexel University College of Medicine, Philadelphia, Pennsylvania
Urinary Tract Infections

Kenneth M. Kaye, MD
Associate Professor, Department of Medicine, Harvard Medical School; Attending Physician, Division of Infectious Diseases, Brigham and Women's Hospital, Boston, Massachusetts
Epstein-Barr Virus (Infectious Mononucleosis, Epstein-Barr Virus–Associated Malignant Diseases, and Other Diseases); Kaposi's Sarcoma–Associated Herpesvirus (Human Herpesvirus 8)

James W. Kazura, MD
Professor of International Health, Center for Global Health and Diseases, Case Western Reserve University School of Medicine, Cleveland, Ohio
Tissue Nematodes (Trichinellosis, Dracunculiasis, Filariasis, Loiasis, and Onchocerciasis)

Jay S. Keystone, MD, MSc (CTM)
Professor of Medicine, University of Toronto; Senior Staff Physician, Tropical Disease Unit, Toronto General Hospital, Toronto, Canada
Cyclospora cayetanensis, Cystoisospora (Isospora) belli, Sarcocystis Species, *Balantidium coli,* and *Blastocystis* Species

Yury Khudyakov, PhD
Division of Viral Hepatitis, National Center for HIV/AIDS, Viral Hepatitis, STD, and TB Prevention, Centers for Disease Control and Prevention, Atlanta, Georgia
Hepatitis A Virus

Rose Kim, MD
Associate Professor of Medicine, Division of Infectious Diseases, Cooper Medical School of Rowan University, Cooper University Hospital, Camden, New Jersey
Other Coryneform Bacteria and Rhodococci

Charles H. King, MD
Professor of International Health, Center for Global Health and Diseases, Case Western Reserve University, Cleveland, Ohio
Tapeworms (Cestodes)

Louis V. Kirchhoff, MD, MPH
Professor of Internal Medicine, University of Iowa; Staff Physician, Medical Service, Department of Veterans Affairs Medical Center, Iowa City, Iowa; Professor of Medicine, State University of New York Upstate Medical University, Syracuse, New York
Trypanosoma Species (American Trypanosomiasis, Chagas' Disease): Biology of Trypanosomes; Agents of African Trypanosomiasis (Sleeping Sickness)

Jerome O. Klein, MD
Professor, Department of Pediatrics, Boston University School of Medicine; Former Director, Division of Pediatric Infectious Diseases, Boston Medical Center, Boston, Massachusetts
Otitis Externa, Otitis Media, and Mastoiditis

Michael Klompas, MD, MPH
Associate Professor of Population Medicine, Harvard Medical School and Harvard Pilgrim Health Care Institute; Associate Hospital Epidemiologist, Brigham and Women's Hospital, Boston, Massachusetts
Nosocomial Pneumonia

Bettina M. Knoll, MD, PhD
Assistant Professor of Medicine, Warren Alpert Medical School of Brown University; Physician, Miriam Hospital and Rhode Island Hospital, Providence, Rhode Island
Prosthetic Valve Endocarditis

Kirk U. Knowlton, MD
Professor of Medicine, Chief of Cardiology,
University of California San Diego School of
Medicine, La Jolla, California
Myocarditis and Pericarditis

Jane E. Koehler, MA, MD
Professor of Medicine, Division of Infectious
Diseases, University of California San Francisco,
San Francisco, California
Bartonella, Including Cat-Scratch Disease

Stephan A. Kohlhoff, MD
Assistant Professor of Pediatrics and Medicine,
State University of New York Downstate College
of Medicine; Co-Director, Division of Pediatric
Infectious Diseases, State University of New York
Downstate Medical Center, Brooklyn, New York
Chlamydia pneumoniae

Dimitrios P. Kontoyiannis, MD
Frances King Black Endowed Professor,
Department of Infectious Diseases, Deputy Head,
Division of Internal Medicine, University of Texas
MD Anderson Cancer Center, Houston, Texas
*Agents of Mucormycosis and
Entomophthoramycosis*

Igor J. Koralnik, MD
Professor of Neurology, Harvard Medical School;
Chief, Division of Neuro-Virology, Director,
HIV/Neurology Center, Beth Israel Deaconess
Medical Center, Boston, Massachusetts
*JC, BK, and Other Polyomaviruses: Progressive
Multifocal Leukoencephalopathy (PML)*

Anita A. Koshy, MD
Assistant Professor, Departments of Neurology
and Immunobiology, University of Arizona,
Tucson, Arizona
Free-Living Amebae

Joseph A. Kovacs, MD
Senior Investigator, Head, AIDS Section, Critical
Care Medicine Department, National Institute of
Health Clinical Center, Bethesda, Maryland
Toxoplasma gondii

Phyllis Kozarsky, MD
Professor of Medicine, Division of Infectious
Diseases, Emory University School of Medicine;
Medical Director, TravelWell, Emory University
Hospital, Atlanta, Georgia
*Cyclospora cayetanensis, Cystoisospora (Isospora)
belli, Sarcocystis Species, Balantidium coli, and
Blastocystis Species*

John Krieger, MD
Professor, Department of Urology, University of
Washington; Chief, Urology Section, Veterans
Affairs Puget Sound Health Care System, Seattle,
Washington
Prostatitis, Epididymitis, and Orchitis

Matthew J. Kuehnert, MD
Director, Office of Blood, Organ, and Other
Tissue Safety, Division of Healthcare Quality
Promotion, Centers for Disease Control and
Prevention, Atlanta, Georgia
*Transfusion- and Transplantation-Transmitted
Infections*

Nalin M. Kumar, DPhil
Professor, Department of Ophthalmology and
Visual Sciences, College of Medicine, University
of Illinois at Chicago, Chicago, Illinois
Microbial Conjunctivitis

Paul N. Levett, PhD, DSc
Assistant Clinical Director, Saskatchewan Disease
Control Laboratory, Regina, Saskatchewan,
Canada
Leptospira Species (Leptospirosis)

Donald P. Levine, MD
Professor of Medicine, Associate Vice Chair for
Continuing Medical Education and Community
Affairs, Department of Medicine, Wayne State
University, Detroit, Michigan
Infections in Injection Drug Users

Matthew E. Levison, MD
Professor of Public Health, Drexel University
School of Public Health; Adjunct Professor of
Medicine, Drexel University College of Medicine,
Philadelphia, Pennsylvania
Peritonitis and Intraperitoneal Abscesses

Russell E. Lewis, PharmD
Associate Professor, Department of Medical
Sciences and Surgery, University of Bologna
Infectious Diseases Unit, S. Orsola Malpighi
Hospital, Bologna, Italy
*Agents of Mucormycosis and
Entomophthoramycosis*

Aldo A. M. Lima, MD, PhD
Professor, Institute of Biomedicine, Federal
University of Ceara, Fortaleza, Ceará, Brazil
Bacterial Inflammatory Enteritides

Ajit P. Limaye, MD
Professor, Division of Allergy and Infectious
Diseases, University of Washington School of
Medicine, Seattle, Washington
Infections in Solid-Organ Transplant Recipients

W. Ian Lipkin, MD
Director, Center for Infection and Immunity,
Mailman School of Public Health, Columbia
University, New York, New York
Zoonoses

Contributors

Nathan Litman, MD
Professor of Pediatrics, Albert Einstein College
of Medicine; Vice Chair, Clinical Affairs,
Department of Pediatrics, Chief, Division of
Pediatric Infectious Diseases, Children's Hospital
at Montefiore, Bronx, New York
Mumps Virus

Bennett Lorber, MD, DSc (Hon)
Thomas M. Durant Professor of Medicine,
Professor of Microbiology and Immunology,
Temple University School of Medicine,
Philadelphia, Pennsylvania
Bacterial Lung Abscess; *Listeria monocytogenes*

Rob Roy MacGregor, MD
Professor, Department of Medicine, Division of
Infectious Diseases, University of Pennsylvania
School of Medicine, Philadelphia, Pennsylvania
Corynebacterium diphtheriae (Diphtheria)

Philip A. Mackowiak, MD, MBA
Professor and Vice Chairman, Department of
Medicine, University of Maryland School of
Medicine; Chief, Medical Care Clinical Center,
Veterans Affairs Maryland Health Care System,
Baltimore, Maryland
Fever of Unknown Origin

Lawrence C. Madoff, MD
Professor of Medicine, University of
Massachusetts Medical School; Director, Division
of Epidemiology and Immunization,
Massachusetts Department of Public Health;
Division of Infectious Disease and Immunology,
University of Massachusetts Memorial Medical
Center, Worcester, Massachusetts
Infections of the Liver and Biliary System (Liver
Abscess, Cholangitis, Cholecystitis); Splenic
Abscess

Alan J. Magill, MD
Director, Malaria, Bill and Melinda Gates
Foundation, Seattle, Washington
Leishmania Species: Visceral (Kala-Azar),
Cutaneous, and Mucosal Leishmaniasis

James H. Maguire, MD, MPH
Professor of Medicine, Harvard Medical School;
Senior Physician, Division of Infectious Disease,
Brigham and Women's Hospital, Boston,
Massachusetts
Intestinal Nematodes (Roundworms); Trematodes
(Schistosomes and Liver, Intestinal, and Lung
Flukes)

Frank Maldarelli, MD, PhD
Head, Clinical Retrovirology Section, HIV Drug
Resistance Program, National Cancer Institute—
Frederick, National Institutes of Health,
Frederick, Maryland
Diagnosis of Human Immunodeficiency Virus
Infection

Lewis Markoff, MD
Chief, Laboratory of Vector-Borne Virus Diseases,
Office of Vaccines, Center for Biologics
Evaluation and Research, U.S. Food and Drug
Administration, Bethesda, Maryland
Alphaviruses

Jeanne M. Marrazzo, MD, MPH
Associate Professor of Medicine, Division of
Allergy and Infectious Diseases, University of
Washington School of Medicine, Seattle,
Washington
Neisseria gonorrhoeae (Gonorrhea)

Thomas J. Marrie, MD
Dean, Faculty of Medicine, Dalhousie University,
Halifax, Nova Scotia, Canada
Coxiella burnetii (Q Fever)

Thomas Marth, MD
Professor of Internal Medicine, Chief, Division of
Internal Medicine, Krankenhaus Maria Hilf,
Daun, Germany
Whipple's Disease

David H. Martin, MD
Harry E. Dascomb, M.D., Professor of Medicine,
Department of Internal Medicine, Professor of
Microbiology, Immunology, and Parasitology,
Louisiana State University Health Sciences Center,
New Orleans, Louisiana
Genital Mycoplasmas: *Mycoplasma genitalium,
Mycoplasma hominis,* and *Ureaplasma* Species

Gregory J. Martin, MD
Chief, Infectious Diseases—Tropical Medicine,
Office of Medical Services, U.S. Department of
State, Washington, DC; Associate Professor of
Medicine and Preventive Medicine and
Biometrics, Uniformed Services University of the
Health Sciences, Bethesda, Maryland
Bacillus anthracis (Anthrax)

Francisco M. Marty, MD
Associate Professor of Medicine, Department of
Medicine, Harvard Medical School; Brigham and
Women's Hospital, Boston, Massachusetts
Cystic Fibrosis

Henry Masur, MD
Chief, Critical Care Medicine Department,
Clinical Center, National Institutes of Health,
Bethesda, Maryland
Management of Opportunistic Infections
Associated with Human Immunodeficiency Virus
Infection

John T. McBride, MD
Professor of Pediatrics, Northeast Ohio Medical
University, Rootstown, Ohio; Vice Chair,
Department of Pediatrics, Akron Children's
Hospital, Akron, Ohio
Croup in Children (Acute
Laryngotracheobronchitis); Bronchiolitis

William M. McCormack, MD
Distinguished Teaching Professor of Medicine
and of Obstetrics and Gynecology, Emeritus,
Division of Infectious Diseases, Department of
Medicine, SUNY Downstate Medical Center,
Brooklyn, New York
Urethritis; Vulvovaginitis and Cervicitis

Catherine C. McGowan, MD
Associate Professor, Department of Medicine,
Division of Infectious Diseases, Vanderbilt
University School of Medicine, Nashville,
Tennessee
Prostatitis, Epididymitis, and Orchitis

Kenneth McIntosh, MD
Professor of Pediatrics, Harvard Medical School;
Senior Physician, Department of Medicine,
Children's Hospital, Boston, Massachusetts
Coronaviruses, Including Severe Acute Respiratory
Syndrome (SARS) and Middle East Respiratory
Syndrome (MERS)

Paul S. Mead, MD, MPH
Chief, Epidemiology and Surveillance Activity,
Bacterial Disease Branch, National Center for
Zoonotic, Vector-Borne, and Enteric Diseases,
Centers for Disease Control and Prevention, Fort
Collins, Colorado
Yersinia Species (Including Plague)

Malgorzata Mikulska, MD
Division of Infectious Diseases, IRCCS AOU San
Martino-IST; Department of Health Sciences,
University of Genova, Genova, Italy
Prophylaxis and Empirical Therapy of Infection in
Cancer Patients

Robert F. Miller, MBBS
Reader in Clinical Infection, Honorary Professor,
London School of Hygiene and Tropical
Medicine; Honorary Consultant Physician,
Camden Provider Services, Central and North
West London NHS Foundation Trust, and at
University College London Hospitals, University
College London, London, United Kingdom
Pneumocystis Species

Samuel I. Miller, MD
Professor of Medicine, Microbiology, Genome
Sciences, and Immunology, Department of
Immunology, University of Washington School of
Medicine, Seattle, Washington
Salmonella Species

David H. Mitchell, MBBS
Clinical Senior Lecturer, University of Sydney
Faculty of Medicine, Sydney, New South Wales,
Australia; Senior Staff Specialist, Centre for
Infectious Diseases and Microbiology, Westmead
Hospital, Westmead, New South Wales, Australia
Nocardia Species

John F. Modlin, MD
Professor of Pediatrics and Medicine, Chair,
Department of Pediatrics, Senior Advising Dean,
Geisel School of Medicine at Dartmouth; Interim
Director, Children's Hospital at Dartmouth,
Lebanon, New Hampshire
Poliovirus; Coxsackieviruses, Echoviruses, and
Numbered Enteroviruses; Human Parechoviruses

Rajal K. Mody, MD, MPH
Lead, National Surveillance Team, Enteric
Diseases Epidemiology Branch, Division of
Foodborne, Waterborne, and Environmental
Diseases, National Center for Emerging and
Zoonotic Diseases, Centers for Disease Control
and Prevention, Atlanta, Georgia
Foodborne Disease

José G. Montoya, MD
Professor of Medicine, Division of Infectious
Diseases and Geographic Medicine, Stanford
University School of Medicine, Stanford,
California
Toxoplasma gondii

Philippe Moreillon, MD, PhD
Professor and Vice Rector for Research,
Department of Fundamental Microbiology,
University of Lausanne, Lausanne, Switzerland
Staphylococcus aureus (Including Staphylococcal
Toxic Shock Syndrome)

J. Glenn Morris, Jr., MD, MPH&TM
Director, Emerging Pathogens Institute,
University of Florida; Professor of Medicine,
Division of Infectious Diseases, University of
Florida College of Medicine, Gainesville, Florida
Human Illness Associated with Harmful Algal
Blooms

Robert S. Munford, MD
Senior Clinician, Laboratory of Clinical Infectious
Diseases, National Institute of Allergy and
Infectious Diseases, National Institutes of Health,
Bethesda, Maryland
Sepsis, Severe Sepsis, and Septic Shock

Edward L. Murphy, MD, MPH
Professor, Departments of Laboratory Medicine
and Epidemiology/Biostatistics, University of
California School of Medicine; Senior
Investigator, Blood Systems Research Institute,
San Francisco, California
Human T-Lymphotropic Virus (HTLV)

Timothy F. Murphy, MD
SUNY Distinguished Professor, Clinical and
Translational Research Center, University at
Buffalo, State University of New York, Buffalo,
New York
Moraxella catarrhalis, Kingella, and Other
Gram-Negative Cocci; Haemophilus Species,
including H. influenzae and H. ducreyi
(Chancroid)

Barbara E. Murray, MD
J. Ralph Meadows Professor and Director,
Division of Infectious Diseases, Department
of Internal Medicine and Department of
Microbiology and Molecular Genetics, University
of Texas Medical School at Houston, Houston,
Texas
Enterococcus Species, Streptococcus gallolyticus
Group, and Leuconostoc Species

Clinton K. Murray, MD
Chief, Infectious Disease, Brooke Army Medical
Center, Fort Sam Houston, Houston, Texas;
Professor of Medicine, Uniformed Services
University of the Health Sciences, Bethesda,
Maryland; Clinical Professor of Medicine and
Infectious Diseases, University of Texas Health
Sciences Center, San Antonio, Texas
Burns

Daniel M. Musher, MD
Professor of Medicine and of Molecular Virology
and Microbiology, Distinguished Service
Professor, Baylor College of Medicine; Infectious
Disease Section, Michael E. DeBakey Veterans
Affairs Medical Center, Houston, Texas
Streptococcus pneumoniae

Anna Narezkina, MD
Fellow, Division of Cardiology, University of
California San Diego School of Medicine, La Jolla,
California
Myocarditis and Pericarditis

Theodore E. Nash, MD
Head, Gastrointestinal Parasites Section,
Laboratory of Parasitic Diseases, National
Institute of Allergy and Infectious Diseases,
National Institutes of Health, Bethesda, Maryland
Giardia lamblia; Visceral Larva Migrans and Other
Uncommon Helminth Infections

Jennifer L. Nayak, MD
Assistant Professor, Department of Pediatrics,
University of Rochester School of Medicine and
Dentistry, University of Rochester Medical
Center, Rochester, New York
Epiglottitis

Marguerite A. Neill, MD
Associate Professor of Medicine, Warren Alpert
Medical School of Brown University, Providence,
Rhode Island; Attending Physician, Division of
Infectious Diseases, Memorial Hospital of Rhode
Island, Pawtucket, Rhode Island
Other Pathogenic Vibrios

Christopher A. Ohl, MD
Professor of Medicine, Section on Infectious
Diseases, Wake Forest School of Medicine;
Medical Director, Center for Antimicrobial
Utilization, Stewardship, and Epidemiology, Wake
Forest Baptist Medical Center, Winston-Salem,
North Carolina
Infectious Arthritis of Native Joints

Pablo C. Okhuysen, MD
Professor, Department of Infectious Diseases,
Infection Control and Employee Health, MD
Anderson Cancer Center, Houston, Texas
Sporothrix schenckii

Andrew B. Onderdonk, PhD
Professor of Pathology, Harvard Medical School;
Microbiology Laboratory, Brigham and Women's
Hospital, Boston, Massachusetts
Gas Gangrene and Other Clostridium-Associated
Diseases; Bacteroides, Prevotella, Porphyromonas,
and Fusobacterium Species (and Other Medically
Important Anaerobic Gram-Negative Bacilli)

Douglas R. Osmon, MD
Professor of Medicine, Division of Infectious
Diseases, Mayo Clinic, Rochester, Minnesota
Osteomyelitis

Michael N. Oxman, MD
Professor of Medicine and Pathology, University
of California San Diego School of Medicine, La
Jolla, California; Staff Physician, Infectious
Diseases, Veterans Affairs San Diego Healthcare
System, San Diego, California
Myocarditis and Pericarditis

Slobodan Paessler, DVM, PhD
Professor, Department of Pathology, Director,
Preclinical Studies Core, Director, Animal
Biosafety Level 3, Galveston National Laboratory,
Institute for Human Infections and Immunity,
University of Texas Medical Branch, Galveston,
Texas
Lymphocytic Choriomeningitis, Lassa Fever, and
the South American Hemorrhagic Fevers
(Arenaviruses)

Raj Palraj, MBBS
Instructor of Medicine, Mayo Clinic College of
Medicine; Senior Associate Consultant, Infectious
Diseases, Mayo Clinic, Rochester, Minnesota
Prosthetic Valve Endocarditis

Peter G. Pappas, MD
Professor of Medicine, Division of Infectious
Diseases, University of Alabama at Birmingham,
Birmingham, Alabama
Chronic Pneumonia

Mark S. Pasternack, MD
Chief, Pediatric Infectious Disease Unit,
Massachusetts General Hospital, Boston,
Massachusetts
Cellulitis, Necrotizing Fasciitis, and Subcutaneous
Tissue Infections; Myositis and Myonecrosis

Thomas F. Patterson, MD
Professor, Department of Medicine, Division of
Infectious Diseases, University of Texas Health
Science Center and South Texas Veterans Health
Care System, San Antonio, Texas
Aspergillus Species

Deborah Pavan-Langston, MD
Professor, Department of Ophthalmology,
Harvard Medical School; Attending Physician,
Massachusetts Eye and Ear Infirmary, Boston,
Massachusetts
Microbial Conjunctivitis; Microbial Keratitis

David A. Pegues, MD
Professor of Medicine, Division of Infectious
Diseases, Perelman School of Medicine at the
University of Pennsylvania; Medical Director,
Healthcare Epidemiology, Infection Prevention
and Control; Antimicrobial Management
Program, Hospital of the University of
Pennsylvania, Philadelphia, Pennsylvania
Salmonella Species

Robert L. Penn, MD
Professor of Medicine, Infectious Diseases
Section, Louisiana State University School of
Medicine in Shreveport; Physician, Infectious
Diseases Section, Overton Brooks Veterans
Affairs Medical Center, Shreveport, Louisiana
Francisella tularensis (Tularemia)

John R. Perfect, MD
James B. Duke Professor of Medicine, Chief,
Infectious Diseases, Department of Medicine,
Duke University Medical Center, Durham, North
Carolina
Cryptococcosis (*Cryptococcus neoformans* and
Cryptococcus gattii)

Stanley Perlman, MD, PhD
Professor, Department of Microbiology and
Pediatrics, University of Iowa Carver College of
Medicine, Iowa City, Iowa
Coronaviruses, Including Severe Acute Respiratory
Syndrome (SARS) and Middle East Respiratory
Syndrome (MERS)

Brett W. Petersen, MD, MPH
Medical Officer, Poxvirus and Rabies Branch,
Division of High-Consequence Pathogens and
Pathology, Centers for Disease Control and
Prevention, Atlanta, Georgia
Orthopoxviruses: Vaccinia (Smallpox Vaccine),
Variola (Smallpox), Monkeypox, and Cowpox;
Other Poxviruses That Infect Humans:
Parapoxviruses (Including Orf Virus), Molluscum
Contagiosum, and Yatapoxviruses

Phillip K. Peterson, MD
Professor of Medicine, Director, International
Medical Education and Research, University of
Minnesota Medical School, Minneapolis,
Minnesota
Infections in the Elderly

William A. Petri, Jr., MD, PhD
Wade Hampton Frost Professor of Epidemiology,
University of Virginia; Chief, Division of
Infectious Disease and International Health,
University of Virginia Health System,
Charlottesville, Virginia
Entamoeba Species, Including Amebic Colitis and
Liver Abscess

Cathy A. Petti, MD
CEO, HealthSpring Global, Inc., Bradenton,
Florida
Streptococcus anginosus Group

Michael Phillips, MD
Associate Professor (Clinical), Associate Director
for Clinical Affairs, Division of Infectious Disease
and Immunology, New York University School of
Medicine; Hospital Epidemiologist and Director
of Infection Prevention and Control, NYU
Langone Medical Center, New York, New York
Acinetobacter Species

Yok-Ai Que, MD, PhD
Instructor and Researcher, University of Lausanne
School of Medicine; Attending Physician,
Department of Critical Care Medicine, Centre
Hospitalier Universitaire Vaudois Lausanne,
Lausanne, Switzerland
Staphylococcus aureus (Including Staphylococcal
Toxic Shock Syndrome)

Justin D. Radolf, MD
Professor, Departments of Medicine, Pediatrics, Immunology, Genetics & Developmental Biology, and Molecular Biology and Biophysics, University of Connecticut Health Center, Farmington, Connecticut; Senior Scientific Advisor, Connecticut Children's Medical Center, Hartford, Connecticut
Syphilis (Treponema pallidum)

Didier Raoult, MD, PhD
Professor and President, Aix Marseille Université; Director, Clinical Microbiology Laboratory for the University Hospitals; Founder, WHO Collaborative Center; President, Universite de la Mediteranee in Marseille, Marseille, France
Rickettsia akari (Rickettsialpox); Coxiella burnetii (Q Fever); Orientia tsutsugamushi (Scrub Typhus)

Stuart C. Ray, MD
Professor of Medicine, Department of Medicine, Division of Infectious Diseases, Johns Hopkins University School of Medicine, Baltimore, Maryland
Hepatitis C

Annette C. Reboli, MD
Founding Vice Dean, Professor of Medicine, Division of Infectious Diseases, Cooper Medical School of Rowan University, Cooper University Hospital, Camden, New Jersey
Other Coryneform Bacteria and Rhodococci; Erysipelothrix rhusiopathiae

Marvin S. Reitz, Jr., PhD
Professor, Institute of Human Virology, University of Maryland School of Medicine, Baltimore, Maryland
Human Immunodeficiency Viruses

Cybèle A. Renault, MD, DTM&H
Clinical Assistant Professor, Department of Internal Medicine, Division of Infectious Diseases, Stanford University School of Medicine, Stanford, California; Attending Physician, Veterans Affairs Palo Alto Health Care, Palo Alto, California
Mycobacterium leprae (Leprosy)

Angela Restrepo, MSc, PhD
Senior Researcher, Medical and Experimental Mycology Unit, Corporación para Investigaciones Biológicas, Medellín, Antioquia, Colombia
Paracoccidioidomycosis

John H. Rex, MD
Adjunct Professor of Medicine, Department of Internal Medicine, Division of Infectious Diseases, Center for the Study of Emerging and Reemerging Pathogens, University of Texas Medical School, Houston, Texas; Head of Infection, Global Medicines Development, AstraZeneca Pharmaceuticals, Waltham, Massachusetts
Sporothrix schenckii

Elizabeth G. Rhee, MD
Director, Clinical Research, Department of Clinical Pharmacology, Merck Research Laboratories, Kenilworth, New Jersey
Adenoviruses

José R. Romero, MD
Horace C. Cabe Professor of Infectious Diseases, Department of Pediatrics, University of Arkansas for Medical Sciences; Director, Pediatric Infectious Diseases Section, Department of Pediatrics, Arkansas Children's Hospital; Director, Clinical Trials Research, Arkansas Children's Hospital Research Institute, Little Rock, Arkansas
Poliovirus; Coxsackieviruses, Echoviruses, and Numbered Enteroviruses; Human Parechoviruses

Alan L. Rothman, MD
Research Professor, Institute for Immunology and Informatics and Department of Cell and Molecular Biology, University of Rhode Island, Providence, Rhode Island
Flaviviruses (Dengue, Yellow Fever, Japanese Encephalitis, West Nile Encephalitis, St. Louis Encephalitis, Tick-Borne Encephalitis, Kyasanur Forest Disease, Alkhurma Hemorrhagic Fever, Zika)

Craig R. Roy, PhD
Professor, Department of Microbial Pathogenesis, Yale University School of Medicine, New Haven, Connecticut
Legionnaires' Disease and Pontiac Fever

Mark E. Rupp, MD
Professor and Chief, Infectious Diseases, University of Nebraska Medical Center; Medical Director, Infection Control and Epidemiology, The Nebraska Medical Center, Omaha, Nebraska
Mediastinitis; Staphylococcus epidermidis and Other Coagulase-Negative Staphylococci

Charles E. Rupprecht, VMD, PhD
Research Coordinator at Global Alliance for Rabies Control, Atlanta, Georgia; Professor, Ross University School of Veterinary Medicine, Basseterre St. Kitts, West Indies
Rabies (Rhabdoviruses)

Thomas A. Russo, MD, CM
Professor of Medicine and Microbiology, Division of Infectious Diseases, State University of New York at Buffalo School of Medicine and Biomedical Sciences; Staff Physician, Veterans Affairs Western New York Health Care System, Buffalo, New York
Agents of Actinomycosis

William A. Rutala, MS, PhD, MPH
Professor of Medicine, Director, Statewide Program for Infection Control and Epidemiology, University of North Carolina at Chapel Hill School of Medicine; Director, Hospital Epidemiology, Occupational Health and Safety, University of North Carolina Health Care, Chapel Hill, North Carolina
The Acutely Ill Patient with Fever and Rash

Edward T. Ryan, MD
Professor of Medicine, Harvard Medical School; Professor of Immunology and Infectious Diseases, Harvard School of Public Health; Director, Tropical Medicine, Massachusetts General Hospital, Boston, Massachusetts
Enteric Fever and Other Causes of Fever and Abdominal Symptoms; Vibrio cholerae

Amar Safdar, MD, MBBS
Associate Professor of Medicine, Division of Infectious Diseases and Immunology, New York University School of Medicine; Director, Transplant Infectious Diseases, Department of Medicine, NYU Langone Medical Center, New York, New York
Stenotrophomonas maltophilia and Burkholderia cepacia

Juan C. Salazar, MD, MPH
Professor and Chairman, Department of Pediatrics, University of Connecticut School of Medicine, Farmington, Connecticut; Physician-in-Chief, Head of Division of Pediatric Infectious Diseases and Immunology, Connecticut Children's Medical Center, Hartford, Connecticut
Syphilis (Treponema pallidum)

Maria C. Savoia, MD
Dean for Medical Education, Professor of Medicine, University of California San Diego School of Medicine, La Jolla, California
Myocarditis and Pericarditis

Paul E. Sax, MD
Professor of Medicine, Harvard Medical School; Clinical Director, Division of Infectious Diseases and Human Immunodeficiency Virus Program, Brigham and Women's Hospital, Boston, Massachusetts
Pulmonary Manifestations of Human Immunodeficiency Virus Infection

W. Michael Scheld, MD
Gerald L. Mandell–Bayer Professor of Infectious Diseases, Professor of Medicine, University of Virginia School of Medicine; Clinical Professor of Neurosurgery, Director, Pfizer Initiative in International Health, University of Virginia Health System, Charlottesville, Virginia
Endocarditis and Intravascular Infections; Acute Meningitis

Joshua T. Schiffer, MD, MSc
Assistant Professor, Department of Medicine, University of Washington; Assistant Member, Vaccine and Infectious Diseases Division, Clinical Research Division, Fred Hutchinson Cancer Research Center, Seattle, Washington
Herpes Simplex Virus

David Schlossberg, MD
Professor, Department of Medicine, Temple University School of Medicine; Medical Director, Tuberculosis Control Program, Philadelphia Department of Public Health, Philadelphia, Pennsylvania
Psittacosis (Due to Chlamydia psittaci)

Thomas Schneider, MD, PhD
Professor of Infectious Diseases, Charité University Hospital, Benjamin Franklin Campus, Berlin, Germany
Whipple's Disease

Jane R. Schwebke, MD
Professor of Medicine, Medicine/Infectious Diseases, University of Alabama at Birmingham, Birmingham, Alabama
Trichomonas vaginalis

Leopoldo N. Segal, MD
Assistant Professor, Department of Medicine, New York University School of Medicine, New York, New York
Acute Exacerbations of Chronic Obstructive Pulmonary Disease

Parham Sendi, MD
Consultant and Lecturer, Basel University Medical Clinic, Liestal, Switzerland; Department of Infectious Diseases, University Hospital and Institute for Infectious Diseases, University of Bern, Bern, Switzerland
Orthopedic Implant–Associated Infections

Kent A. Sepkowitz, MD
Deputy Physician-in-Chief, Quality and Safety, Memorial Sloan Kettering Cancer Center; Professor of Medicine, Weill Cornell Medical College, New York, New York
Health Care–Acquired Hepatitis

Edward J. Septimus, MD
Clinical Professor, Department of Internal
Medicine, Texas A&M Health Science Center,
Houston, Texas; Medical Director, Infection
Prevention and Epidemiology, Clinical Services
Group, HCA, Inc., Nashville, Tennessee
Pleural Effusion and Empyema

Alexey Seregin, PhD
Research Scientist, Department of Pathology,
University of Texas Medical Branch, Galveston,
Texas
Lymphocytic Choriomeningitis, Lassa Fever, and
the South American Hemorrhagic Fevers
(Arenaviruses)

Stanford T. Shulman, MD
Virginia H. Rogers Professor of Pediatric
Infectious Diseases, Northwestern University
Feinberg School of Medicine; Chief, Division of
Infectious Diseases, Department of Pediatrics,
Ann & Robert H. Lurie Children's Hospital of
Chicago, Chicago, Illinois
Nonsuppurative Poststreptococcal Sequelae:
Rheumatic Fever and Glomerulonephritis

George K. Siberry, MD, MPH
Medical Officer, Maternal and Pediatric Infectious
Disease Branch, Eunice Kennedy Shriver National
Institute of Child Health and Human
Development, National Institutes of Health,
Bethesda, Maryland
Pediatric Human Immunodeficiency Virus
Infection

Omar K. Siddiqi, MD
Clinical Instructor, Department of Neurology,
Beth Israel Deaconess Medical Center, Boston,
Massachusetts; Honorary Lecturer, Department
Medicine, University of Zambia School of
Medicine, Lusaka, Zambia
Neurologic Diseases Caused by Human
Immunodeficiency Virus Type 1 and Opportunistic
Infections

Costi D. Sifri, MD
Associate Professor of Medicine, Division of
Infectious Diseases and International Health,
University of Virginia School of Medicine;
Attending Physician, Department of Medicine,
University of Virginia Health System,
Charlottesville, Virginia
Infections of the Liver and Biliary System (Liver
Abscess, Cholangitis, Cholecystitis)

Michael S. Simberkoff, MD
Professor of Medicine, Department of Medicine,
Division of Infectious Diseases and Immunology,
New York University School of Medicine, New
York, New York
Mycoplasma pneumoniae and Atypical
Pneumonia

Francesco R. Simonetti, MD
Guest Researcher, HIV Drug Resistance Program,
National Cancer Institute—Frederick, National
Institutes of Health, Frederick, Maryland
Diagnosis of Human Immunodeficiency Virus
Infection

Kamaljit Singh, MD, D(ABMM)
Associate Professor, Departments of Medicine
and Pathology, Rush University Medical Center,
Chicago, Illinois
Rabies (Rhabdoviruses)

Nina Singh, MD
Professor of Medicine, Department of Medicine,
Division of Infectious Diseases, University of
Pittsburgh and VA Pittsburgh Healthcare System,
Pittsburgh, Pennsylvania
Infections in Solid-Organ Transplant Recipients

Upinder Singh, MD
Associate Professor of Medicine, Departments of
Infectious Diseases and Microbiology &
Immunology, Stanford School of Medicine,
Stanford, California
Free-Living Amebae

Scott W. Sinner, MD
Hyperbaric Medical Director, Mercy-Clermont
Hospital, Batavia, Ohio
Viridans Streptococci, Nutritionally Variant
Streptococci, Groups C and G Streptococci, and
Other Related Organisms

Leonard N. Slater, MD
Professor of Infectious Diseases, Department of
Internal Medicine, College of Medicine,
University of Oklahoma, Oklahoma City,
Oklahoma
Bartonella, Including Cat-Scratch Disease

A. George Smulian, MB BCh, MSc
Associate Professor, University of Cincinnati
College of Medicine; Chief, Infectious Disease
Section, Veterans Affairs Cincinnati Medical
Center, Cincinnati, Ohio
Pneumocystis Species

Jack D. Sobel, MD
Professor of Medicine, Division of Infectious
Diseases, Wayne State University School of
Medicine, Detroit, Michigan
Urinary Tract Infections

M. Rizwan Sohail, MD
Associate Professor of Medicine, Divisions of
Infectious Diseases and Cardiovascular Diseases,
Department of Medicine, Mayo Clinic College of
Medicine, Rochester, Minnesota
Infections of Nonvalvular Cardiovascular Devices

David E. Soper, MD
Professor and Vice Chairman, Department of
Obstetrics and Gynecology, Medical University of
South Carolina, Charleston, South Carolina
Infections of the Female Pelvis

Tania C. Sorrell, AM, MD, MBBS
Professor and Director, Marie Bashir Institute for
Infectious Diseases and Biosecurity, University of
Sydney, Sydney, New South Wales, Australia;
Director, Centre for Infectious Diseases and
Microbiology and Service Director, Infectious
Diseases and Sexual Health, Westmead, New
South Wales, Australia
Nocardia Species

James M. Steckelberg, MD
Professor of Medicine, Consultant, Division of
Infectious Diseases, Mayo Clinic, Rochester,
Minnesota
Osteomyelitis

Allen C. Steere, MD
Professor of Medicine, Harvard Medical School,
Harvard University; Director, Translational
Research in Rheumatology, Massachusetts
General Hospital, Boston, Massachusetts
Lyme Disease (Lyme Borreliosis) Due to *Borrelia
burgdorferi*

James P. Steinberg, MD
Professor of Medicine, Division of Infectious
Diseases, Emory University School of Medicine;
Chief Medical Officer, Emory University Hospital
Midtown, Atlanta, Georgia
Other Gram-Negative and Gram-Variable Bacilli

David S. Stephens, MD
Stephen W. Schwarzmann Distinguished
Professor of Medicine, Chair, Department of
Medicine, Emory University School of Medicine;
Vice President for Research, Robert W. Woodruff
Health Sciences Center, Emory University,
Atlanta, Georgia
Neisseria meningitidis

Timothy R. Sterling, MD
Professor of Medicine, Division of Infectious
Diseases, Vanderbilt University School of
Medicine, Nashville, Tennessee
General Clinical Manifestations of Human
Immunodeficiency Virus Infection (Including Acute
Retroviral Syndrome and Oral, Cutaneous, Renal,
Ocular, Metabolic, and Cardiac Diseases);
Mycobacterium tuberculosis

Dennis L. Stevens, MD, PhD
Associate Chief of Staff, Research and
Development Service, Veterans Affairs Medical
Center, Boise, Idaho; Professor of Medicine,
Department of Medicine, University of
Washington, Seattle, Washington
Streptococcus pyogenes

Charles W. Stratton IV, MD
Associate Professor of Pathology and Medicine,
Vanderbilt University School of Medicine;
Director, Clinical Microbiology Laboratory,
Vanderbilt University Medical Center, Nashville,
Tennessee
Streptococcus anginosus Group

Anthony F. Suffredini, MD
Senior Investigator, Critical Care Medicine
Department, Clinical Center, National Institutes
of Health, Bethesda, Maryland
Sepsis, Severe Sepsis, and Septic Shock

Kathryn N. Suh, MD, MSc
Associate Professor of Medicine, University of
Ottawa; Division of Infectious Diseases, The
Ottawa Hospital, Ottawa, Canada
*Cyclospora cayetanensis, Cystoisospora (Isospora)
belli, Sarcocystis* Species, *Balantidium coli,* and
Blastocystis Species

Mark S. Sulkowski, MD
Professor of Medicine, Medical Director, Viral
Hepatitis Center Divisions of Infectious Diseases
and Gastroenterology/Hepatology, Johns Hopkins
University School of Medicine, Baltimore,
Maryland
Gastrointestinal, Hepatobiliary, and Pancreatic
Manifestations of Human Immunodeficiency Virus
Infection

Morton N. Swartz, MD†
Associate Firm Chief, Infectious Diseases Unit,
Massachusetts General Hospital, Boston,
Massachusetts
Cellulitis, Necrotizing Fasciitis, and Subcutaneous
Tissue Infections; Myositis and Myonecrosis

Thomas R. Talbot, MD, MPH
Associate Professor of Medicine and Health
Policy, Vanderbilt University School of Medicine;
Chief Hospital Epidemiologist, Vanderbilt
University Medical Center, Nashville, Tennessee
Surgical Site Infections and Antimicrobial
Prophylaxis

C. Sabrina Tan, MD
Assistant Professor of Medicine, Harvard Medical
School, Beth Israel Deaconess Medical Center,
Boston, Massachusetts
JC, BK, and Other Polyomaviruses: Progressive
Multifocal Leukoencephalopathy (PML)

Ming Tan, MD
Professor of Medicine, Microbiology and
Molecular Genetics, University of California at
Irvine School of Medicine, Irvine, California
Chlamydia trachomatis (Trachoma, Genital
Infections, Perinatal Infections, and
Lymphogranuloma Venereum)

†Deceased.

Chloe Lynne Thio, MD
Associate Professor of Medicine, Department of
Internal Medicine, Division of Infectious
Diseases, Johns Hopkins University School of
Medicine, Baltimore, Maryland
Hepatitis B Virus and Hepatitis Delta Virus

David L. Thomas, MD, MPH
Professor of Medicine, Director, Division of
Infectious Diseases, Johns Hopkins University
School of Medicine, Baltimore, Maryland
Hepatitis C

Stephen J. Thomas, MD
Director, Viral Diseases Branch, Walter Reed
Army Institute of Research, Silver Spring,
Maryland
Flaviviruses (Dengue, Yellow Fever, Japanese
Encephalitis, West Nile Encephalitis, St. Louis
Encephalitis, Tick-Borne Encephalitis, Kyasanur
Forest Disease, Alkhurma Hemorrhagic Fever,
Zika)

Anna R. Thorner, MD
Assistant Clinical Professor of Medicine,
Department of Medicine, Harvard Medical
School; Associate Physician, Division of
Infectious Disease, Brigham and Women's
Hospital, Boston, Massachusetts
Zoonotic Paramyxoviruses: Nipah, Hendra, and
Menangle

Angela María Tobón, MD
Director, Chronic Infectious Diseases Unit,
Department of Internal Medicine, Corporación
para Investigaciones Biológicas, Medellín,
Colombia
Paracoccidioidomycosis

Edmund C. Tramont, MD
Associate Director, Special Projects, Division of
Clinical Research, National Institute of Allergy
and Infectious Diseases, National Institutes of
Health, Bethesda, Maryland
Syphilis (Treponema pallidum)

John J. Treanor, MD
Chief, Division of Infectious Diseases,
Department of Medicine, University of Rochester
Medical Center, Rochester, New York
Influenza (Including Avian Influenza and Swine
Influenza); Noroviruses and Sapoviruses
(Caliciviruses); Astroviruses and Picobirnaviruses

Athe M. N. Tsibris, MD, MS
Assistant Professor in Medicine, Division of
Infectious Diseases, Harvard Medical School;
Brigham and Women's Hospital, Boston,
Massachusetts
Antiretroviral Therapy for Human
Immunodeficiency Virus Infection

Allan R. Tunkel, MD, PhD, MACP
Professor of Medicine, Associate Dean for
Medical Education, Warren Alpert Medical
School of Brown University, Providence, Rhode
Island
Acute Meningitis; Brain Abscess; Subdural
Empyema, Epidural Abscess, and Suppurative
Intracranial Thrombophlebitis; Cerebrospinal Fluid
Shunt and Drain Infections; Viridans Streptococci,
Nutritionally Variant Streptococci, Groups C and
G Streptococci, and Other Related Organisms

Ronald B. Turner, MD
Professor of Pediatrics, University of Virginia
School of Medicine, Charlottesville, Virginia
The Common Cold; Rhinovirus

Kenneth L. Tyler, MD
Reuler-Lewin Family Professor of Neurology and
Professor of Medicine and Microbiology,
University of Colorado Denver School of
Medicine, Aurora, Colorado; Chief, Neurology
Service, Denver Veterans Affairs Medical Center,
Denver, Colorado
Encephalitis; Orthoreoviruses and Orbiviruses;
Coltiviruses and Seadornaviruses; Prions and Prion
Diseases of the Central Nervous System
(Transmissible Neurodegenerative Diseases)

Ahmet Uluer, DO, MS
Assistant Professor of Pediatrics, Department of
Medicine, Harvard Medical School; Boston
Children's Hospital, Boston, Massachusetts
Cystic Fibrosis

Diederik van de Beek, MD, PhD
Professor, Department of Neurology, Center of
Infection and Immunity Amsterdam (CINIMA),
Academic Medical Center, University of
Amsterdam, Amsterdam, The Netherlands
Acute Meningitis

Edouard G. Vannier, PharmD, PhD
Assistant Professor of Medicine, Division of
Geographic Medicine and Infectious Diseases,
Tufts Medical Center and Tufts University School
of Medicine, Boston, Massachusetts
Babesia Species

Trevor C. Van Schooneveld, MD
Assistant Professor of Infectious Diseases,
Department of Internal Medicine, University of
Nebraska Medical Center, Omaha, Nebraska
Mediastinitis

Claudio Viscoli, MD
Division of Infectious Diseases, IRCCS AOU San
Martino-IST; Department of Health Sciences,
University of Genova, Genova, Italy
Prophylaxis and Empirical Therapy of Infection in
Cancer Patients

Ellen R. Wald, MD
Alfred Dorrance Daniels Professor on Diseases of Children, University of Wisconsin School of Medicine and Public Health; Pediatrician-in-Chief, American Family Children's Hospital, Madison, Wisconsin
Sinusitis

Matthew K. Waldor, MD, PhD
Edward H. Kass Professor of Medicine, Harvard Medical School; Division of Infectious Diseases, Brigham and Women's Hospital, Boston, Massachusetts
Vibrio cholerae

David H. Walker, MD
Professor, Department of Pathology, University of Texas Medical Branch; Executive Director, Center for Biodefense and Emerging Infectious Diseases, Galveston, Texas
Rickettsia rickettsii and Other Spotted Fever Group Rickettsiae (Rocky Mountain Spotted Fever and Other Spotted Fevers); *Rickettsia prowazekii* (Epidemic or Louse-Borne Typhus); *Rickettsia typhi* (Murine Typhus); *Ehrlichia chaffeensis* (Human Monocytotropic Ehrlichiosis), *Anaplasma phagocytophilum* (Human Granulocytotropic Anaplasmosis), and Other Anaplasmataceae

Richard J. Wallace, Jr., MD
Chairman, Department of Microbiology, University of Texas Health Northeast, Tyler, Texas
Infections Caused by Nontuberculous Mycobacteria Other than *Mycobacterium avium* Complex

Edward E. Walsh, MD
Professor of Medicine, Department of Infectious Diseases, University of Rochester School of Medicine and Dentistry, Rochester, New York
Acute Bronchitis; Respiratory Syncytial Virus (RSV)

Stephen R. Walsh, MD
Assistant Professor of Medicine, Harvard Medical School; Beth Israel Deaconess Medical Center, Boston, Massachusetts
Hepatitis E Virus

Peter D. Walzer, MD, MSc
Emeritus Professor of Medicine, University of Cincinnati; Retired Associate Chief of Staff for Research, Cincinnati VA Medical Center, Cincinnati, Ohio
Pneumocystis Species

Christine A. Wanke, MD
Professor, Department of Medicine, Associate Chair, Department of Public Health and Community Medicine, Tufts University School of Medicine, Boston, Massachusetts
Tropical Sprue: Enteropathy

Cirle A. Warren, MD
Assistant Professor, Infectious Diseases and International Health, University of Virginia School of Medicine, Charlottesville, Virginia
Bacterial Inflammatory Enteritides

Ronald G. Washburn, MD
Associate Chief of Staff for Research and Development, Medical Research, Chief of Infectious Diseases, Medical Service, Shreveport Veterans Affairs Medical Center; Professor of Medicine, Infectious Diseases Section, Louisiana State University Health Sciences Center, Shreveport, Louisiana
Rat-Bite Fever: *Streptobacillus moniliformis* and *Spirillum minus*

Valerie Waters, MD, MSc
Associate Professor, Department of Pediatric Infectious Diseases, Hospital for Sick Children, Toronto, Ontario, Canada
Bordetella pertussis

David J. Weber, MD, MPH
Professor of Medicine, Pediatrics, and Epidemiology, University of North Carolina at Chapel Hill School of Medicine; Associate Chief of Staff and Medical Director, Hospital Epidemiology and Occupational Health, University of North Carolina Health Care, Chapel Hill, North Carolina
The Acutely Ill Patient with Fever and Rash

Michael D. Weiden, MD
Associate Professor, Departments of Medicine and Environmental Medicine, New York University School of Medicine, Langone Medical Center, New York, New York
Acute Exacerbations of Chronic Obstructive Pulmonary Disease

Geoffrey A. Weinberg, MD
Professor of Pediatrics, Department of Pediatrics, University of Rochester School of Medicine and Dentistry; Director, Pediatric HIV Program, Golisano Children's Hospital, University of Rochester Medical Center, Rochester, New York
Epiglottitis; Pediatric Human Immunodeficiency Virus Infection

Daniel J. Weisdorf, MD
Professor of Medicine, Division of Hematology, Oncology, and Transplantation, Director, Adult Blood and Marrow Transplant Program, University of Minnesota Medical School, Minneapolis, Minnesota
Infections in Recipients of Hematopoietic Stem Cell Transplants

Contributors

Louis M. Weiss, MD, MPH
Professor, Departments of Pathology and
Medicine, Albert Einstein College of Medicine,
Bronx, New York
Microsporidiosis

David F. Welch, PhD
Clinical Consultant, Medical Microbiology
Consulting, LLC, Dallas, Texas
Bartonella, Including Cat-Scratch Disease

Thomas E. Wellems, MD, PhD
Chief, Laboratory of Malaria and Vector
Research, Chief, Malaria Genetics Section,
Laboratory of Malaria and Vector Research,
National Institute of Allergy and Infectious
Diseases, Rockville, Maryland
Malaria (*Plasmodium* Species)

A. Clinton White, Jr., MD
Paul R. Stalnaker Distinguished Professor,
Director, Division of Infectious Diseases,
Department of Internal Medicine, University of
Texas Medical Branch, Galveston, Texas
Cryptosporidiosis (*Cryptosporidium* Species)

Richard J. Whitley, MD
Distinguished Professor of Pediatrics, Loeb
Eminent Scholar Chair in Pediatrics, Professor of
Microbiology, Medicine, and Neurosurgery,
Department of Pediatrics, University of Alabama
at Birmingham, Birmingham, Alabama
Chickenpox and Herpes Zoster (Varicella-Zoster
Virus)

Walter R. Wilson, MD
Professor of Medicine and Assistant Professor of
Microbiology, Mayo Clinic College of Medicine;
Consultant, Infectious Diseases, Mayo Clinic,
Rochester, Minnesota
Prosthetic Valve Endocarditis

William F. Wright, DO, MPH
Assistant Professor of Medicine and Microbiology,
Division of Infectious Diseases and Travel
Medicine, Georgetown University School of
Medicine, Washington, DC
Fever of Unknown Origin

Jo-Anne H. Young, MD
Professor of Medicine, Division of Infectious
Disease and International Medicine, Medical
Director of the Program in Adult Transplant
Infectious Disease University of Minnesota,
Minneapolis, Minnesota; Editor-in-Chief, Clinical
Microbiology Reviews, American Society of
Microbiology, Washington, DC
Infections in Recipients of Hematopoietic Stem
Cell Transplants

Vincent B. Young, MD, PhD
Associate Professor, Department of Internal
Medicine, Division of Infectious Diseases,
Department of Microbiology and Immunology,
University of Michigan Medical School, Ann
Arbor, Michigan
Clostridium difficile Infection

Nadezhda Yun, MD
Assistant Professor, Department of Pathology,
Assistant Director, Preclinical Studies Core,
Galveston National Laboratory, University of
Texas Medical Branch, Galveston, Texas
Lymphocytic Choriomeningitis, Lassa Fever, and
the South American Hemorrhagic Fevers
(Arenaviruses)

Werner Zimmerli, MD
Professor, Basel University Medical Clinic, Liestal,
Switzerland
Orthopedic Implant–Associated Infections

John J. Zurlo, MD
Professor of Medicine, Department of Medicine/
Infectious Diseases, Penn State Hershey Medical
Center, Hershey, Pennsylvania
Pasteurella Species

Preface

This handbook is an introduction to *Mandell, Douglas, and Bennett's Principles and Practice of Infectious Diseases*, also known as *PPID*, which is the detailed, authoritative reference book for the field. The handbook consists of "short view summaries" that introduce 241 of the 324 chapters in the 8th edition of *PPID* and that appear at the beginning of each chapter in a template format. The summaries are accompanied by tables and figures that illustrate the material contained therein. In addition, this handbook reflects the annual updates that appear in the electronic version of *PPID*.

The field of infectious disease is undergoing an extraordinary expansion of knowledge, with dramatic advances in diagnosis, therapy, and prevention of infectious diseases, as well as recognition of novel pathogens and diseases. The handbook is intended to provide information on these topics in an easy-to-use form, and to facilitate access to further information as needed. In this regard,

the handbook is organized on the same basis as the parent textbook, *PPID*. Information is presented according to major infectious clinical syndromes, and individual pathogens are addressed in more detail subsequently. Examples of topics in which important new developments have occurred include hepatitis B and C, Ebola, influenza, *Clostridium difficile,* methicillin-resistant *Staphylococcus aureus* (MRSA), tuberculosis, human immunodeficiency virus, and Middle East respiratory syndrome (MERS).

We hope this handbook will be a convenient, useful, and current source of information for those interested in infectious diseases, and that it will serve as an introduction to the more detailed and comprehensive material that can be found in the parent text, *PPID*.

John E. Bennett, MD, MACP
Raphael Dolin, MD
Martin J. Blaser, MD

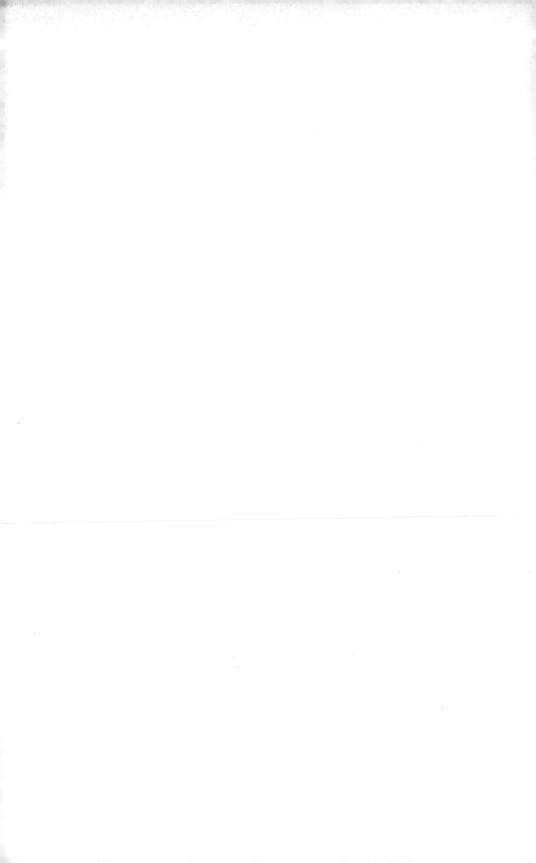

Contents

II INFECTIOUS DISEASES AND THEIR ETIOLOGIC AGENTS

Contents

Major Clinical Syndromes

1 Fever of Unknown Origin

William F. Wright and Philip A. Mackowiak

DEFINITION

- Occurrence of several occasions of fever higher than 38.3°C (101°F) with a duration greater than at least 3 weeks despite 1 week of hospital evaluation is still recognized as the classic definition for fever of unknown origin (FUO).
- The advent of improved diagnostic testing modalities coupled with an increasing number of immunocompromised patients led to a revised definition in which cases of FUO are currently codified into four distinct subclasses: classic FUO, health care–associated FUO, immune-deficient FUO, and human immunodeficiency virus (HIV)-related FUO.

ETIOLOGY AND EPIDEMIOLOGY

- Infections, neoplasms, connective tissue diseases, miscellaneous causes, and undiagnosed fevers remain the most common causes of classic FUO.
- The frequency with which infections and neoplasms have been identified as the causes of classic FUO has decreased steadily, whereas the proportion of miscellaneous causes and undiagnosed conditions has risen in recent years.

DIAGNOSIS

- A comprehensive medical history with verification of fever and a detailed physical examination are essential in directing formal laboratory testing.

THERAPY

- Empirical therapeutic trials of antimicrobial agents continue to have a limited role in the management of patients with FUO.
- Owing to the relatively high prevalence of serious bacterial infections responsible for fevers in patients with neutropenia, such patients should receive broad-spectrum antipseudomonal therapy immediately after samples for appropriate cultures have been obtained.

PROGNOSIS

- Although the prognosis of an FUO is determined by its etiology and underlying diseases, most patients with prolonged undiagnosed FUO generally have a favorable outcome.

2 The Acutely Ill Patient with Fever and Rash

David J. Weber, Myron S. Cohen, and William A. Rutala

DEFINITION
- Skin lesions are frequently present in acutely ill patients with serious infectious diseases and may provide important clues that aid in early diagnosis and treatment.

EPIDEMIOLOGY
- Acutely ill patients with a potential infectious disease and skin lesions (or rash) should have a history obtained that elicits the following: recent drug ingestion; travel outside the local area; potential occupational exposures; recent immunizations; risk factors for sexually transmitted infections, including human immunodeficiency virus infection; factors affecting host resistance or immunocompromising conditions; prior allergies to antibiotics; recent exposures to febrile or ill persons; exposure to rural habits, insects, arthropods, and wild animals; and exposure to pets or animals.
- Patients with skin lesions or rashes consistent with a communicable infectious disease (e.g., invasive meningococcal infection) should be immediately placed on appropriate isolation precautions (i.e., contact, droplet, or airborne).
- Infectious disease physicians should be familiar with the skin lesions (or rash) that might accompany a patient with disease that could be the result of the intentional use of a bioweapon (e.g., anthrax, smallpox, plague, viral hemorrhagic fevers).

MICROBIOLOGY
- Serious bacterial infections with skin lesions include *Staphylococcus aureus* (toxic shock syndrome, scalded skin syndrome), *Streptococcus pyogenes* (toxic shock syndrome), *Salmonella enterica* serotype Typhi, *Neisseria meningitidis,* and *Rickettsia rickettsii.*
- Potentially serious viral infections with skin lesions include measles, rubella, Epstein-Barr infection, cytomegalovirus, human herpesvirus 6, and viral hemorrhagic fevers (e.g., Ebola, Marburg, Lassa).
- Life-threatening drug reactions may result from antibiotic therapy for disorders such as Stevens-Johnson syndrome/toxic epidermolysis necrosis and from drug reaction with eosinophilia and systemic symptoms (DRESS).

DIAGNOSIS
- Key aspects of skin lesions that aid in a proper diagnosis include (1) primary type(s) of skin lesions, (2) distribution of the lesions, (3) pattern of progression of the rash, and (4) timing of onset of the rash relative to the onset of fever and other systemic signs.
- The appearance of skin lesions may be very useful in the diagnosis of specific infectious diseases. Maculopapular rashes are usually seen in viral illnesses, drug eruptions, and immune complex–mediated diseases. Nodular lesions are suggestive of mycobacteria or fungal infections. Diffuse erythema suggests scarlet fever, toxic shock syndrome, Kawasaki disease, or Stevens-Johnson syndrome/toxic epidermal necrolysis. Bullous lesions suggest streptococcal erysipelas with necrotizing fasciitis, ecthyma gangrenosum, and *Vibrio*

3

infections. Petechial eruptions suggest gram-negative sepsis, invasive *Neisseria meningitidis* infection, and rickettsial infections.
- Consideration should be given to biopsy of skin lesions, if present, in acutely ill immuno-compromised patients for appropriate stains (e.g., Gram stain, fungal stain) and cultures and for pathologic study.

THERAPY
- Empirical therapy should often be initiated in acutely ill patients with skin lesions based on the clinical diagnosis.
- Most acutely ill patients with skin lesions will require systemic therapy.

PREVENTION
- Standard vaccines should be provided to children and adults because many vaccine-preventable diseases produce rashes (e.g., measles, rubella, varicella).
- Underlying noninfectious diseases that lead to disruption of skin should be treated because the damaged skin serves as risk factor for infection.

3 The Common Cold

Ronald B. Turner

DEFINITION

- The common cold is an upper respiratory illness that includes rhinorrhea and nasal obstruction as prominent symptoms.

EPIDEMIOLOGY

- Common cold illnesses occur 5 to 7 times per year in children and 2 to 3 times per year in adults.
- Illnesses occur most commonly between the early fall and late spring in temperate climates.
- Transmission of the viral pathogens causing the common cold may occur via direct contact, large-particle aerosol, or small-particle aerosol.

MICROBIOLOGY

- The rhinoviruses are responsible for the majority of common cold illnesses.
- Coronavirus, respiratory syncytial virus, and metapneumovirus may also be associated with the common cold syndrome.
- Other respiratory viruses may cause common cold symptoms but are frequently associated with lower respiratory symptoms in addition to the upper respiratory illness.
- Coinfection with more than one pathogen is common in these illnesses.

DIAGNOSIS

- The diagnosis of the common cold is a clinical diagnosis.
- The responsible pathogen(s) can be determined by polymerase chain reaction assay, but this is rarely useful in the management of the patient.

THERAPY

- There are no specific antiviral agents that are useful for treatment of the common cold.
- Management depends on symptomatic therapy with treatment directed at the most bothersome symptoms.

PREVENTION

- There are no proven interventions for prevention of the common cold.

4 Pharyngitis

Anthony R. Flores and Mary T. Caserta

DEFINITION
- Pharyngitis is defined as the triad of sore throat, fever, and pharyngeal inflammation.
- Generally a primary disease, pharyngitis may be associated with systemic disorders.

EPIDEMIOLOGY
- Pharyngitis is one of the most common disorders in adults and children, with more than 10 million ambulatory visits per year.
- The highest burden of disease is found in children and young adults, with 50% of cases identified between the ages of 5 to 24 years.
- In temperate climates, most cases occur in winter months, corresponding with peaks in respiratory viruses.

MICROBIOLOGY
- Viruses are the single most common cause of pharyngitis, with adenovirus being the most commonly identified (see Table 4-1).
- Group A *Streptococcus* (GAS) is the bacterial cause for which ample evidence exists for antibiotic therapy to prevent postinfectious sequelae.
- *Fusobacterium necrophorum* has been recently recognized as a cause of pharyngitis with potential severe complications (i.e., Lemierre syndrome), especially in young adults.

DIAGNOSIS
- Essential to diagnosis is the identification of treatable causes (e.g., GAS) to prevent complications.
- Signs and symptoms of GAS pharyngitis include acute onset of sore throat with tonsillar or pharyngeal exudates, tender anterior cervical lymphadenopathy, and fever (see Table 4-2).
- Signs and symptoms consistent with viral etiologies include conjunctivitis, coryza, oral ulcers, cough, and diarrhea.
- Testing for GAS pharyngitis should not be pursued in those with signs and symptoms indicative of a viral etiology (see Table 4-3).
- Rapid antigen detection tests (RADTs) alone are sufficient for the diagnosis of GAS in adults, but negative results should be backed up by throat culture in children.
- Specific techniques should be used to identify other causes where appropriate.

TABLE 4-1 Microbial Causes of Acute Pharyngitis

PATHOGEN	ASSOCIATED DISORDER(S)
Bacteria	
Streptococcus, group A	Pharyngitis, tonsillitis, scarlet fever
Streptococcus, groups C and G	Pharyngitis, tonsillitis
Mixed anaerobes	Vincent's angina
Fusobacterium necrophorum	Pharyngitis, tonsillitis, Lemierre syndrome
Neisseria gonorrhoeae	Pharyngitis, tonsillitis
Corynebacterium diphtheria	Diphtheria
Arcanobacterium haemolyticum	Pharyngitis, scarlatiniform rash
Yersinia pestis	Plague
Francisella tularensis	Tularemia, oropharyngeal form
Treponema pallidum	Secondary syphilis
Viruses	
Rhinovirus	Common cold
Coronavirus	Common cold
Adenovirus	Pharyngoconjunctival fever
Herpes simplex type 1 and 2	Pharyngitis, gingivostomatitis
Parainfluenza	Cold, croup
Enteroviruses	Herpangina, hand-foot-mouth disease
Epstein-Barr virus	Infectious mononucleosis
Cytomegalovirus	CMV mononucleosis
Human immunodeficiency virus	Primary HIV infection
Influenza A and B	Influenza
Respiratory syncytial virus	Cold, bronchiolitis, pneumonia
Human metapneumovirus	Cold, bronchiolitis, pneumonia
Mycoplasma	
Mycoplasma pneumoniae	Pneumonia, bronchitis, pharyngitis
Chlamydia	
Chlamydia psittaci	Acute respiratory disease, pneumonia
Chlamydia pneumoniae	Pneumonia, pharyngitis

CMV, cytomegalovirus; HIV, human immunodeficiency virus.
Modified from Alcaide ML, Bisno AL. Pharyngitis and epiglottitis. *Infect Dis Clin North Am.* 2007;21:449-469, vii; with permission.

THERAPY

- Treatment of pharyngitis is focused on prevention of postinfectious sequelae (e.g., acute rheumatic fever) from GAS.
- Penicillin and its derivatives remain the primary treatment for GAS pharyngitis (see Table 4-4).
- Antimicrobial therapy should not be used to prevent GAS pharyngitis except in special circumstances.
- Given the potential severity of complications from pharyngitis caused by *F. necrophorum*, signs of bacteremia or neck swelling warrant expansion of antibiotic therapy and further evaluation.

TABLE 4-2 Clinical and Epidemiologic Findings Associated with Group A *Streptococcus* Pharyngitis

Suggestive of Group A *Streptococcus*

Sudden onset
Sore throat
Fever
Headache
Nausea, vomiting, and abdominal pain
Inflammation of pharynx and tonsils
Patchy discrete exudates
Tender, enlarged anterior cervical nodes
Patient aged 5-15 yr
Presentation in winter or early spring
History of exposure

Suggestive of Viral Etiology

Conjunctivitis
Coryza
Cough
Diarrhea
Discrete ulcerative lesions

Suggestive of Complications of Pharyngitis

Dysphagia
Stridor
Drooling
Dysphonia
Marked neck swelling
Respiratory distress
Pharyngeal pseudomembrane
Hemodynamic instability
HIV behavioral risk
Travel to or exposure to individuals from a region endemic for diphtheria
Lack of diphtheria immunization

HIV, human immunodeficiency virus.
Modified from Shulman ST, Bisno AL, Clegg HW, et al. Clinical practice guideline for the diagnosis and management of group A streptococcal pharyngitis: 2012 update by the Infectious Diseases Society of America. *Clin Infect Dis.* 2012;55:e86-e102; and Kociolek LK, Shulman ST. In the clinic. Pharyngitis. *Ann Intern Med.* 2012;157:ITC3-1-ITC3-16; with permission.

TABLE 4-3 Modified Centor Score and Culture Management Approach for Pharyngitis

CRITERIA	POINTS
Temperature >38° C	1
Absence of cough	1
Swollen, tender anterior cervical nodes	1
Tonsillar swelling or exudate	1
Age	
3-14 yr	1
15-44 yr	0
45 yr or older	−1

SCORE	RISK OF STREPTOCOCCAL INFECTION	SUGGESTED MANAGEMENT
≤0	1%-2.5%	No further testing or antibiotic
1	5%-10%	
2	11%-17%	Culture all: antibiotics only for positive culture results
3	28%-35%	
≥4	51%-53%	Treat empirically with antibiotics and/or culture

From McIsaac WJ, Kellner JD, Aufricht P, et al. Empirical validation of guidelines for the management of pharyngitis in children and adults. *JAMA.* 2004;291:1587-1595; with permission.

TABLE 4-4   Antimicrobial Therapy for Group A Streptococcal Pharyngitis

DRUG	DOSE	DURATION
Oral Regimens		
Penicillin V	Children: 250 mg bid or tid Adolescents and adults: 250 mg tid or qid or 500 mg bid	10 days
Amoxicillin	50 mg/kg once daily (maximum 1000 mg) Alternative: 25 mg/kg bid (maximum 500 mg)	10 days
For Penicillin-Allergic Patients		
Erythromycin	Varies with formulation	10 days
First-generation cephalosporins	Varies with agent	10 days
Intramuscular Regimens		
Benzathine penicillin G	600,000 units for patients <27 kg	1 dose
	1.2 million units for patients ≥27 kg	1 dose
Mixtures of benzathine and procaine penicillin G	Varies with formulation	1 dose

Modified from Alcaide ML, Bisno AL. Pharyngitis and epiglottitis. *Infect Dis Clin North Am.* 2007;21:449-469, vii; with permission.

5 Acute Laryngitis

Mary T. Caserta

DEFINITION

- Acute laryngitis is a clinical syndrome characterized by a hoarse voice with decreased phonation and voice projection, usually occurring after an upper respiratory tract infection with cough.

EPIDEMIOLOGY

- Approximately 1% of medical care claims are due to dysphonia, with 42% of those classified as acute laryngitis.
- Two percent of individuals with acute respiratory symptoms are diagnosed with acute laryngitis.
- Acute laryngitis is diagnosed more frequently in women (mean age, 36 years) than men (mean age, 41 years).
- More cases are diagnosed in the colder months of the year.

MICROBIOLOGY

- A viral upper respiratory tract infection is often associated (see Table 5-1).
- Bacterial infections of the upper respiratory tract have also been implicated.
- Unusual causes include tuberculosis, blastomycosis, histoplasmosis, coccidiomycosis, cryptococcosis, and herpesvirus infections of the larynx.

DIAGNOSIS

- Clinical diagnosis is based on the appropriate history and changes of the voice.
- Visualization of the larynx reveals edema and vascular engorgement of the mucous membranes with hyperemic and erythematous vocal folds.

THERAPY

- Treatment is based on the underlying cause of the laryngeal pathologic process.
- Often, symptomatic therapy with voice rest, analgesics, and humidification is sufficient.

TABLE 5-1 Frequency of Laryngitis Associated with Common Respiratory Pathogens

PATHOGEN	FREQUENCY (%)
Rhinovirus	25-29
Influenza	28-35
Parainfluenza	8.5
Adenovirus	22-35
Coronavirus	25
Mycoplasma pneumoniae	3-37
Chlamydia pneumoniae	30
Group A β-hemolytic streptococcus	2.3-19
Human metapneumovirus	3-91

6 Croup in Children (Acute Laryngotracheobronchitis)

John Bower and John T. McBride

DEFINITION

- Croup is an acute viral infection of the upper airway presenting as stridor and a brassy cough.
- Most children develop croup only once, but a few children develop recurrent episodes called spasmodic croup.

EPIDEMIOLOGY

- Croup can be sporadic but usually occurs in epidemics in the fall that in temperate climates recently have been worse in odd-numbered years.

ETIOLOGY AND MICROBIOLOGY

- Parainfluenza type 1 virus infection is the most common cause of viral croup.
- The other parainfluenza viruses, respiratory syncytial virus (RSV), adenovirus, and measles are a few of the other agents associated with viral croup.
- Bacterial infections of the airway, including epiglottitis (*Haemophilus influenzae* type b) and tracheitis *(Staphylococcus aureus, Streptococcus),* represent medical emergencies and should be rapidly discriminated from viral croup.
- Diphtheria should be considered in the developing world and in nonimmunized populations.

DIAGNOSIS

- Diagnosis is clinical, although radiographs of the upper airway may be helpful.
- Children with epiglottitis and bacterial tracheitis are typically toxic and have difficulty swallowing and usually lack the brassy cough and harsh stridor.
- Recurrent (spasmodic) croup may be more common in children with atopy or gastroesophageal reflux.

THERAPY

- Home remedies including mist and cold air have not been proven to be effective.
- A single dose of a systemic corticosteroid decreases the severity and length of croup.

7 Otitis Externa, Otitis Media, and Mastoiditis

Jerome O. Klein

DEFINITION

Otitis Externa

- Otitis externa is an infection and inflammation of the external auditory canal.

Otitis Media

- Acute otitis media (AOM) is an acute illness marked by the presence of fluid in the middle ear and inflammation of the mucosa lining the middle ear space. Fluid may persist in the middle ear for weeks to months after appropriately treated AOM and is termed otitis media with effusion.

Mastoiditis

- Mastoiditis is infection and inflammation of the mastoid air cells and usually results from episodes of severe AOM.

EPIDEMIOLOGY

Otitis Externa

- Acute diffuse otitis externa or swimmer's ear occurs in hot humid weather.
- Invasive or malignant otitis externa occurs in diabetic, immunocompromised, and debilitated patients.
- Children are prone to place foreign objects in the external ear canal, which may cause maceration and infection of the skin lining the external canal.

Otitis Media

- Otitis media occurs at all ages, but the peak age group is children in the first 3 years of life.
- Children at risk for severe and recurrent otitis media are more frequently male, have a genetic predisposition to ear infections, and may be in large-group daycare exposed to frequent respiratory viruses and bacterial pathogens.

Mastoiditis

- The epidemiology of mastoiditis parallels that of otitis media.

MICROBIOLOGY

Otitis Externa

- The microbial microbiota of the external ear canal responsible for otitis externa is similar to that of skin elsewhere, including staphylococcal species and anaerobic bacteria.
- *Pseudomonas aeruginosa* is a frequent cause of swimmer's ear and malignant otitis externa.

Otitis Media

- *Streptococcus pneumoniae* and nontypeable *Haemophilus influenzae* are the most frequent bacterial pathogens in all age groups.
- *Moraxella catarrhalis,* group A *Streptococcus* and *Staphylococcus aureus* are less frequent causes of AOM.
- Respiratory viruses are frequent causes of AOM alone or associated with bacterial pathogens.

Mastoiditis

- The microbiology of mastoiditis is similar to that of AOM.
- Patients with persistent perforation of the tympanic membrane may have invasion of the mastoid by organisms present in the external ear canal, including S. *aureus* and P. *aeruginosa*.

DIAGNOSIS

Otitis Externa

- Acute localized otitis externa may occur as a pustule or furuncle that is visualized in the canal.
- Swimmer's ear is identified by edema, swelling, and erythema of the canal wall.
- Malignant otitis externa is associated with severe pain and tenderness of the tissues around the pinna and mastoid; pus may be present in the canal.

Otitis Media

- AOM is an acute illness with fluid in the middle ear and bulging or decreased mobility and inflammation of the tympanic membrane.

Mastoiditis

- The signs of mastoiditis include swelling, redness, and tenderness over the mastoid bone.
- The pinna is displaced downward and outward, and a purulent discharge may emerge through a perforation of the tympanic membrane.

THERAPY

Otitis Externa

- Swimmer's ear may be managed with gentle cleansing and irrigation of the external canal.
- Antibiotic solutions, including fluoroquinolone eardrops, are effective in localized infections.
- Systemic antimicrobial therapy, including activity against P. *aeruginosa*, is necessary to manage invasive external otitis.

Otitis Media

- High-dose amoxicillin is the preferred drug for patients with AOM.
- If amoxicillin fails, amoxicillin-clavulanate or parenteral ceftriaxone is preferred.
- Some children with AOM improve without use of antimicrobial agents.
- Placement of tympanostomy tubes may be warranted for children with severe and recurrent episodes of AOM.

Mastoiditis

- Antimicrobial therapy is similar to that of AOM.
- Incision and drainage may be necessary when abscesses form in the mastoid air cells.

PREVENTION

Otitis Externa

- Patients should be dissuaded from placing foreign objects, including cotton-tipped applicators, in the external canal.

Otitis Media

- Chemoprophylaxis may be of value for prevention of episodes of AOM in children with severe and recurrent disease.
- Pneumococcal conjugate vaccines have been effective in reducing episodes of AOM due to vaccine serotypes.
- Influenza virus vaccines reduce the incidence of AOM during the winter respiratory season.

Mastoiditis

- Prevention is similar to that of AOM.

8 Sinusitis

Gregory P. DeMuri and Ellen R. Wald

DEFINITION

- Sinusitis is defined as an inflammatory disorder of the paranasal sinuses.

EPIDEMIOLOGY

- Bacterial infection of the sinuses is estimated to occur in 0.5% to 2% of cases of viral upper respiratory infection (URI) in adults and 6% to 13% of children.

MICROBIOLOGY

- Classic studies of the bacteriology of sinusitis have obtained a specimen of sinus secretions by puncture of the maxillary antrum to reduce the risk of nasal contamination.
- *Streptococcus pneumoniae* is the most frequently isolated organism, followed by nontypeable *Haemophilus influenzae* and *Moraxella catarrhalis.*
- *Staphylococcus aureus* is not likely a significant cause of acute sinusitis but does play a role in the complications of sinusitis.
- The frequency of isolation of *S. pneumoniae* is decreasing recently with an increase in β-lactamase–producing *H. influenzae.*

DIAGNOSIS

- Imaging studies are not indicated for the routine diagnosis of acute sinusitis but may be useful when complications are suspected.
- The following three clinical presentations will identify patients with acute bacterial sinusitis:
  - Onset with *persistent* symptoms or signs, lasting at least 10 days without evidence of clinical improvement
  - Onset with severe symptoms or signs of high fever (≥39° C) and purulent nasal discharge lasting for 3 to 4 consecutive days
  - Onset with worsening symptoms or signs characterized by the new development of fever, headache, or increased nasal discharge after a typical viral URI that lasted 5 to 6 days with initial improvement

THERAPY

- For most adults and children, amoxicillin with or without clavulanate remains an excellent first-line agent for the treatment of sinusitis.
- Second-line agents include fluoroquinolones, cefdinir, cefuroxime, or the combination of cefixime with either clindamycin or linezolid.
- The duration of therapy should be for 7 days after the patient becomes free of signs and symptoms.
- Adjunctive therapies such as antihistamines, decongestants, nasal steroids, and nasal washes have provided minimal improvement in acute sinusitis.
- Surgical drainage is indicated for the complications of acute bacterial sinusitis.

9 Epiglottitis

Jennifer L. Nayak and Geoffrey A. Weinberg

EPIDEMIOLOGY AND ETIOLOGY

- *Pediatric epiglottitis:* a localized, invasive *Haemophilus influenzae* type b infection of the supraglottic area, including the epiglottis, that can be associated with bacteremia (60% to 98%); routine conjugate vaccination has largely eliminated this form of epiglottitis.
- *Adult epiglottitis:* often involves more of the supraglottic structures (aryepiglottic folds, vallecula, tongue base) and is not associated with bacteremia (<15%); when a bacterial pathogen is identified, it is more likely to be *Streptococcus pneumoniae, Streptococcus pyogenes,* or *Neisseria meningitidis.*
- Before routine infant immunization with *H. influenzae* type b conjugate vaccines 65% to 75% of all patients with epiglottitis were children 1 to 4 years of age; currently, 90% to 95% are adults.
- Incidence of adult epiglottitis in the United States and Europe is approximately 2/100,000 population.

CLINICAL MANIFESTATIONS

- *Pediatric epiglottitis:* an abrupt illness in a febrile young child with a toxic appearance, dysphagia or sore throat, a muffled or hoarse voice, stridor, drooling, and often a distinctive posture—the "tripod position," comprising apprehension, sitting very still, preferring to lean forward with hyperextension of the neck, and protrusion of the chin. Cough is distinctly uncommon.
- *Adult epiglottitis:* 80% to 95% have odynophagia and sore throat; only 20% to 40% have fever, drooling, or stridor.

DIAGNOSIS

- Airway management should be promptly evaluated as soon as the diagnosis is considered. Laboratory and radiologic testing in a child with suspected epiglottitis should be performed only in a safe environment (i.e., in the operating room, emergency department, or intensive care unit, with an individual trained in pediatric airway intubation), because of the propensity to develop acute airway obstruction (although airway obstruction is much less common in adults).
- Peripheral leukocytosis is common but not universal. Lateral and anteroposterior neck radiographs show enlargement of the epiglottis (the "thumb sign," as opposed to the "pencil-point narrowing" of the airway in viral croup).
- Direct or indirect laryngoscopy and fiberoptic nasopharyngeal endoscopy are the definitive diagnostic tests.

DIFFERENTIAL DIAGNOSIS

- Stridor with toxicity and drooling but lack of cough favors epiglottitis; stridor, barking cough, and lack of drooling favors viral croup (laryngotracheobronchitis). Other conditions that mimic infectious epiglottitis include bacterial tracheitis, thermal epiglottitis (scald burn from smoke or hot beverages), possibly angioneurotic edema, retropharyngeal or peritonsillar abscesses, uvulitis, and diphtheria.

THERAPY

- *Pediatric epiglottitis:* Ideally, diagnosis is confirmed by visualization at the time the airway is secured by intubation, at which time laryngeal and blood cultures and complete blood cell counts may be obtained. Emergent tracheotomy or cricothyroidotomy is rarely required.
- *Adult epiglottitis:* In contrast to children, adults with epiglottitis generally tolerate direct visualization of the epiglottis for diagnosis. Hospitalization in an intensive care unit during the acute phase of the illness is suggested; however, in most adults (75% to 80%) the infection is successfully managed without endotracheal intubation or tracheotomy.
- Empirical therapy for epiglottitis includes intravenous cefotaxime, ceftriaxone, or ampicillin-sulbactam to treat streptococci, pneumococci, *H. influenzae,* and meningococci. In areas with a high proportion of drug-resistant pneumococci, empirical therapy should be broadened.
- Therapy directed against *Staphylococcus aureus* should be considered if bacterial tracheitis cannot be excluded.

PREVENTION

- Chemoprophylaxis for household contacts of children with *H. influenzae* type b epiglottitis should be given for those households containing underimmunized or nonimmunized children younger than 4 years of age or immunocompromised children.
- Contacts of adults with epiglottitis are unlikely to require any prophylaxis, except in the rare instance of proven *H. influenzae* type b or meningococcal infection.

10 Infections of the Oral Cavity, Neck, and Head

Anthony W. Chow

DEFINITION

- Infections of the oral cavity, neck, and head are diverse in etiology and clinical presentation.
- Although uncommon in the postantibiotic era, deep fascial space infections and vascular complications are potentially life-threatening. These include Lemierre syndrome and Ludwig's angina.
- A clear understanding of their interrelationships, anatomic routes of spread, and salient clinical features is critical to diagnosis and management.

EPIDEMIOLOGY

- Infections of the oral cavity are most commonly odontogenic in origin and include dental caries, periodontal disease, and deep fascial space infections.
- Nonodontogenic infections of the oral cavity include those of the oral mucosa and infections of the major salivary glands.
- Miscellaneous infections of the head and neck most commonly result from human or animal bites, irradiation, or surgical procedures but may also arise from suppurative adenitis, infected embryologic cysts, and suppurative thyroiditis.

MICROBIOLOGY

- The microbiota associated with odontogenic infections generally reflect the indigenous oral microbiota and are typically polymicrobial involving both strict anaerobes and facultative bacteria.
- Dental caries originate from "cariogenic" bacteria residing within the supragingival plaque, whereas periodontal disease arises from "periodontopathic" bacteria residing within the subgingival plaque.
- Important differences within these complex bacterial compositions support the concept of the "specific" plaque hypothesis of dental caries and periodontal disease.

DIAGNOSIS

- Microbiologic investigation requires proper specimen collection, taking care to minimize contamination by resident commensal microbiota.
- Needle aspiration of loculated pus by an extraoral approach is desirable, and specimens should be transported immediately to the laboratory under anaerobic conditions.
- Tissue biopsy specimens should be routinely examined for histopathologic evidence of acute or chronic inflammation and infection.
- Immunofluorescence staining and rapid molecular diagnostic tools such as DNA probes or polymerase chain reaction are valuable for the detection of fastidious or noncultivable pathogens.
- Computed tomography (CT) with contrast is the most effective tool for localizing and evaluating the extent of deep space infections of the oral cavity, head, and neck.

17

- Magnetic resonance imaging (MRI) with or without angiography is more sensitive than CT for assessing soft tissue and bone involvement, as well as vascular complications.
- Technetium bone scans in combination with gallium- or indium-labeled white blood cells may be useful for the diagnosis of acute or chronic osteomyelitis.

THERAPY

- Surgical drainage of loculated infection and removal of necrotic tissue are the keys to management of deep fascial space infections of the oral cavity, head, and neck.
- Antimicrobial therapy is important in halting the local spread of infection and in preventing hematogenous dissemination.
- Choice of antimicrobial regimens is empirical, depending on the primary source (e.g., odontogenic or oropharyngeal vs. rhinogenic or otogenic), anticipated causative microorganisms, and immunity of the host (see Tables 10-1 and 10-2).

PREVENTION

- Oral hygiene and dental treatment to prevent caries and advanced periodontal disease
- Dietary counseling and use of topical fluorides and chlorhexidine oral rinses for patients at high risk for dental caries
- Behavioral modification of risk factors such as tobacco smoking

TABLE 10-1 Antimicrobial Regimens for Various Odontogenic and Nonodontogenic Orofacial Infections

CLINICAL ENTITY	COMMON CAUSATIVE ORGANISMS	ANTIMICROBIAL REGIMENS
Odontogenic		
Supragingival dental plaque and dental caries prevention	*Streptococcus mutans*, other streptococci, *Actinomyces* spp.	Fluoride-containing toothpaste or oral rinses (e.g., sodium fluoride 1.1% or stannous fluoride 0.4%) two or three times daily
		with or without
		Fluoride-containing varnishes (e.g., sodium fluoride 5%) applied three or four times yearly
		with or without
		Chlorhexidine 0.12% oral rinses
Acute simple gingivitis	Streptococci, *Actinomyces* spp., oral spirochetes	Penicillin G, 2-4 MU IV q4-6h (or penicillin V, 500 mg q8h) *plus* metronidazole, 500 mg PO or IV q8h
		or
		Ampicillin-sulbactam, 1.5-3 g IV q6-8h
		or
		Amoxicillin-clavulanate, 500 mg PO q8h
		or
		Clindamycin, 450 mg PO q6-8h or 600 mg IV q6-8h
Acute necrotizing ulcerative gingivitis (ANUG), or Vincent's angina	*Prevotella intermedia, Fusobacterium* spp., *Tannerella forsythensis, Treponema denticola*, other oral spirochetes	Metronidazole, 500 mg PO or IV q8h
		or
		Amoxicillin-clavulanate, 500 mg PO q8h
		or
		Ampicillin-sulbactam, 1.5-3 g IV q6h
		or
		Clindamycin, 450 mg PO q6h or 600 mg IV q6-8h

TABLE 10-1 Antimicrobial Regimens for Various Odontogenic and Nonodontogenic Orofacial Infections—cont'd

CLINICAL ENTITY	COMMON CAUSATIVE ORGANISMS	ANTIMICROBIAL REGIMENS
Early-onset, "aggressive," or "localized juvenile" periodontitis	*Aggregatibacter actinomycetemcomitans, Porphyromonas gingivalis, Treponema denticola, Prevotella intermedia*	Doxycycline, 200 mg PO or IV q12h (only in patients ≥8 yr of age) *or* Metronidazole, 500 mg PO or IV q8h
Adult or "established" periodontitis	*Treponema denticola,* other oral spirochetes, black-pigmented *Bacteroides* spp. (*Porphyromonas gingivalis* and *Prevotella melaninogenica*), *Tannerella forsythensis*	Topical application of minocycline microspheres (Arestin) *or* Topical application of doxycycline hyclate periodontal extended-release liquid (Atridox)
Nonodontogenic		
Gangrenous stomatitis (noma)	*Fusobacterium nucleatum, Borrelia vincentii, Prevotella melaninogenica,* other oral anaerobes	Penicillin G, 2-4 MU IV q4-6h *plus* metronidazole, 500 mg PO or IV q8h *or* Ampicillin-sulbactam, 1.5-3 g IV q6-8h *or* Amoxicillin-clavulanate, 500 mg PO q8h *or* Clindamycin, 450 mg PO q6-8h or 600 mg IV q6-8h
Severe oral mucositis in immunocompromised hosts	Viridans and other streptococci, *Bacteroides* spp., *Peptostreptococcus* spp., and other oral anaerobes, facultative gram-negative bacilli	Topical chlorhexidine (0.1%) mouth rinses TID *plus one of the following:* Cefotaxime, 2 g IV q6h *or* Ticarcillin-clavulanate, 3.1 g IV q4h *or* Piperacillin-tazobactam, 3.375 g IV q6h *or* Imipenem, 500 mg IV q6h *or* Meropenem, 1 g IV q8h
Sialadenitis and suppurative parotitis	*Staphylococcus aureus,* * *Streptococcus viridans* and other streptococci, *Bacteroides* spp., *Peptostreptococcus* spp., and other oral anaerobes	Nafcillin, 2 g IV q4h, or vancomycin, 1 g IV q12h *plus either* Metronidazole, 0.5 g IV q6h *or* Clindamycin, 600 mg IV q6h

IV, intravenously; MU, million units; PO, orally; TID, three times a day.

*For *Staphylococcus aureus* infections in which methicillin-resistant *S. aureus* is suspected, replace nafcillin with vancomycin, 1 g IV q12h; in immunosuppressed hosts, cefotaxime or ceftriaxone or imipenem, as described in the table, can be added.

TABLE 10-2 Initial Empirical Antimicrobial Regimens for Suppurative Infections of the Head and Neck

INFECTION	USUAL CAUSATIVE ORGANISMS	ANTIBIOTIC REGIMENS, NORMAL HOST*
Suppurative orofacial odontogenic infections, including Ludwig's angina	*Streptococcus viridans* and other streptococci, *Peptostreptococcus* spp., *Bacteroides* spp., and other oral anaerobes	Penicillin G, 2-4 MU IV q4-6h *plus* metronidazole, 0.5 g IV q6h *or* Ampicillin-sulbactam, 2 g IV q4h *or* Clindamycin, 600 mg IV q6h *or* Cefoxitin, 1-2 g IV q6h
Lateral pharyngeal or retropharyngeal space infections		
Odontogenic	*S. viridans* and other streptococci, *Staphylococcus* spp., *Peptostreptococcus* spp., *Bacteroides* spp., and other oral anaerobes	Penicillin G, 2-4 MU IV q4-6h *plus* metronidazole 0.5 g IV q6h *or* Ampicillin-sulbactam 2 g IV q4h *or* Clindamycin 600 mg IV q6h
Rhinogenic	*Streptococcus pneumoniae, Haemophilus influenzae,* viridans and other streptococci, *Bacteroides* spp., *Peptostreptococcus* spp., and other oral anaerobes	One of the following: (1) Penicillin G, 2-4 MU IV q4-6h, or levofloxacin, 500 mg IV q24h, or ciprofloxacin, 750 mg IV q12h *plus* Metronidazole, 0.5 g IV q6h, *or* clindamycin, 600 mg IV q6h *or* (2) Moxifloxacin, 400 mg IV q24h
Otogenic	Same as for rhinogenic space infections	Same as for rhinogenic space infections
Suppurative cervical adenitis and infected embryologic cysts	*Streptococcus pyogenes, Peptostreptococcus* spp., *Fusobacterium* spp., oral anaerobes	One of the following: (1) Penicillin G, 2-4 MU IV q4h, *plus* metronidazole, 500 mg IV q6h *or* (2) Ampicillin-sulbactam, 2 g IV q4h *or* (3) Clindamycin, 600 mg IV q6h *or* (4) Cefoxitin, 1-2 g IV q6h
Suppurative thyroiditis	*S. aureus, S. pyogenes, S. pneumoniae, Haemophilus influenzae, Streptococcus viridans* and other streptococci, oral anaerobes	Nafcillin, 2 g IV q4-6h, or vancomycin, 1 g IV q12h *plus either* Metronidazole, 500 mg IV q6h *or* Clindamycin, 600 mg IV q6h
Cervicofacial actinomycosis	*Actinomyces israelii, Arachnia propionica, Actinobacillus actinomycetemcomitans*	One of the following: (1) Penicillin G, 2-4 MU IV q4-6h *or* (2) Doxycycline, 200 mg PO or IV q12h *or* (3) Clindamycin, 450 mg PO q6h or 600 mg IV q6h

TABLE 10-2 Initial Empirical Antimicrobial Regimens for Suppurative Infections of the Head and Neck—cont'd

INFECTION	USUAL CAUSATIVE ORGANISMS	ANTIBIOTIC REGIMENS, NORMAL HOST*
Human or animal bites	S. pyogenes, S. aureus, Eikenella corrodens, oral anaerobes Pasteurella multocida	One of the following: (1) Ampicillin-sulbactam, 2 g IV q4h or (2) Amoxicillin-clavulanate, 500 mg PO q8h or (3) Moxifloxacin, 400 mg IV or PO q12h
Maxillofacial trauma, postsurgical wound infections	S. aureus, S. pyogenes, Peptostreptococcus spp., other oral anaerobes, Pseudomonas aeruginosa, Enterobacteriaceae spp.	Nafcillin, 2 g IV q4h, or vancomycin, 1 g IV q12h plus one of the following: (1) Ticarcillin-clavulanate, 3.1 g IV q4h or (2) Piperacillin-tazobactam, 3.375 g IV q6h or (3) Imipenem-cilastatin, 500 mg IV q6h or (4) Meropenem, 1 g IV q8h or (5) Moxifloxacin, 400 mg IV or PO q24h or (6) Tigecycline, 100 mg IV, then 50 mg IV q12h
Suppurative jugular thrombophlebitis (Lemierre syndrome)	Fusobacterium necrophorum; same as for odontogenic space infections	Same as for odontogenic space infections
Suppurative cavernous sinus thrombosis	Same as for odontogenic, rhinogenic, or otogenic space infections	Same as for odontogenic, rhinogenic, or otogenic space infections
Mandibular osteomyelitis	Same as for odontogenic space infections	Clindamycin, 600 mg IV q6h or Moxifloxacin, 400 mg PO or IV q24h
Extension of osteomyelitis from prevertebral space infection	Staphylococcus aureus,[†] facultative gram-negative bacilli	Either nafcillin, 2 g IV q4h, or vancomycin, 1 g IV q12h plus Either tobramycin, 1.7 mg/kg IV q8h, or ciprofloxacin, 400 mg IV q12h

IV, intravenously; MU, million units; PO, orally.

*For immunocompromised hosts, consider replacing penicillin G with one of the following: cefotaxime, 2 g IV q4h; ceftriaxone, 1 g IV q12h; or cefepime, 2 g IV q12h. Other regimens to consider are ticarcillin-clavulanate, 3.1 g IV q64h; piperacillin/tazobactam, 3.375 g IV q6h; imipenem, 500 mg IV q6h; meropenem, 1 g IV q8h; moxifloxacin, 400 mg IV q24h; or tigecycline, 100 mg IV, then 50 mg IV q12h.

[†]For Staphylococcus aureus infections in which methicillin-resistant S. aureus is suspected, replace nafcillin with vancomycin, 1 g IV q12h; in immunosuppressed hosts, cefotaxime or ceftriaxone or imipenem, as described in the table, can be added.

11 Acute Bronchitis

Edward E. Walsh

DEFINITION

- Acute bronchitis is a self-limited syndrome characterized by acute cough with or without sputum but without signs of pneumonia.

EPIDEMIOLOGY

- Acute bronchitis occurs year-round and is caused by a large number of respiratory pathogens according to the typical epidemiology of each pathogen.

MICROBIOLOGY

- Acute bronchitis is primarily caused by viral infections. Most common are rhinovirus, influenza viruses, respiratory syncytial virus, metapneumovirus, coronaviruses, and adenovirus. Fewer than 10% of cases are caused by *Mycoplasma pneumoniae, Chlamydia pneumoniae,* and Bordetella pertussis.

DIAGNOSIS

- Diagnosis is primarily made by the clinical presentation in the absence of signs and symptoms of pneumonia.

THERAPY

- Therapy is symptomatic because antibiotics are uncommonly required and unnecessary in the majority of cases.

PREVENTION

- Prevention is directed at specific pathogens when possible (e.g., influenza and pertussis vaccination).

12 Acute Exacerbations of Chronic Obstructive Pulmonary Disease

Leopoldo N. Segal, Michael D. Weiden, and Harold W. Horowitz

DEFINITION

- Chronic lung disease with irreversible airflow limitation with reduced forced expiratory volume in 1 second (FEV_1) and FEV_1/forced vital capacity (FVC) ratio
- Acute exacerbation indicated by acute change from a patient's baseline with increased dyspnea, sputum volume, or sputum purulence; number of changes clinically defines severity

EPIDEMIOLOGY

- Prevalence expected to reach 10% of the overall population and 50% of smokers; fourth leading cause of death worldwide
- Increased risk for acute exacerbation in winter
- Risk factors: cigarette smoking, environmental particulate matter, genetic predisposition

PATHOGENESIS

- Intermittent progressive airway inflammation; remodeling and loss of lung function
- Ciliary dysfunction; excess mucus production; impaired phagocytosis leading to bacterial colonization

MICROBIOLOGY

- Airways of patients with stable disease are frequently colonized with *Streptococcus pneumoniae, Haemophilus influenzae,* and *Moraxella catarrhalis;* respiratory syncytial virus is most frequent colonizing virus.
- Microaspiration in stable disease introduces oral anaerobes (e.g., *Prevotella* and *Veillonella* spp.) into lower airway.
- During acute exacerbation, bacteria or viruses or both may be isolated, with more gram-negative rods found with worsening lung function. "Atypical" bacteria are not frequently isolated. Acquisition of new pathogen is associated with exacerbation.

DIAGNOSIS

- Acute exacerbation is defined by increased sputum purulence, volume, and dyspnea.

THERAPY

- Use of bronchodilators has increased for mild exacerbation without antibiotic therapy.
- Oral or intravenously administered corticosteroids and early empirical antibiotic therapy are advised for moderate to severe exacerbations.

PREVENTION

- Avoid exposure to particulate matter and cease smoking.
- Administer influenza, pneumococcal, and pertussis vaccines.
- Prescribe prophylactic daily azithromycin in patients with advanced disease with a history of exacerbation and no cardiac risk factors.

13 Bronchiolitis

John Bower and John T. McBride

DEFINITION

- Bronchiolitis is small airway inflammation/obstruction most frequently caused by infection with respiratory syncytial virus (RSV) in the first years of life.

EPIDEMIOLOGY

- RSV bronchiolitis occurs in winter epidemics in temperate climates and sporadically in the tropics.
- Bronchiolitis is a leading cause of hospitalization in the first year of life in the developed world.

MICROBIOLOGY

- Many other respiratory viruses may cause bronchiolitis, including human metapneumovirus, influenza, parainfluenza, adenovirus, coronavirus, and bocavirus.

DIAGNOSIS

- Diagnosis is clinically based on presence of RSV in the community, initial episode of wheezing, and evidence of upper respiratory infection.
- Other causes of wheezing in early childhood should be excluded, such as congenital heart disease with failure, foreign-body aspiration, dysphagia, and asthma.
- Apnea may occur early in the course of viral bronchiolitis, usually in infants younger than 44 weeks' postconceptional age.

THERAPY

- Therapy is supportive and includes hydration, oxygen, and respiratory support as needed.
- Corticosteroids and bronchodilators are not generally beneficial.
- Hypertonic saline aerosols delivered three times daily may hasten recovery but have not been widely adopted.
- Respiratory support by high-flow nasal cannula may prevent or delay intubation in patients with apnea or respiratory failure.

PREVENTION

- Careful attention to hand sanitation is important in limiting spread of RSV infection during epidemics.
- Monoclonal antibody prophylaxis may prevent or mitigate infection in high risk infants.

14 Acute Pneumonia

Richard T. Ellison III and Gerald R. Donowitz

EPIDEMIOLOGY AND ETIOLOGY

- Pneumonia is the most common cause of infection-related death.
- Predominant pathogens of community-acquired pneumonia (CAP) in adults include *Streptococcus pneumoniae, Haemophilus influenzae, Mycoplasma pneumoniae,* and *Chlamydia pneumoniae.*
- *Legionella* species, *Staphylococcus aureus,* and enteric gram-negative bacilli are less frequent causes that can produce more severe disease.
- Predominant pathogens of patients recently hospitalized or nursing home residents include *S. aureus,* aerobic gram-negative rods, including *Pseudomonas aeruginosa,* and mixed aerobic/anaerobic organisms.

DIAGNOSIS

- Typical clinical manifestations are cough—the sine qua non of pneumonia—sputum production, dyspnea, chest pain, fever, fatigue, sweats, headache, nausea, myalgia, and occasionally abdominal pain and diarrhea.
- Gram stain and culture of sputum samples remain valuable diagnostic assays.
- Blood cultures should be obtained in all patients who are immunocompromised, have health care–associated (HCAP) or hospital-acquired pneumonia (HAP), or are hospitalized with severe CAP.
- Chest radiographs should be obtained on all patients with suspected pneumonia.
- Several biomarkers, including procalcitonin and C-reactive protein, are under assessment as discriminatory assays to define populations with a higher likelihood of bacterial infection that could benefit from antibiotic therapy, but the clinical utility of such assays has not yet been established.

THERAPY

- One of three severity index scores (PSI, CURB-65, or CRB-65) can be used to assess the need for hospitalization in immunocompetent patients with CAP, and similar indices can be used to define the need for intensive care unit admission.
- Antibiotic therapy for pneumonia should be started as soon as the diagnosis is considered likely.

- Advanced macrolides, respiratory fluoroquinolones, and β-lactam agents are the principal antibiotics used for the treatment of CAP. Coverage for *S. aureus* and mixed anaerobes should be considered in select situations (see Table 14-1 for suggested agents and dosages).
- Antibiotic treatment for HCAP should include coverage for potentially drug-resistant *S. aureus* and aerobic gram-negative bacilli and in most settings includes coverage for *Pseudomonas aeruginosa* (see Table 14-1 for suggested agents and dosages).
- The duration of intravenous treatment, inpatient hospitalization, and total intravenous and oral antibiotic therapy for CAP should be guided by the patient's clinical stability.

PREVENTION

- Provide immunization as appropriate with influenza and pneumococcal vaccines.
- Encourage cessation of tobacco smoking.

TABLE 14-1 Guide to Empirical Choice of Antimicrobial Agent for Treating Adult Patients with Community-Acquired Pneumonia or Health Care–Acquired Pneumonia

PATIENT CHARACTERISTICS	PREFERRED TREATMENT OPTIONS
Outpatient *Previously Healthy*	
No recent antibiotic therapy	Macrolide[a] or doxycycline (100 mg 2 times/day)
Recent antibiotic therapy[b]	A respiratory fluoroquinolone[c] alone, an advanced macrolide[d] plus oral β-lactam[e]
Comorbidities (COPD, Diabetes, Renal Failure or Congestive Heart Failure, or Malignancy)	
No recent antibiotic therapy	An advanced macrolide plus oral β-lactam or a respiratory fluoroquinolone
Recent antibiotic therapy	A respiratory fluoroquinolone alone or an advanced macrolide plus a β-lactam
Suspected aspiration with infection	Amoxicillin-clavulanate or clindamycin (600 mg IV q8h or 300 mg PO q6h)
Influenza with bacterial superinfection	Vancomycin, linezolid, or other coverage for MRSA, including community-acquired MRSA[f]
Inpatient *Medical Ward*	
No recent antibiotic therapy	A respiratory fluoroquinolone alone or an advanced macrolide plus an intravenous β-lactam[g]
Recent antibiotic therapy	An advanced macrolide plus an intravenous β-lactam, or a respiratory fluoroquinolone alone (regimen selected will depend on nature of recent antibiotic therapy)
Intensive Care Unit (ICU)	
Pseudomonas infection is not a concern	A β-lactam[g] plus either an advanced macrolide or a respiratory fluoroquinolone
Pseudomonas infection is not a concern but patient has a β-lactam allergy	A respiratory fluoroquinolone, with or without clindamycin
Pseudomonas infection is a concern[h] (cystic fibrosis, impaired host defenses)	Either (1) an antipseudomonal β-lactam[i] plus ciprofloxacin (400 mg IV q8h or 750 mg PO q12h), or (2) an antipseudomonal agent plus an aminoglycoside[j] plus a respiratory fluoroquinolone or a macrolide
Pseudomonas infection is a concern but the patient has a β-lactam allergy	Aztreonam (2 g IV q8h) plus aminoglycoside plus a respiratory fluoroquinolone

TABLE 14-1 Guide to Empirical Choice of Antimicrobial Agent for Treating Adult Patients with Community-Acquired Pneumonia or Health Care–Acquired Pneumonia—cont'd

PATIENT CHARACTERISTICS	PREFERRED TREATMENT OPTIONS
Health Care–Associated Pneumonia[k]	
—	Either (1) an antipseudomonal β-lactam plus ciprofloxacin or levofloxacin or (2) an antipseudomonal agent plus an aminoglycoside plus a respiratory fluoroquinolone or a macrolide plus vancomycin or linezolid (for MRSA coverage)

COPD, chronic obstructive pulmonary disease; MRSA, methicillin-resistant *S. aureus*.

Note: All dosages are usual adult doses and may require adjustment in relation to renal or hepatic function, a patient's body mass index, or drug-drug interactions.

[a]Azithromycin, clarithromycin, or erythromycin.

[b]That is, the patient was given a course of antibiotic(s) for treatment of any infection within the past 3 months, excluding the current episode of infection. Such treatment is a risk factor for drug-resistant *Streptococcus pneumoniae* and possibly for infection with gram-negative bacilli. Depending on the class of antibiotics recently given, one or another of the suggested options may be selected. Recent use of a fluoroquinolone should dictate selection of a nonfluoroquinolone regimen and vice versa.

[c]Moxifloxacin (400 mg once daily), gemifloxacin (320 mg once daily), or levofloxacin (750 mg once daily).

[d]Azithromycin (500 mg once daily), clarithromycin (250-500 mg twice daily), erythromycin (250-500 mg four times a day).

[e]High-dose amoxicillin (1 g three times a day), high-dose amoxicillin-clavulanate (2 g twice daily), cefpodoxime (200 mg twice daily), or cefuroxime (500 mg twice daily).

[f]Vancomycin dosing should target a vancomycin trough level of 15 to 20 μg/mL; linezolid (600 mg twice daily).

[g]Cefotaxime (1-2 g IV q4-8h), ceftriaxone (1 g IV daily), ampicillin (1-2 g IV q4-6h), ampicillin-sulbactam (1.5-3 g IV q6h), or ertapenem (1 g IV daily).

[h]Risk factors for *Pseudomonas* infection include severe structural lung disease (e.g., bronchiectasis) and recent antibiotic therapy, health care–associated exposures or stay in hospital (especially in the ICU). For patients with community-acquired pneumonia in the ICU, coverage for *S. pneumoniae* and *Legionella* species must always be considered.

[i]Piperacillin (3 g IV q4h), piperacillin-tazobactam (3.375 g IV q6h), imipenem (500-1000 mg IV q6h), meropenem (1-2 g IV q8h), ceftazidime (2 g IV q6-8h), or cefepime (1-2 g IV q8h) are excellent β-lactams and are adequate for most *S. pneumoniae* and *H. influenzae* infections. They may be preferred when there is concern for relatively unusual pathogens of community-acquired pneumonia, such as *P. aeruginosa, Klebsiella* species, and other gram-negative bacteria.

[j]Data suggest that older adults receiving aminoglycosides have worse outcomes. Traditionally dosed aminoglycosides should achieve peak levels of at least 8 μg/mL for gentamicin or tobramycin and 25-35 μg/mL for amikacin and troughs less than 2 μg/mL for gentamicin and tobramycin and less than 10 μg/mL for amikacin. Once-daily dosing for gentamicin or tobramycin is 7 mg/kg IV with trough target <1 μg/mL, and 20 mg/kg IV for amikacin with trough target <4 μg/mL.

[k]Pneumonia developing in patients who have been hospitalized for 2 or more days within 90 days of developing infection; patients attending hospital or hemodialysis clinics; patients receiving intravenous antibiotic therapy, wound care, or chemotherapy at home within 30 days of developing infection; and residents of long-term care facilities or nursing homes.

Modified from Mandell LA, Wunderink RG, Anzueto A, et al. Infectious Diseases Society of America/American Thoracic Society consensus guidelines on the management of community-acquired pneumonia in adults. *Clin Infect Dis.* 2007;44(suppl 2):S27-S72; and American Thoracic Society, Infectious Diseases Society of America. Guidelines for the management of adults with hospital-acquired, ventilator-associated, and healthcare-associated pneumonia. *Am J Respir Crit Care Med.* 2005;171:388-416.

15 Pleural Effusion and Empyema

Edward J. Septimus

DIAGNOSIS

- Fluid in the pleural space may be transudative or exudative (see Table 15-1). An exudative effusion with pus in the pleural space is called an *empyema*. Computed tomography (CT) is better than a chest radiograph for distinguishing pleural fluid from pneumonia and may allow visualization of stranding or loculation within an empyema.

THORACENTESIS

- For pleural fluid suspected of empyema, send fluid in capped syringe for pH, inoculate aerobic and anaerobic blood culture bottles directly at bedside, moisten syringe with preservative-free heparin because clotting interferes with white blood cell count (WBC), cytology, and Gram stain. Laboratory studies: WBC, differential, protein, glucose, lactate dehydrogenase (LDH), Gram stain, culture for bacteria, cytology, mycobacteria and fungi. Send blood for LDH and protein to determine pleural fluid–to-serum ratio.
- Special studies on pleural fluid: immunochromatographic test for *Streptococcus pneumoniae* antigen, polymerase chain reaction (PCR) targeting 16S ribosomal DNA, modified acid-fast stain for *Nocardia*, PCR, or nucleic acid amplification test or adenosine deaminase or culture of pleural biopsy for *Mycobacterium tuberculosis*
- Source of empyema affects the most common organisms:
  - Community-acquired pneumonia: *S. pneumoniae, Staphylococcus aureus*
  - Community-acquired empyema: *Streptococcus anginosus* group, *Prevotella, Bacteroides*
  - Post-trauma or postoperative hemothorax: *Staphylococcus aureus*
  - Complication of viral influenza: *S. pneumoniae, S. aureus, Streptococcus pyogenes*
  - Esophageal rupture: mixed aerobic and anaerobic bacteria, *Candida*
  - Hematogenous seeding of serous effusion: gram-negative bacilli
  - Spread across diaphragm: amebiasis, mixed aerobic-anaerobic

TREATMENT

- Systemic antibiotics plus adequate drainage is necessary for empyema. Empirical antibiotic choices for a presumed bacterial empyema include ampicillin-sulbactam, piperacillin-tazobactam, imipenem, ertapenem, doripenem, meropenem, or combination of a third- or fourth-generation cephalosporin and either clindamycin or metronidazole. Indications for drainage include cloudy fluid, pH <7.2, glucose <60 mg/dL, protein >3 g/dL, LDH >1000, or ratio of pleural fluid to serum for protein >0.5 or LDH >0.6.
- Video-assisted thoracoscopy is being used earlier in empyema treatment, particularly in children, and in adults with empyema not responding to CT- or ultrasound-guided catheter tube drainage. Fibrinolytic therapy still has advocates, although it is contraindicated if bronchopleural fistula is present.

TABLE 15-1 Features Differentiating Exudative from Transudative Pleural Effusion

FEATURE	TRANSUDATE	EXUDATE
Appearance	Serous	Cloudy
Leukocyte count	$<10,000/mm^3$	$>50,000/mm^3$
pH	>7.2	<7.2
Protein	<3.0 g/dL	>3.0 g/dL
Ratio of pleural fluid protein to serum	<0.5	>0.5
Lactate dehydrogenase (LDH)	<200 IU/L	>200 IU/L
Ratio of pleural fluid LDH to serum	<0.6	>0.6
Glucose	≥60 mg/dL	<60 mg/dL

16 Bacterial Lung Abscess

Bennett Lorber

DEFINITION
- Localized necrosis of lung tissue caused by microbial infection. One or more cavities.

EPIDEMIOLOGY
- Primary lung abscess: bad teeth, altered consciousness, aspiration. Secondary: airway obstruction or immunosuppression.

MICROBIOLOGY
- Polymicrobial. Predominantly mouth anaerobes and streptococci. *Klebsiella* or *Staphylococcus aureus* uncommonly.

DIAGNOSIS
- Radiograph or computed tomography (CT): thick-walled cavity with air-fluid level. Putrid sputum in half of cases.

THERAPY
- β-Lactam/β-lactamase combination or clindamycin.

PREVENTION
- Maintain oral hygiene. Elevate head of bed for those with altered consciousness.

17 Chronic Pneumonia

Peter G. Pappas

DEFINITION

- Persistent or progressive cough, dyspnea, often with chronic sputum production, with or without fever, lasting weeks or months rather than days
- Always associated with abnormal chest radiography
- Constitutional symptoms, including weight loss and anorexia, are typical
- Definition does not include asymptomatic solitary pulmonary nodules
- May be infectious or noninfectious

EPIDEMIOLOGY

- Age, race/ethnicity, and gender are important considerations
- Underlying health issues and comorbid conditions
- Current and past residence, occupation, travel, and recreation history may be important
- Recent hospitalization or history of imprisonment
- Drug and alcohol history
- Recent prescription drug exposure

MICROBIOLOGY

- Bacterial: anaerobes, microaerophilic and viridans streptococci; *Staphylococcus aureus;* selected community-acquired and nosocomial gram-negative bacilli; *Burkholderia pseudomallei*
- Higher-order bacteria: *Mycobacterium tuberculosis, Mycobacterium kansasii,* and other non-tuberculous mycobacteria; *Nocardia* spp.; *Rhodococcus equi; Actinomyces* spp.
- Fungi: *Histoplasma capsulatum, Blastomyces dermatitidis, Coccidioides immitis/posadasii, Paracoccidioides brasiliensis, Cryptococcus neoformans,* and *Cryptococcus gattii, Aspergillus* spp., *Scedosporium* spp.
- Parasites: *Dirofilaria, Echinococcus granulosus, Paragonimus westermani,* filariasis
- Noninfectious causes: vasculitides, neoplasia, drug induced, sarcoidosis, pulmonary alveolar proteinosis, and a host of other conditions

DIAGNOSIS

- Careful clinical assessment, including detailed history, is essential.
- Clinical findings are generally nonspecific; rash, osteoarticular findings, and mucocutaneous and neurologic findings may provide helpful clues.
- Radiographic imaging, including routine chest radiograph or chest computed tomography, or both, are critical to diagnosis.
- Routine microbiologic studies, including sputum examination by Gram stain, potassium hydroxide, acid-fast stain, and preparations for ova and parasites, are important.
- Culture for routine bacteria, fungi, and acid-fast bacilli when possible.
- Biopsy and culture of nonpulmonary specimens (e.g., skin, bone, or brain biopsy) in clinically relevant settings. Potentially important serologic studies include the quantiFERON gold

assay for tuberculosis; *Histoplasma* antigen; cryptococcal antigen; and serum and bronchoal-veolar lavage galactomannan.
- Bronchoalveolar lavage for acid-fast, modified acid-fast, and Gram stain; wet mount or calcofluor stain; cultures for bacteria, mycobacteria, and fungi; galactomannan assay; and cytopathology.

THERAPY
- Specific therapy is entirely dependent on the most likely etiologies, of which there are many possibilities, usually including antimicrobials.

PREVENTION
- In this broad category of disease, prevention generally entails the recognition and avoidance of circumstances, which increase the likelihood of developing chronic pneumonia. In selected settings, such as high-risk patients receiving chemotherapy, prophylactic antimicrobials may be warranted.

18 Cystic Fibrosis

Ahmet Uluer and Francisco M. Marty

DEFINITION
- Cystic fibrosis (CF) is a genetically inherited autosomal-recessive disease resulting from mutations to the cystic fibrosis transmembrane conductance regulator gene (*CFTR,* located on the long arm of chromosome 7), and although it is a multisystem disorder, respiratory and gastrointestinal manifestations predominate.

EPIDEMIOLOGY
- *Staphylococcus aureus* and *Pseudomonas aeruginosa* (PA) are the most common CF-associated pathogens. The prevalence of other bacterial infections varies between countries and CF clinics.

MICROBIOLOGY
- Chronic airway infection and inflammation, most commonly associated with PA, are strongly associated with morbidity and mortality. Many other pathogens, including methicillin-resistant *S. aureus, Burkholderia cepacia* complex organisms, and *Stenotrophomonas maltophilia,* are also implicated in chronic progressive lung disease.

DIAGNOSIS
- Newborn screening is now available in the United States and other countries.
- Sweat chloride testing and *CFTR* gene mutation analysis are the mainstay for diagnosing CF, along with immunoreactive trypsinogen associated with newborn screening.
- Acute pulmonary exacerbations are usually linked to progression of disease (see Table 18-1). Respiratory viruses may trigger pulmonary exacerbations.

THERAPY
- Maintenance therapy includes mucolytics, airway hydrating agents, chest physiotherapy, anti-inflammatories, and a combination of oral and inhaled antibiotics (see Table 18-2).
- Acute pulmonary exacerbation may be treated with oral and nebulized antibiotics as needed, whereas more serious exacerbations usually require intravenous antibiotics, intense airway clearance accompanying mucolytics and airway hydrating agents, and aggressive nutritional management while monitoring for complications (see Table 18-2).
- Selection of antibiotics is guided by current and previous patient respiratory cultures. Severity of exacerbation will determine whether oral or intravenous antibiotics will be used.
- CF patients require higher doses of many hydrophilic antibiotics because of CF-associated increased volume of distribution and clearance. These include aminoglycosides, penicillins, and cephalosporins.
- In addition to the CFTR modulator ivacaftor—U.S. Food and Drug Administration [FDA] approved for those with at least one gating defect mutation (e.g., G551D)—and R117H, Orkambi, a combination of ivacaftor and lumacaftor, has also been approved by the FDA for therapy of patients homozygous for the F508del mutation.

TABLE 18-1 Summary of Recommendations for Chronic Pulmonary Therapies for Patients with Cystic Fibrosis, 2013

TREATMENT	RECOMMENDATION	CERTAINTY OF NET BENEFIT	ESTIMATE OF NET BENEFIT	RECOMMENDATION
Inhaled tobramycin—moderate to severe disease*	For individuals with CF, 6 yr of age and older, with moderate to severe lung disease and *Pseudomonas aeruginosa* persistently present in culture of the airways, the CF Foundation strongly recommends the chronic use of inhaled tobramycin to improve lung function, improve quality of life, and reduce exacerbations.	High	Substantial	A
Dornase alfa—moderate to severe disease*	For individuals with CF, 6 yr of age and older, with moderate to severe lung disease, the CF Foundation strongly recommends the chronic use of dornase alfa to improve lung function, improve quality of life, and reduce exacerbations.	High	Substantial	A
Ivacaftor†	For individuals with CF, 6 yr of age and older, with at least one G551D *CFTR* mutation, the Pulmonary Clinical Practice Guidelines Committee strongly recommends the chronic use of ivacaftor to improve lung function, improve quality of life, and reduce exacerbations.	High	Substantial	A
Inhaled aztreonam—moderate to severe disease*	For individuals with CF, 6 yr of age and older, with moderate to severe lung disease and *P. aeruginosa* persistently present in cultures of the airways, the CF Foundation strongly recommends the chronic use of inhaled aztreonam to improve lung function and quality of life.	High	Substantial	A
Dornase alfa—mild disease*	For individuals with CF, 6 yr of age and older, with asymptomatic or mild lung disease, the CF Foundation recommends the chronic use of dornase alfa to improve lung function and reduce exacerbations.	High	Moderate	B
Azithromycin with *P. aeruginosa*	For individuals with CF, 6 yr of age and older, with *P. aeruginosa* persistently present in cultures of the airways, the CF Foundation recommends the chronic use of azithromycin to improve lung function and reduce exacerbations.	High	Moderate	B
Inhaled tobramycin—mild disease*	For individuals with CF, 6 yr of age and older, with mild lung disease and *P. aeruginosa* persistently present in cultures of the airways, the CF Foundation recommends the chronic use of inhaled tobramycin to reduce exacerbations.	Moderate	Moderate	B
Inhaled hypertonic saline	For individuals with CF, 6 yr of age and older, the CF Foundation recommends the chronic use of inhaled hypertonic saline to improve lung function, improve quality of life, and reduce exacerbations.	Moderate	Moderate	B
Inhaled aztreonam—mild disease†	For individuals with CF, 6 yr of age and older, with mild lung disease and *P. aeruginosa* persistently present in cultures of the airways, the CF Foundation recommends the chronic use of inhaled aztreonam to improve lung function and quality of life.	Moderate	Moderate	B
Chronic use of ibuprofen (age < 18 yr)	For individuals with CF, between 6 and 17 yr of age, with an FEV_1 ≥60% predicted, the CF Foundation recommends the chronic use of oral ibuprofen, at a peak plasma concentration of 50-100 µg/mL, to slow the loss of lung function.	Moderate	Moderate	B

TABLE 18-1 Summary of Recommendations for Chronic Pulmonary Therapies for Patients with Cystic Fibrosis, 2013—cont'd

TREATMENT	RECOMMENDATION	CERTAINTY OF NET BENEFIT	ESTIMATE OF NET BENEFIT	RECOMMENDATION
Azithromycin without *P. aeruginosa*	For individuals with CF, 6 yr of age and older, without *P. aeruginosa* persistently present in cultures of the airways, the CF Foundation recommends the chronic use of azithromycin should be considered to reduce exacerbations.	Moderate	Small	C
Inhaled corticosteroids	For individuals with CF, 6 yr of age and older, without asthma or allergic bronchopulmonary aspergillosis, the CF Foundation recommends against the routine use of inhaled corticosteroids to improve lung function or quality of life and reduce pulmonary exacerbations.	High	Zero	D
Oral corticosteroids	For individuals with CF, 6 yr of age and older, without asthma or allergic bronchopulmonary aspergillosis, the CF Foundation recommends against the chronic use of oral corticosteroids to improve lung function, quality of life, or reduce exacerbations.	High	Negative	D
Other inhaled antibiotics	For individuals with CF, 6 yr of age and older, with *P. aeruginosa* persistently present in cultures of the airways, the CF Foundation concludes that the evidence is insufficient to recommend for or against the chronic use of other inhaled antibiotics (i.e., carbenicillin, ceftazidime, colistin, gentamicin) to improve lung function and quality of life or reduce exacerbations.	Low	—	I
Oral antipseudomonal antibiotics	For individuals with CF, 6 yr of age and older, with *P. aeruginosa* persistently present in the culture of the airways, the CF Foundation concludes that the evidence is insufficient to recommend for or against the routine use of chronic oral antipseudomonal antibiotics to improve lung function and quality of life or reduce exacerbations	Low	—	I
Leukotriene modifiers	For individuals with CF, 6 yr of age and older, the CF Foundation concludes that the evidence is insufficient to recommend for or against the routine chronic use of leukotriene modifiers to improve lung function and quality of life or reduce exacerbations.	Low	—	I
Inhaled or oral N-acetylcysteine, or inhaled glutathione	For individuals with CF, 6 yr of age and older, the CF Foundation concludes that the evidence is insufficient to recommend for or against the chronic use of inhaled or oral N-acetylcysteine or inhaled glutathione to improve lung function and quality of life or reduce exacerbations.	Low	—	I
Inhaled anticholinergics	For individuals with CF, 6 yr of age or older, the CF Foundation concludes that the evidence is insufficient to recommend for or against the chronic use of inhaled anticholinergic bronchodilators to improve lung function and quality of life or reduce exacerbations.	Low	—	I
Chronic use of ibuprofen (age ≥ 18 yr)	For individuals with CF, 18 years of age and older, the CF Foundation concludes that the evidence is insufficient to recommend for or against the chronic use of oral ibuprofen to slow the loss of lung function or reduce exacerbations.	Low	—	I

Continued

TABLE 18-1 Summary of Recommendations for Chronic Pulmonary Therapies for Patients with Cystic Fibrosis, 2013—cont'd

TREATMENT	RECOMMENDATION	CERTAINTY OF NET BENEFIT	ESTIMATE OF NET BENEFIT	RECOMMENDATION
Chronic inhaled β₂-adrenergic receptor agonists	For individuals with CF, 6 yr of age and older, the CF Foundation concludes that the evidence is insufficient to recommend for or against chronic use of inhaled β₂-adrenergic receptor agonists to improve lung function and quality of life or reduce exacerbations.	Low	—	I
Oral antistaphylococcal antibiotics, chronic use	For individuals with CF, 6 yr of age and older, with *Staphylococcus aureus* persistently present in cultures of the airways, the CF Foundation concludes that the evidence is insufficient to recommend for or against the chronic use of oral antistaphylococcal antibiotics to improve lung function and quality of life or reduce exacerbations.	Low	—	I

A, substantial; B, moderate; C, small; CF, cystic fibrosis; D, zero negative; FEV_1, forced expiratory volume in 1 second; I, the committee concludes that the current evidence is insufficient to assess the balance of benefits, and harms of the service. Evidence is lacking, of poor quality, or conflicting, and the balance and harms cannot be determined.

*Severity of lung disease is defined by FEV_1% predicted as follows: normal, >90% predicted; mildly impaired, 70%-89% predicted; moderately impaired, 50%-69% predicted; and severely impaired, <40% predicted (1).

†CF Foundation personnel did not participate in any activity related to ivacaftor.

From Mogayzel PJ, Naureckas ET, Robinson KA. Cystic fibrosis pulmonary guidelines. *Am J Respir Crit Care Med.* 2013;187:680-689.

TABLE 18-2 Acute Pulmonary Exacerbations in Cystic Fibrosis*

Increase in sputum volume or color
New or increased hemoptysis
Increased cough
Increased dyspnea
Malaise
Fatigue or lethargy
Temperature >38° C
Anorexia or weight loss
Sinus pain or tenderness
Change in sinus discharge
Change in physical examination of the chest
Decrease in FEV_1 by 10% or more
Radiographic changes in support of a pulmonary infection

FEV_1, forced expiratory volume in 1 second.

*Generally defined as the presence of four of the above.

From Cystic Fibrosis Foundation. Treatment of pulmonary exacerbations of cystic fibrosis. In: *Clinical Practice Guidelines for Cystic Fibrosis.* Bethesda, MD: Cystic Fibrosis Foundation; 1997.

PREVENTION

- Strictly adhere to infection control measures to prevent transmission of CF-associated pathogens among CF patients.
- Early eradication will prevent chronic airway infection with PA and other pathogens associated with chronic progressive lung disease.

19 Urinary Tract Infections

Jack D. Sobel and Donald Kaye

PATHOLOGIC CHARACTERISTICS
- With acute pyelonephritis there is suppurative necrosis or abscess formation.
- With chronic pyelonephritis there is uneven scarring.
- With papillary necrosis one or more pyramids may slough.

PATHOGENESIS
- Most urinary tract infections (UTIs) are the result of retrograde ascending infection, consequent to numerous behavioral factors.
- Because of efficient host defense mechanisms, bacterial pathogens capable of causing UTIs (uropathogens) are selected by virtue of genetically determined virulence factors.
- Virulence factors facilitate microorganism persistence in the urinary tract.
- Virulence factors include adhesins, bacterial capsules, aerobactin, cytotoxic necrotizing factors, hemolysins, and siderophore receptors.
- In functional and structurally compromised urinary tracts, there is reduced requirement for virulence factors in order to produce infection.

HOST DEFENSES
- Nonimmune mechanisms, especially antibacterial activity of urine, shearing force of micturition, and urine flow, are highly effective in reducing UTI frequency.
- Adaptive immunity, both antibody- and cell-mediated mechanisms, has a limited protective role.
- Innate immunity based on uroepithelial cells and response to adherent microbes reflects a complex recognition and reactive proinflammatory response consisting of multiple cytokines and inflammatory cells.
- Protective cytokine response is genetically determined and influences outcome spectrum from asymptomatic bacteriuria to suppurative renal disease.
- Genetic susceptibility to UTI is still minimally recognized and understood.

EPIDEMIOLOGY AND NATURAL HISTORY
- *Escherichia coli* is the most common infecting organism.
- Resistant *E. coli* and other resistant bacteria are increased in health care–related infection compared with community infection.
- Resistant bacteria are increased in complicated UTI.
- Asymptomatic bacteriuria is common and of little consequence except in a few groups.
- UTIs occur in 1% to 2% of infants, about 5% of girls, and 0.5% or less of boys.
- Renal damage is related to vesicoureteral reflux, which occurs in 30% to 50% of preschool children with infection; structural or functional obstruction also causes damage.
- UTIs are much more common in women than men and are most often asymptomatic.
- Up to 60% of women have symptomatic UTIs during their lifespan, and 10% of women have UTIs each year.
- Two to five percent of women have recurrent UTIs with a genetic predisposition.

- UTI in men is uncommon but often associated with structural or functional abnormality.
- Renal infection rarely causes end-stage renal disease without other underlying disease.

DIAGNOSIS

- Urine dipsticks for pyuria and bacteriuria are useful screening tests.
- A negative test for pyuria makes UTI unlikely.
- Negative tests for bacteriuria are common in UTI because of low titers of bacteria.
- Two urine cultures with greater than or equal to 10^5 of the same uropathogen/mL urine are required for diagnosis of asymptomatic bacteriuria.
- One culture with 10^2/mL or more of a gram-negative bacillary uropathogen is diagnostic in symptomatic UTI.
- One third of young women with cystitis have fewer than 10^5 bacteria/mL urine.

MANAGEMENT AND TREATMENT (SEE TABLE 19-1)

- All symptomatic UTI is usually treated for relief of symptoms.
- Most asymptomatic infection should be neither sought nor treated because of lack of benefit; exceptions are pregnancy and those who are to have traumatic urologic procedures. Controversial exceptions are some young children and after renal transplantation.
- Nonantimicrobial prevention measures are directed at reinfections and reducing risk factors. They include avoidance of spermicidal jellies and catheterization and investigational use of estrogens, cranberry products, and probiotics.
- Treatment for infants younger than 3 months involves a β-lactam and aminoglycoside intravenously.
- Treatment for infants older than 3 months is as mentioned above for those seriously ill and oral β-lactam or trimethoprim-sulfamethoxazole (TMP-SMX) for others.
- Treatment for acute, uncomplicated pyelonephritis in nonpregnant women is a urine culture and then fluoroquinolone.
- Treatment for uncomplicated cystitis in women is short-course therapy with nitrofurantoin, TMP-SMX, fosfomycin, pivmecillinam, or fluoroquinolone.
- Treatment for complicated UTI is urine culture and then fluoroquinolone. Cystitis nitrofurantoin and fosfomycin are options.
- Treatment of relapses is prolonged therapy or chronic suppression. Complicated UTI or prostatitis is possible.
- Reinfections can be self-treated per episode or prevented using single-dose prophylaxis for intercourse or long-term prophylaxis.

PREGNANCY

- Asymptomatic bacteriuria of pregnancy requires therapy and post-treatment surveillance to reduce the risk of maternal pyelonephritis, hypertension, and preterm delivery.
- UTI treatment options are reduced given lack of availability of quinolones, tetracyclines, and sulfonamides (at term) as treatment options.

IMAGING

- The ever-improving quality and availability of renal ultrasonography has facilitated the diagnosis of renal complications and underlying urologic abnormalities. Excretory urography (intravenous pyelography) has fast disappeared, replaced by computed tomography scan and magnetic resonance imaging examinations.
- The use of imaging studies in infants and preschool children with febrile UTIs remains controversial with reduced reliance on cystourethrography and the preference shifting to a "top-down" approach selecting children who would most benefit from investigation.

TABLE 19-1 Recommendations for Initial Therapy of Urinary Tract Infection in Adults

PARAMETER	ORAL*	PARENTERAL (SWITCH TO ORAL WHEN RESPONSE)
Uncomplicated Pyelonephritis		
GNB or no urine Gram stain available	CP 7 days, LV 5 days; if cannot use FQ, TMP-SMX 14 days ± 1 dose CT or AM	FQ 7 days or extended spectrum β-lactam (e.g., CT), 14 days ± AM
GPC in chains	Amoxicillin, 14 days	Ampicillin, 14 days
GPC in clusters	Linezolid or TMP-SMX, 14 days	Vancomycin, 14 days
Complicated Pyelonephritis		
Nonpregnant women or men	As for uncomplicated pyelonephritis	FQ, 7 days plus extended spectrum β-lactam initially ± AM
Pregnant women	Extended spectrum β-lactam; TMP-SMX[†] only if known sensitive both for 14 days	Extended spectrum β-lactam ± AM for 14 days
Uncomplicated Cystitis		
Nonpregnant women	Nitrofurantoin, 5 days or fosfomycin, 1 dose, or TMP-SMX, 3 days, or pivmecillinam, 3-7 days; FQ in reserve, 3 days	
Complicated Cystitis		
Women or men	FQ or nitrofurantoin, 7 days or fosfomycin, 1 dose	
Pregnant women	Cephalexin, 3-5 days or fosfomycin, 1 dose or nitrofurantoin, 7 days or TMP-SMX,[†] 3 days if sensitive	

GNB, gram-negative bacilli; GPC, gram-positive cocci.
Drugs and Doses:
    CP, ciprofloxacin orally 500 mg twice/day or 1000 mg once/day.
    LV, levofloxacin orally 750 mg once/day.
    TMP-SMX, trimethoprim-sulfamethoxazole orally 160/800 mg twice/day.
    CT, ceftriaxone parenterally 1 g/day.
    FQ, fluoroquinolone parenterally—ciprofloxacin 500 mg twice/day or levofloxacin 750 mg once/day.
    FQ, fluoroquinolone orally—ciprofloxacin 500 mg twice/day or 1000 once/day or levofloxacin 750 mg once/day.
    AM, aminoglycoside parenterally (e.g., gentamicin 5 mg/kg/day).
    Amoxicillin orally 875 mg twice/day.
    Ampicillin parenterally 2 g every 4 hr.
    Linezolid orally 600 mg twice/day.
    Vancomycin parenterally 15 mg/kg twice/day.
    Nitrofurantoin orally 100 mg twice/day.
    Fosfomycin orally 3 g once.
    Pivmecillinam orally 400 mg twice/day.
    Cephalexin orally 500 mg four times/day.
*Preferred if the patient is reliable, compliant, hemodynamically stable, and able to take oral therapy.
[†]TMP-SMX should be avoided in the third trimester.

20 Sepsis, Severe Sepsis, and Septic Shock

Robert S. Munford and Anthony F. Suffredini

DEFINITIONS
- Sepsis is the body's harmful systemic reaction to microbial infection.
- Severe sepsis is organ dysfunction complicating infection; if hypotension is present, it can be reversed with intravenous fluids.
- Septic shock is sepsis-associated hypotension that requires pharmacologic reversal.

EPIDEMIOLOGY
- Most commonly affected persons are the very young and older adults.
- Major outcome determinants are age and comorbidity, especially immunosuppressive illness.

MICROBIOLOGY
- Virtually any microbe can trigger sepsis.
- Most cases today occur in previously morbid individuals and are caused by opportunists from the patient's own microbiome.

DIAGNOSIS
- Usual signs: tachycardia, tachypnea, leukocytosis or leukopenia, fever or hypothermia
- Frequent, suggestive: thrombocytopenia, lactatemia, delirium, respiratory alkalosis, hyperbilirubinemia

THERAPY
- Prompt administration of antimicrobial drugs that can kill the patient's offending microbe (see Table 20-1)
- Intravenous fluids and pressor support as needed
- Source control: eliminating the local site of infection, usually with surgery or removal of indwelling device
- Supportive care

PREVENTION
- Hospital infection control
- Vaccination

TABLE 20-1 Empirical Antibiotic Options for Patients with Severe Sepsis or Septic Shock

		SUSPECTED SOURCE			
	LUNG	ABDOMEN	SKIN/SOFT TISSUE	URINARY TRACT	SOURCE UNCERTAIN
Major Community-Acquired Pathogens	*Streptococcus pneumoniae* *Haemophilus influenzae* *Legionella* *Chlamydia pneumoniae*	*Escherichia coli* *Bacteroides fragilis*	*Streptococcus pyogenes* *Staphylococcus aureus* Polymicrobial	*E. coli* *Klebsiella* species *Enterobacter* species *Proteus* spp. Enterococci	
Empirical Antibiotic Therapy	Moxifloxacin *or* levofloxacin *or* azithromycin *plus* cefotaxime *or* ceftazidime *or* cefepime *or* piperacillin-tazobactam	Imipenem *or* meropenem *or* doripenem *or* piperacillin-tazobactam ± aminoglycoside If biliary source: piperacillin-tazobactam, ampicillin-sulbactam, *or* ceftriaxone with metronidazole	Vancomycin *or* daptomycin *plus either* imipenem *or* meropenem *or* piperacillin-tazobactam; ± clindamycin	Ciprofloxacin *or* levofloxacin (if gram-positive cocci, use ampicillin *or* vancomycin ± gentamicin)	Vancomycin *plus either* doripenem *or* ertapenem *or* imipenem *or* meropenem
Major Commensal or Nosocomial Microorganisms	Aerobic gram-negative bacilli	Aerobic gram-negative rods Anaerobes *Candida* spp.	*Staphylococcus aureus* (? MRSA) Aerobic gram-negative rods	Aerobic gram-negative rods Enterococci	Consider MDRO if in area of high prevalence Consider echinocandin if neutropenic or indwelling intravascular catheter
Empirical Antibiotic Therapy	Imipenem *or* meropenem *or* doripenem *or* cefepime (if *Acinetobacter baumanii* or carbapenem-resistant *Klebsiella* in ICU, add colistin)	Imipenem *or* meropenem ± aminoglycoside (consider echinocandin)	Vancomycin *or* daptomycin *plus* imipenem-cilastatin *or* meropenem *or* cefepime, ± clindamycin	Vancomycin *plus* imipenem *or* meropenem *or* cefepime	Cefepime *plus* vancomycin ± caspofungin

Dosages for intravenous administration (normal renal function):
  *Imipenem-cilastatin, 0.5-1.0 g q6-8h
  *Meropenem, 1-2 g q8h
  *Doripenem, 0.5 g q8h
  Piperacillin-tazobactam, 3.375 g q4h or 4.5 g q6h
  Vancomycin, load 25-30 mg/kg, then 15-20 q8-12h
  Cefepime, 1-2 g q8h
  Levofloxacin, 750 mg q24h
  Ciprofloxacin, 400 mg q8-12h
  Moxifloxacin, 400 mg qd
  Ceftriaxone, 2.0 g q24h
  Caspofungin, 70 mg, followed by 50 mg q24h
  Colistin: loading dose = 5 mg/kg body weight. For maintenance dosing, see University of California, Los Angeles Dosing Protocol: www.infectiousdiseases-ucla-affiliated.org/Intranet/FILES/ColistinDosing.pdf
ICU, intensive care unit; MDRO, multidrug-resistant organisms; MRSA, methicillin-resistant *Staphylococcus aureus*. For MDRO, resistance usually includes carbapenems.
*Carbapenems are less susceptible to extended-spectrum β-lactamases; base choice on local resistance pattern.

21 Peritonitis and Intraperitoneal Abscesses

Matthew E. Levison and Larry M. Bush

DEFINITION

- Infection in the abdominal cavity encompasses a wide spectrum of entities and may involve any intra-abdominal organ or space.
- Peritonitis is an inflammatory response within the peritoneal cavity as the result of contamination with microorganisms, chemicals, or both.
- Infective peritonitis is classified as either diffuse or localized, primary *(spontaneous)*, secondary, or tertiary and is further characterized as "uncomplicated" or "complicated."
- In primary peritonitis, there is no intra-abdominal source, whereas in secondary, there is an intra-abdominal source of infection.
- Uncomplicated infections are contained within a single organ without anatomic disruption, whereas complicated infections involve extension beyond the organ, either localized or generalized peritonitis, with spillage of microorganisms into the sterile peritoneal space.
- Peritonitis is a common complication occurring in patients undergoing continuous ambulatory peritoneal dialysis (CAPD).
- Intraperitoneal abscesses are focal collections of pus complicating either primary or secondary peritonitis, with locations generally related to the site of primary disease and the direction of dependent peritoneal drainage.
- The majority of intra-abdominal infections (80%) are "community acquired" and are graded from "mild to moderate" to "more severe" on the basis of physiologic scoring systems (Acute Physiology and Chronic Health Evaluation II [APACHE II]), the patient's comorbid conditions, underlying immune status, and an inability to achieve adequate source control.
- Health care–associated intra-abdominal infections are most commonly acquired as complications of previous elective or emergency abdominal surgeries.

EPIDEMIOLOGY

- Primary peritonitis accounts for approximately 1% of all peritonitis cases.
- Adult patients usually have cirrhosis and ascites and are at greater risk if there is a coexisting gastrointestinal hemorrhage, previous episode, or low ascitic protein concentration.
- Secondary peritonitis is the most common intra-abdominal infection (80% to 90%), caused by microbial or chemical contamination of the sterile peritoneal cavity from multiple disease processes (see Table 21-1).
- Tertiary peritonitis refers to a persistent or recurrent infection without a surgically treatable focus, may be due to disturbance in the host's immune response, and often is associated with less virulent and potentially resistant microorganisms.
- CAPD peritonitis is the major complication of peritoneal dialysis and most often is due to touch contamination or catheter-related infection.
- It recurs in 20% to 30% and is the primary reason for a switch to hemodialysis.
- Intraperitoneal abscesses occur secondarily as a consequence of diseased organs, penetrating trauma, or a surgical procedure.

TABLE 21-1	Causes of Secondary Peritonitis
Distal esophagus	Boerhaave syndrome Malignancy Trauma Iatrogenic*
Stomach	Peptic ulcer perforation Malignancy Trauma Iatrogenic*
Duodenum	Peptic ulcer perforation Trauma Iatrogenic*
Biliary tract	Cholecystitis Stone perforation from gallbladder or common duct Malignancy Trauma Iatrogenic*
Pancreas	Pancreatitis (e.g., alcohol, drugs, gallstones) Trauma Iatrogenic*
Small bowel	Ischemic bowel Incarcerated hernia Crohn's disease Malignancy Meckel's diverticulum Trauma
Large bowel and appendix	Ischemic bowel Diverticulitis Malignancy Ulcerative colitis and Crohn's disease Appendicitis Volvulus Trauma (mostly penetrating) Iatrogenic*
Uterus, salpinx, and ovaries	Pelvic inflammatory disease (e.g., salpingo-oophoritis, tubo-ovarian abscess, ovarian cyst) Trauma Malignancy Iatrogenic*

*Dehiscence of surgical anastomosis or inadvertent injury during a procedure (e.g., endoscopy).
 Modified from Solomkin JS, Mazuski JE, Bradley JS, et al. Diagnosis and management of complicated intra-abdominal infection in adults and children: guidelines by the Surgical Infection Society and the Infectious Diseases Society of America. *Clin Infect Dis.* 2010;50:133-164.

MICROBIOLOGY

- Primary peritonitis is a monomicrobial infection with more than 60% of episodes in cirrhotic patients caused by gram-negative enteric bacteria.
- In children, hematogenous spread of *Streptococcus pneumoniae* and other streptococcal species is more frequent.
- *Staphylococcus aureus* is rarely isolated in primary peritonitis.
- Variants of primary peritonitis include ascites that grows a single type of organism but has fewer than 250 polymorphonuclear white blood cells (PMN WBCs)/mm^3 (monomicrobial non-neutrocytic bacterascites) or has more than 250 PMN WBCs/mm^3 with negative cultures (culture-negative neutrophilic ascites).
- Secondary peritonitis is characteristically polymicrobial (see Table 21-2) and depends upon the microflora associated with the primary disease process, which may be altered by previous antibiotic therapy, other medications, and specific host factors.
- Enterococci and *Candida* spp. can often be isolated, the significance of which is controversial.

TABLE 21-2 Organisms Causing Complicated Intra-abdominal Infections	
ORGANISM	**PATIENTS (%)**
Facultative and Aerobic Gram-Negative Bacilli	
Escherichia coli	71
Klebsiella spp.	14
Pseudomonas aeruginosa	14
Proteus mirabilis	5
Enterobacter spp.	5
Anaerobic	
Bacteroides fragilis	35
Other Bacteroides spp.	71
Clostridium spp.	29
Prevotella spp.	12
Peptostreptococcus spp.	17
Fusobacterium spp.	9
Eubacterium spp.	17
Gram-Positive Aerobic Cocci	
Streptococcus spp.	38
Enterococcus faecalis	12
Enterococcus faecium	3
Enterococcus spp.	8
Staphylococcus aureus	4

Modified from Solomkin JS, Mazuski JE, Bradley JS, et al. Diagnosis and management of complicated intra-abdominal infection in adults and children: guidelines by the Surgical Infection Society and the Infectious Diseases Society of America. *Clin Infec Dis.* 2010;50:133-164.

- CAPD peritonitis is caused by gram-positive organisms (*Staphylococcus epidermidis, S. aureus,* and *Streptococcus* spp.) in 60% to 80% of cases.
- Gram-negative bacteria (e.g., Enterobacteriaceae, *Pseudomonas* spp., and *Acinetobacter* spp.) make up 15% to 30% of cases, often derived from urinary tract, bowel, skin, or contaminated water.
- Fungal and mycobacterial species are occasionally involved.
- Polymicrobial peritonitis in CAPD is assumed to be secondary to an intestinal process (e.g., bowel perforation).
- Intraperitoneal abscesses are mostly polymicrobial and involve the same microorganisms that cause secondary peritonitis.
- Pathogens include obligate anaerobic species (e.g., *Bacteroides fragilis,* anaerobic cocci, and *Clostridia*) along with facultative gram-negative bacilli (e.g., *Escherichia coli* and *Proteus* and *Klebsiella* spp.)

DIAGNOSIS
- Primary peritonitis is diagnosed by excluding a primary source of intra-abdominal infection.
- Ascitic fluid studies include WBC count with differential, protein concentration, Gram stain, and culture.
- The difference between serum and ascitic fluid albumin concentration is greater than 1.1 g/dL, which is correlated with portal hypertension.
- Ascitic fluid glucose, amylase, and lactate dehydrogenase measurements may help to distinguish primary from secondary peritonitis.
- Patients suspected of having secondary peritonitis or an intraperitoneal abscess on the basis of clinical findings or peritoneal fluid examination require radiologic evaluation with a computed tomography scan and/or ultrasonography.

TABLE 21-3 Primary Peritonitis: Indications for Initiation of Therapy

Temperature >37.8°C (100°F)
Abdominal pain and/or tenderness
An unexplained change in mental status
Laboratory abnormalities suggestive of infection (e.g., renal failure, acidosis, or peripheral leukocytosis)
Peritoneal fluid neutrophil count ≥250 cells/mm³

TABLE 21-4 Recommended Agents for Treatment of Complicated Intra-abdominal Infections

TYPE OF THERAPY[a]	FOR MILD TO MODERATELY SEVERE INFECTIONS[b]	FOR HIGHLY SEVERE COMMUNITY-ACQUIRED, HEALTH CARE–ASSOCIATED, AND TERTIARY INFECTIONS[c]
Single Agent		
β-lactam/β-lactamase inhibitor combinations	Ticarcillin-clavulanic acid	Piperacillin-tazobactam[d]
Fluoroquinolone[e]	Moxifloxacin[f]	Moxifloxacin[f]
Carbapenems	Ertapenem	Imipenem-cilastatin[d] or meropenem or doripenem
Glycylcyclines	Tigecycline[f]	Tigecycline[f]
Combination Therapy		
Cephalosporin based	Cefazolin, cefuroxime, cefotaxime, ceftriaxone plus metronidazole	Third- or fourth-generation cephalosporin (ceftazidime or cefepime) plus metronidazole Ceftazidime/avibactam plus metronidazole[g] Ceftolozane/tazobactam plus metronidazole
Fluoroquinolone based[e]	Ciprofloxacin or levofloxacin, each in combination with metronidazole[g]	Ciprofloxacin in combination with metronidazole[h]
Monobactam based		Aztreonam plus vancomycin[f] or clindamycin plus metronidazole

[a]Empirical antimicrobial regimens should be adjusted according to culture and susceptibility reports to ensure activity against the predominant pathogens isolated in culture.
[b]Applies mainly to community-acquired intra-abdominal infections.
[c]Applies to health care–associated and tertiary peritonitis cases, as well as some severe community-acquired intra-abdominal infections. **However, tigecycline should NOT be used as empirical therapy for health care–associated or tertiary infection due to inactivity of tigecycline against Pseudomonas aeruginosa.**
[d]In vitro activity may be less, compared to alternative antibiotics.
[e]Fluoroquinolone-resistant Escherichia coli has become common in some communities, and fluoroquinolones should not be used unless hospital surveys indicate at least 90% susceptibility of E. coli to fluoroquinolones.
[f]Risk of mortality may be greater compared with alternative antimicrobials.
[g]Clinical cure rates were lower than those achieved with meropenem in a phase III trial, with baseline creatinine clearance (CrCL) of 30 to 50 mL/min. However, patients treated with ceftazidime/avibactam received a 33% lower daily dose than is currently recommended for patients with this CrCL.
[h]Because Bacteroides strains are resistant to these fluoroquinolones, addition of metronidazole is necessary.

- When clinically suspected, CAPD peritonitis is confirmed by finding greater than 100 WBCs/mm³ (predominantly PMN cells) in mostly cloudy dialysate, together with the isolation of a microorganism (90% to 95% of cases).

THERAPY

- Pending confirmatory studies, empirical antibiotic therapy for suspected primary peritonitis should be initiated (see Table 21-3) on the basis of the most likely pathogens.
- Five days of antibiotic therapy is sufficient in most instances, and oral antibiotic therapy may be an option in selected cases.
- The treatment of secondary peritonitis requires antibiotic therapy (see Tables 21-4 and 21-5), along with appropriate medical support, source control, and removal of a diseased organ,

TABLE 21-5 Antibiotic Dosage for Peritonitis during Peritoneal Dialysis

DRUG	INTERMITTENT (PER EXCHANGE, ONCE DAILY)	CONTINUOUS (ALL EXCHANGES)
Aminoglycosides		
Gentamicin	0.6 mg/kg	LD: 8 mg/L MD: 4 mg/L
Tobramycin	0.6 mg/kg	LD: 8 mg/L MD: 4 mg/L
Cephalosporins		
Cefazolin	15 mg/kg	LD: 500 mg/L MD: 125 mg/L
Cefepime	1 g	LD: 500 mg/L MD: 125 mg/L
Ceftazidime	1-1.5 g	LD: 500 mg/L MD: 125 mg/L
Cefotaxime	1 g	LD: 500 mg/L MD: 125 mg/L
Penicillins		
Ampicillin	ND	MD: 125 mg/L
Oxacillin	ND	MD: 125 mg/L
Penicillin G	ND	LD: 50,000 U MD: 25,000 U
Piperacillin	ND	LD: 500 mg/L MD: 250 mg/L
Quinolones		
Ciprofloxacin	ND	LD: 50 mg/L MD: 25 mg/L
Others		
Vancomycin	15-30 mg/kg every 5-7 days	LD: 1000 mg/L MD: 25 mg/L
Aztreonam	ND	LD: 1000 mg/L MD: 250 mg/L
Trimethoprim-sulfamethoxazole	ND	LD: 320/1600 mg/L PO MD: 80/400 mg/L PO daily
Combinations		
Ampicillin-sulbactam	2 g every 12 hr	LD: 1000 mg/L MD: 100 mg/L
Imipenem-cilastatin	1 g every 12 hr	LD: 500 mg/L MD: 200 mg/L
Antifungals		
Amphotericin B	NA	1.5 mg/L
Fluconazole	ND	200 mg/L IP or PO daily

IP, intraperitoneal; LD, loading dose; MD, maintenance dose; NA, not applicable; ND, no data; PO, orally.
Modified from Piraino B, Bailie GR, Bernardini J, et al. Peritoneal dialysis-related infections recommendations: 2005 update. *Perit Dial Int.* 2005;25:107-131.

TABLE 21-6 CAPD Peritonitis: Indications for Catheter Removal

Persistent infection at skin exit site or tunnel
Relapsing peritonitis with same organism—within 4 wk
Refractory peritonitis—failure to respond within 5 days
Fungal, mycobacterial, *Pseudomonas aeruginosa* peritonitis
Intraperitoneal abscess
Catheter malfunction

CAPD, continuous ambulatory peritoneal dialysis.

necrotic tissue, purulence, blood, feces, and other intraperitoneal foreign material, when present.
- CAPD peritonitis is treated with intraperitoneal antibiotics (see Table 21-6) usually for 10 to 21 days.
- Peritoneal dialysis catheter removal is necessary in 10% to 20% of patients, particularly with fungal and nontuberculous mycobacterial infections (see Table 21-6).
- Intraperitoneal abscesses require drainage (percutaneous catheter or surgical), antibiotic therapy (see Tables 21-4 and 21-5), and possibly source control.

PREVENTION
- Primary peritonitis prophylaxis is recommended in cirrhotic patients with ascites who are having a gastrointestinal hemorrhage.
- Long-term antibiotic prophylaxis (e.g., norfloxacin or trimethoprim-sulfamethoxazole) is indicated in patients with one or more episodes of primary peritonitis, as well as in cirrhotic patients with ascitic fluid protein concentrations less than 1.5 g/dL.

22 Infections of the Liver and Biliary System (Liver Abscess, Cholangitis, Cholecystitis)

Costi D. Sifri and Lawrence C. Madoff

DEFINITION

- A pyogenic liver abscess is the end result of a number of pathologic processes resulting in a focal, purulent bacterial collection in the liver.
- An amebic liver abscess is an invasive complication of intestinal amebiasis resulting in a focal collection of nonpurulent fluid in the liver.
- Cholecystitis: Inflammation/bacterial infection of the gallbladder often resulting from obstructing gallstones. Acalculous cholecystitis is a similar process in the absence of gallstones.
- Cholangitis is inflammation/infection of the bile ducts.

EPIDEMIOLOGY

- An estimated 10 to 20 cases of pyogenic liver abscess occur per 100,000 hospital admissions, or 11 cases per million persons per year.
- Amebic liver abscesses are rarer, about 1 per million persons, but more common in endemic regions. They affect men about 10 times more frequently than women.
- Tens of millions in the United States have gallstones; 1% to 3% are complicated by acute cholecystitis.
- Approximately 120,000 cholecystectomies occur each year in the United States.
- Between 2% and 15% of cases occur without gallstones, known as "acalculous cholecystitis."
- In endemic regions, parasites such as *Ascaris* and *Clonorchis* may cause biliary disease.

MICROBIOLOGY

- Pyogenic liver abscesses may be monomicrobial, especially when caused by bacteremia, or polymicrobial involving aerobic gram-negative bacilli and anaerobes.
- *Klebsiella pneumoniae* (typically K1 and K2 strains) are now an important cause of pyogenic liver abscess, particularly in parts of Asia, but increasingly elsewhere.
- Amebic liver abscesses are caused by invasive strains of *Entamoeba histolytica*.

DIAGNOSIS

- Symptoms are often nonspecific, and a high index of suspicion is required.
- Diagnostic imaging, especially by ultrasonography, radionuclide cholescintigraphy, or computed tomography, is essential. For pyogenic liver abscesses, it is often coupled with diagnostic/therapeutic aspiration.

THERAPY

- Some pyogenic processes require prompt recognition and urgent image-guided drainage or definitive surgery.
- Antibiotics directed at the suspected pathogens play an important role as adjuncts to surgery or, in limited cases, may be the sole form of therapy (e.g., small pyogenic liver abscesses, amebic liver abscess).

23 Pancreatic Infection

Miriam Baron Barshak

DEFINITION

- Infection of pancreatic tissue.
- Most commonly develops as a complication of acute pancreatitis (AP), in tissue that has been damaged by inflammation (see Table 23-1).
- Pancreatic abscess is a circumscribed collection of pus usually in or near the pancreas, arising as a consequence of AP or pancreatic trauma.

EPIDEMIOLOGY

- Approximately 185,000 cases of AP per year in the United States, 20% of which may have significant pancreatic necrosis.
- Up to 70% of patients with pancreatic necrosis may develop pancreatic infection.

MICROBIOLOGY

- Gastrointestinal bacterial flora most common (aerobes and anaerobes, gram-positive, and gram-negative).
- Use of preemptive antibiotics may select for more resistant bacterial species and fungal pathogens.

DIAGNOSIS

- Must be distinguished from sterile pancreatic necrosis, which can be associated with a sepsis-like syndrome.
- Tissue sampling is required to identify infection.

THERAPY

- Antimicrobial therapy targeting organisms identified in cultures of the infected site, in combination with catheter drainage and/or surgical removal of the infected material (see Table 23-2).
- Delay in surgery for infected pancreatic necrosis may allow for a more stable patient with better-demarcated areas of necrotic tissue.
- Newer surgical approaches include video-assisted retroperitoneal débridement and endoscopic transgastric necrosectomy.

PREVENTION

- Avoid too-early enteral feeding.
- A consensus favoring use of early (preemptive) systemic antibiotics emerged in the 1990s and 2000s, using carbapenem alone or quinolone plus metronidazole as first-choice therapy.
- More recent randomized controlled studies have not demonstrated a benefit from this practice, and some guidelines no longer recommend preemptive antibiotics for patients with AP.

Part I Major Clinical Syndromes

TABLE 23-1 Definitions Derived from the International Symposium on Acute Pancreatitis, 1992

TERM	DEFINITION
Acute pancreatitis	Acute inflammatory process of the pancreas with variable involvement of other regional tissues or remote organ systems
Severe acute pancreatitis	Association with organ failure or local complications, or both, such as necrosis, abscess, or pseudocyst
Acute fluid collection	Occurs early in the course of AP, located in or near the pancreas, always lacking a wall of granulation or fibrous tissue; bacteria variably present; occurs in 30%-50% of severe AP; most acute fluid collections regress, but some progress to pseudocyst or abscess
Pancreatic necrosis	Diffuse or focal area(s) of nonviable pancreatic parenchyma, typically associated with peripancreatic fat necrosis, diagnosed by computed tomography scan with intravenous contrast enhancement
Acute pseudocyst	Collection of pancreatic juice enclosed by a wall of fibrous or granulation tissue that arises as a consequence of AP, pancreatic trauma, or chronic pancreatitis; formation requires 4 or more weeks from onset of AP
Pancreatic abscess	Circumscribed intraabdominal collection of pus usually in or near the pancreas, containing little or no pancreatic necrosis, arises as a consequence of AP or pancreatic trauma

AP, acute pancreatitis.
Note: The use of terms such as phlegmon, infected pseudocyst, hemorrhagic pancreatitis, and persistent acute pancreatitis is explicitly discouraged.
From Bradley EL. A clinically based classification system for acute pancreatitis. *Arch Surg.* 1993;128:586-590.

TABLE 23-2 Pancreatic Infection Incidence and Mortality Rate in Controlled Trials with Antibiotics and Meta-Analyses

AUTHOR	ANTIBIOTIC	NO. OF PATIENTS	PANCREATIC INFECTION RATE (%) CONTROL/CASE	MORTALITY RATE (%) CONTROL/CASE	COMMENTS
Luiten et al	SGD: enteral colistin, norfloxacin, and amphotericin B, until clinical recovery plus IV cefotaxime until gram-negative bacteria are eliminated from the oral cavity	102 severe AP	38/18*	35/22	Nonblinded. Necrosis not defined. Mortality difference statistically significant when disease severity differences between the groups are taken into account. Predominant effect on gram-negative pancreatic infection (8% in SGD group vs. 33% in conventional treatment group). Treatment with intravenous cefuroxime as well as enteral SGD obscures interpretation of the effect of enteral treatments alone.
Pederzoli et al	Imipenem, 500 mg IV tid, 14 days	74 necrotizing pancreatitis, mostly of biliary origin	30/12*	12/7	Not placebo-controlled. Nonpancreatic infections also reduced (15% vs. 49%, $P < .01$). No change in multiorgan failure rate, need for surgery, or survival compared with no early antibiotic treatment.
Sainio et al	Cefuroxime, 1.5 g IV tid, until clinical recovery and normalization of CRP level	60 severe acute alcoholic pancreatitis and necrosis of at least one third of the pancreas by contrast-enhanced CT	40/30	23/3*	Not placebo-controlled. Reduction in total infections, infections per patient, and operations also statistically significant. Rate of culture-proven sepsis not statistically significant. Only urinary tract infections were reduced significantly.
Delcenserie et al	Ceftazidime, amikacin, and metronidazole IV, 10 days	23 alcohol-induced severe AP	58/0*	25/9	CT with two or more fluid collections, necrosis not defined
Schwarz et al	Ofloxacin and metronidazole IV, 10 days	26 CT-confirmed pancreatic necrosis	53/61	15/0	Not placebo-controlled. FNA performed on days 1, 3, 5, 7, and 10 in all patients; antibiotics given to control patients with evidence of infection. Better clinical course in intervention group, but no effect on development of pancreatic infections.
Bassi et al	Pefloxacin (400 mg bid) vs. imipenem (500 mg tid), 14 days	60 severe necrotizing pancreatitis	Pefloxacin: 33* Imipenem: 10*	Pefloxacin: 24 Imipenem: 10	Nonblinded. CT confirmed at least 50% necrosis.

Continued

TABLE 23-2 Pancreatic Infection Incidence and Mortality Rate in Controlled Trials with Antibiotics and Meta-Analyses—cont'd

AUTHOR	ANTIBIOTIC	NO. OF PATIENTS	PANCREATIC INFECTION RATE (%) CONTROL/CASE	MORTALITY RATE (%) CONTROL/CASE	COMMENTS
Isenmann et al	Ciprofloxacin (400 mg bid) and metronidazole (500 mg bid) IV, or placebo, 14 or 21 days	114 AP plus serum CRP >150 mg/L and/or necrosis on contrast-enhanced CT	12/9	5/7	Randomized, double-blinded, placebo-controlled; 28% of CIP/MET group and 46% of placebo group required open antibiotic treatment; most placebo group switches motivated by extrapancreatic infections; overall mortality and rates of pancreatic infection low, number of patients with pancreatic necrosis low
Golub et al	Meta-analysis of eight controlled trials, including trials from the 1970s				Findings: Early antibiotic administration reduced mortality from AP but only for patients with severe pancreatitis who received broad-spectrum antibiotics reaching therapeutic levels in pancreatic tissue
Sharma et al	Meta-analysis including only randomized, controlled, nonblinded studies evaluating patients with necrotizing pancreatitis who received either no preemptive antibiotics or preemptive treatment with antibiotics reaching therapeutic levels in necrotic pancreatic tissue	84 received antibiotic prophylaxis; 76 did not; of note, the total of 160 patients in the pooled data set is inadequate for detection of a 50% reduction in the rate of infections			Findings: Nonsignificant trend toward decreased local infection in patients given early imipenem, cefuroxime, or ofloxacin. Incidence of sepsis and overall mortality significantly lower (absolute risk reductions, 21.1% and 12.3%, respectively, for a relative risk reduction of 72%) for antibiotic treatment. On this basis, the authors recommend that "all patients with acute necrotizing pancreatitis...be given prophylaxis with an antibiotic with proven efficacy in necrotic pancreatic tissue."
Villatoro et al	Cochrane Review including randomized controlled trials comparing antibiotics with placebo in AP with CT-proven necrosis	294 (from 5 evaluable studies)			Findings: Significantly less mortality with therapy (6%) vs. controls (15.3%). No differences in rates of infected pancreatic necrosis, operative treatment, nonpancreatic infection, and fungal infection. Subgroup analysis of β-lactam treatment: Significantly less mortality (6.3% vs. 16.7%) than in controls, without significant differences in rates of operative treatment or nonpancreatic infections. No significant differences with quinolone plus imidazole treatment. β-Lactams associated with significantly decreased mortality and infected pancreatic necrosis.

Study	Study design	No. of patients			Findings
Rokke et al	Prospective randomized controlled trial, imipenem (500 mg tid for 5-7 days) vs. no antibiotics	73: 36 received imipenem; 37 received no antibiotics	43/14*	11/8	Underpowered study (slow patient accrual). No differences in length of hospital stay, need of intensive care, need of acute interventions, need for surgery, or 30-day mortality rates. Authors conclude that "the study, although underpowered, supports the use of early prophylactic treatment with imipenem in order to reduce the rate of septic complications in patients with severe pancreatitis."
Dellinger et al	Multicenter, prospective, double-blind, placebo-controlled randomized study set in 32 centers within North America and Europe	100 clinically severe, confirmed necrotizing pancreatitis: 50 received meropenem (1g IV q8h); 50 received placebo within 5 days of symptom onset, for 7 to 21 days	12/18	18/20	No statistically significant difference between the treatment groups for pancreatic or peripancreatic infection, mortality, or requirement for surgical intervention.
Jafri et al	Meta-analysis assessing the clinical outcome of patients with severe AP treated with prophylactic antibiotics compared with that of patients not treated with antibiotics	502 (from 8 studies)			Findings: No effect of antibiotics on mortality, rates of infected necrosis, or frequency of surgical intervention. Apparent benefit regarding nonpancreatic infections (RR, 0.60; 95% CI, 0.44-0.82), with a RR reduction of 40% (95% CI, 18%-56%); absolute risk reduction of 15% (95% CI, 6%-23%), and number needed to treat of 7 (95% CI, 4-17).
Villatoro et al	Cochrane Review including randomized controlled trials comparing antibiotics with placebo in AP with CT-proven necrosis	404 (from 7 evaluable studies)			Findings: No benefit of antibiotics in preventing infection of pancreatic necrosis or mortality, except when imipenem was considered on its own, in which case a significant decrease in pancreatic infection was found ($P = .02$; RR, 0.34; 95% CI, 0.13-0.84) without effect on mortality. "None of the studies included in this review were adequately powered. Further better designed studies are needed if the use of antibiotic prophylaxis is to be recommended."

AP, acute pancreatitis; CI, confidence interval; CIP/MET, ciprofloxacin/metronidazole; CRP, C-reactive protein; CT, computed tomography; FNA, fine-needle aspiration; IV, intravenous; RR, relative risk; SGD, selective gut decontamination.
*$P < .05$.
Modified from Toouli J, Brooke-Smith M, Bassi C, et al. Guidelines for the management of acute pancreatitis. J Gastroenterol Hepatol. 2002;17(suppl):S15-S39.

24 Splenic Abscess
Lawrence C. Madoff

DEFINITION
- The abscesses comprise one or more focal collections induced by bacteria, mycobacteria, or fungi in the spleen.
- Predisposing conditions include immunosuppression, trauma, diabetes, hemoglobinopathy, Felty's syndrome, intravenous drug use, and endocarditis.

EPIDEMIOLOGY
- Splenic abscesses are uncommon and have only been reported in small numbers in the medical literature.
- Splenic abscesses are present in 0.2% to 0.7% in general autopsy series.
- Splenic abscesses are a frequent finding in bacterial endocarditis and are present in up to one third of patients at autopsy.
- There is a bimodal age distribution, with peaks in the third and sixth decades of life.

MICROBIOLOGY
- Streptococci, staphylococci, salmonellae, and *Escherichia coli* are important causative agents and, also increasingly, fungi and mycobacteria.
- In specific geographic areas of Asia, *Klebsiella pneumoniae* and *Burkholderia pseudomallei* are important causative agents.
- Anaerobes are rare.

CLINICAL FINDINGS AND DIAGNOSIS
- Fever is present, with abdominal pain in left upper quadrant but a paucity of specific symptoms and findings.
- Ultrasound, computed tomography, and magnetic resonance tomography are used for diagnosis.

THERAPY
- Splenectomy has been the gold standard of treatment, along with antibiotic treatment of underlying infection elsewhere.
- Recent emphasis is on the use of percutaneous drainage with antibiotic treatment or, in some cases, antibiotic treatment alone, in an attempt to reduce morbidity and preserve the spleen.

25 Appendicitis

Costi D. Sifri and Lawrence C. Madoff

DEFINITION

- Appendicitis is acute inflammation of the vermiform appendix that is often related to obstruction and may be complicated by polymicrobial infection.
- Complications include perforation, peritonitis, and intra-abdominal abscesses.

EPIDEMIOLOGY

- Acute appendicitis is a relatively common disease, often presenting in adolescence and early adulthood.
- Lifetime risk for appendicitis is 8.6% in men and 6.7% in women.
- Over 300,000 appendectomies are performed annually in the United States.

MICROBIOLOGY

- The inflammation is usually polymicrobial, frequently involving aerobic and anaerobic gram-negative bacilli.
- A large variety of microbes have been isolated from acute appendicitis and related abscesses.
- Infections by *Yersinia* spp., parasites, including *Entamoeba histolytica,* and viruses may mimic appendicitis (e.g., mesenteric adenitis) or cause obstruction leading to acute appendicitis.

DIAGNOSIS

- Clinical diagnosis is enhanced by the use of imaging, especially computed tomography and ultrasonography.
- Diagnosis is more difficult in women of childbearing age in whom gynecologic processes may mimic appendicitis.

THERAPY

- Surgical removal of the appendix, often done laparoscopically, is curative.
- Adjunctive use of broad-spectrum antibiotics, such as piperacillin-tazobactam, ceftriaxone, and metronidazole, may be required.

26 Diverticulitis and Typhlitis

Costi D. Sifri and Lawrence C. Madoff

DEFINITION

- Diverticulitis is inflammation and infection of the bowel wall, leading to microperforation of colonic diverticula.
- Typhlitis (neutropenic enterocolitis) is characterized by abdominal pain and fever during periods of neutropenia resulting from mucosal inflammation, degeneration, and microbial invasion.

EPIDEMIOLOGY

- Diverticulitis occurs in 10% to 25% of all individuals with diverticulosis, which has a prevalence of 30% to 40% in Western society.
- Diverticulitis leads to 150,000 hospital admissions and 24,000 elective operations annually in the United States.
- The incidence of typhlitis is unknown but has been estimated to be 5% in hospitalized neutropenic adults with cancer.
- Bacteremia or fungemia occurs in 14% to 44% of patients with typhlitis.

MICROBIOLOGY

- Acute diverticulitis is a polymicrobial infection caused by endogenous anaerobic and facultative bacteria, including *Bacteroides* spp., *Peptostreptococcus* spp., *Enterobacteriaceae*, viridans streptococci, and enterococci.
- *Pseudomonas aeruginosa*, *Enterobacteriaceae*, *Bacteroides fragilis*, viridans streptococci, enterococci, and *Candida* spp. are common causes of bloodstream infections in patients with typhlitis.

DIAGNOSIS

- Radiographic imaging (computed tomography and ultrasonography) is essential for the evaluation of suspected diverticulitis and typhlitis.
- More than half of patients with clinically suspected diverticulitis are diagnosed with an alternative condition after diagnostic imaging.
- Radiographic findings of diverticulitis include pericolic fat stranding, diverticula, bowel wall thickening, and phlegmon or abscess formation.
- Typhlitis can be defined as bowel wall thickening greater than 4 mm, usually of the cecum, with neutropenia, fever, and abdominal pain.

THERAPY

- Acute uncomplicated diverticulitis can be safely treated in select outpatients with a short course of oral antibiotics.
- However, the necessity of antibiotic therapy for the treatment of uncomplicated diverticulitis is controversial.
- Complicated diverticulitis or patients with comorbidities or other predictors of worse outcomes should be hospitalized.

- Percutaneous drainage of large abscesses (>5 cm in diameter) can be temporizing in acutely ill patients.
- Management of typhlitis includes bowel rest, intravenous fluids, nutritional support, and broad-spectrum parenteral antibiotics that cover enteric facultative and anaerobic flora, *Pseudomonas aeruginosa*, and perhaps yeast.
- Surgery may be required for patients with diverticulitis or typhlitis with intraperitoneal perforation, uncontrolled sepsis, persistent gastrointestinal bleeding, obstruction, or who fail to respond to medical therapy.

PREVENTION
- High dietary fiber and physical activity may be associated with reduced symptomatic diverticular disease.

27 Endocarditis and Intravascular Infections

Vance G. Fowler, Jr., W. Michael Scheld, and Arnold S. Bayer

DEFINITION

- *Infective endocarditis* (IE) is an infection of the endocardial surface of the heart.

EPIDEMIOLOGY

- It is traditionally associated with heart valves damaged by rheumatic heart disease.
- In the current era, health care contact and injection drug use are the primary risk factors.

MICROBIOLOGY

- *Staphylococcus aureus* is now the leading cause of IE in most of the industrialized world.
- Historically, viridans group streptococci were the most common cause of endocarditis.
- *Bartonella* spp. are the most common cause of culture-negative IE in the United States. Other common causes of culture-negative IE are summarized in Table 27-1.

DIAGNOSIS

- Results of blood cultures remain the cornerstone of diagnosis of endocarditis.
- Clinical evaluation alone is insufficient to exclude the possibility of endocarditis.
- Echocardiography, particularly transesophageal echocardiography, has greatly improved the clinician's ability to identify endocarditis.
- Diagnostic schema, such as the modified Duke Criteria, are useful in establishing the presence of endocarditis.

THERAPY

- Cardiac surgery is required in up to half of patients with endocarditis and improves patient outcome.
- Cardiac surgery is especially important in patients with endocarditis who have heart failure, paravalvular abscess, recurrent embolic events, or ongoing sepsis or who are infected with highly resistant or fungal pathogens.
- Although the timing of cardiac surgery, particularly after embolic events involving the central nervous system, remains controversial, emerging evidence supports the benefit of early valve replacement surgery for endocarditis.
- Antibiotic therapy involves extended courses of antibiotics. Treatment is highly pathogen specific and is summarized in Table 27-2. Guidelines for treatment of IE were published in 2005 and are currently being updated.
- Addition of adjunctive low-dose, short-course gentamicin to standard antibiotic treatment of *S. aureus* native valve IE has been shown to confer high risk for nephrotoxicity without significant improvement in clinical outcomes and is not encouraged.
- Several observational studies support the use of high-dose ceftriaxone in combination with ampicillin for the treatment of ampicillin-susceptible, aminoglycoside-resistant enterococcal endocarditis or for patients with underlying renal disease.

TABLE 27-1 Causes of Culture-Negative Endocarditis

ORGANISM	EPIDEMIOLOGY AND EXPOSURES	DIAGNOSTIC APPROACHES
Aspergillus and other noncandidal fungi	Prosthetic valve	Lysis-centrifugation technique; also culture and histopathologic examination of any emboli
Bartonella spp.	*B. henselae:* exposure to cats or cat fleas *B. quintana:* louse infestation; homelessness, alcohol abuse	Most common cause of culture-negative IE in United States; serologic testing (may cross-react with *Chlamydia* spp.); PCR assay of valve or emboli is best test; lysis-centrifugation technique may be useful
Brucella spp.	Ingestion of unpasteurized milk or dairy products; livestock contact	Blood cultures ultimately become positive in 80% of cases with extended incubation time of 4-6 wk; lysis-centrifugation technique may expedite growth; serologic tests are available
Chlamydia psittaci	Bird exposure	Serologic tests available but exhibit cross-reactivity with *Bartonella;* monoclonal antibody direct stains on tissue may be useful; PCR assay now available
Coxiella burnetii (Q fever)	Global distribution; exposure to unpasteurized milk or agricultural areas	Serologic tests (high titers of antibody to both phase 1 and phase 2 antigens); also PCR assay on blood or valve tissue
HACEK spp.	Periodontal disease or preceding dental work	Although traditionally a cause of culture-negative IE, HACEK species are now routinely isolated from most liquid broth continuous monitoring blood culture systems without prolonged incubation times
Legionella spp.	Contaminated water distribution systems; prosthetic valves	Serology available; periodic subcultures onto buffered charcoal yeast extract medium; lysis-centrifugation technique; PCR assay available
Nutritionally variant streptococci	Slow and indolent course	Supplemented culture media or growth as satellite colonies around *Staphylococcus aureus* streak; antimicrobial susceptibility testing often requires processing specialized microbiology laboratory
Tropheryma whipplei (Whipple's disease)	Typical signs and symptoms include diarrhea, weight loss, arthralgias, abdominal pain, lymphadenopathy, central nervous system involvement; IE may be present without systemic symptoms	Histologic examination of valve with periodic acid–Schiff stain; valve cultures may be done using fibroblast cell lines; PCR assay on vegetation material

HACEK, *Haemophilus* spp., *Aggregatibacter* spp., *Cardiobacterium hominis, Eikenella corrodens,* and *Kingella* spp.; IE, infective endocarditis; PCR, polymerase chain reaction.

PREVENTION

- Prevention of endocarditis involves reduction of bloodstream infections, especially in the health care setting.
- The role of antibiotic prophylaxis for the prevention of endocarditis is controversial. Guidelines have been published from the American Heart Association.

Chapter 27 Endocarditis and Intravascular Infections

Part I Major Clinical Syndromes

TABLE 27-2 Summary of Treatment Options for Endocarditis

ORGANISM/REGIMEN[a]		COMMENTS
Staphylococcus aureus		
Native Valve		
Methicillin-susceptible	Nafcillin or oxacillin, 2 g IV q4h × 4-6 wk *Optional:* gentamicin, 1 mg/kg IV q8h × 3-5 days[b]	Use of gentamicin in native valve *S. aureus* IE is associated with significant nephrotoxicity without clear clinical benefit and therefore is not encouraged
	Cefazolin, 2 g IV q8h × 4-6 wks *Optional:* gentamicin, 1 mg/kg IV q8h × 3-5 days[b]	Acceptable in setting of penicillin allergy other than immediate hypersensitivity. See above cautions about gentamicin use.
Methicillin-resistant	Vancomycin, 15-20 mg/kg IV q8-12h × 6 wk[b]	Also acceptable in setting of immediate hypersensitivity or anaphylaxis to penicillin; goal vancomycin trough level 15-20 µg/mL is recommended
Prosthetic Valve		
Methicillin-susceptible	Nafcillin or oxacillin, 2 g IV q4h × ≥6 wk, *plus* gentamicin, 1 mg/kg IV q8h × 2 wk, *plus* rifampin, 300 mg PO/IV q8h × ≥6 wk	
Methicillin-resistant	Vancomycin, 15-20 mg/kg IV q8-12h × ≥6 wk *plus* gentamicin, 1 mg/kg IV q8h × 2 wk, *plus* rifampin, 300 mg PO/IV q8h × ≥6 wk	Goal vancomycin trough level 15-20 µg/mL is recommended
Injection Drug Use		
Methicillin-susceptible	Nafcillin or oxacillin, 2 g IV q4h × 2 wk; *plus* gentamicin, 1 mg/kg IV q8h × 2 wk	Two-week regimen only for use in injection drug users with infection limited to tricuspid valve, no renal insufficiency, and no extrapulmonary infection. Two weeks of monotherapy with antistaphylococcal penicillin has also been successfully used in these patients.
Methicillin-resistant	Vancomycin, 15-20 mg/kg IV q8-12h × 4 wk	Use of gentamicin in this setting is not recommended. Goal vancomycin trough level 15-20 µg/mL is recommended.
	Daptomycin, 6 mg/kg IV qd × 4-6 wk	Daptomycin is U.S. Food and Drug Administration–approved for treatment of right-sided *S. aureus* IE; for adults, some experts recommend 8-10 mg/kg IV
Coagulase-Negative Staphylococci		
Native Valve		
Methicillin-susceptible	Nafcillin or oxacillin, 2 g IV q4h × 4-6 wk *Optional:* gentamicin, 1 mg/kg IV q8h × 3-5 days	
Methicillin-resistant	Vancomycin, 15-20 mg/kg IV q8-12h × 6 wk	Also acceptable in setting of immediate hypersensitivity or anaphylaxis to penicillin. Goal vancomycin trough level 15-20 µg/mL is recommended.
Prosthetic Valve		
Methicillin-susceptible	Nafcillin or oxacillin, 2 g IV q4h × ≥6 wk, *plus* gentamicin, 1 mg/kg IV q8h × 2 wk, *plus* rifampin, 300 mg PO/IV q8h × ≥6 wk	
Methicillin-resistant	Vancomycin, 15-20 mg/kg IV q8-12h × ≥6 wk, *plus* gentamicin, 1 mg/kg IV q8h × 2 wk, *plus* rifampin, 300 mg PO/IV q8h × ≥6 wk	Goal vancomycin trough level 15-20 µg/mL is recommended

TABLE 27-2 Summary of Treatment Options for Endocarditis—cont'd

	ORGANISM/REGIMEN[a]	COMMENTS
Penicillin-Susceptible Viridans Streptococci (MIC ≤0.1 μg/mL) and _Streptococcus bovis_ (S. gallolyticus)		
	Penicillin, 2-3 million units IV q4h × 4 wk, _or_ ampicillin, 2 g IV q4h × 4wk	Also effective for other penicillin-susceptible nonviridans streptococci (e.g., group A streptococci)
	Ceftriaxone, 2 g IV qd × 4 wk	For penicillin allergy; patients with uncomplicated viridans streptococcal IE are candidates for outpatient therapy
	Penicillin, 2-3 million units IV q4h × 2 wk, _plus_ gentamicin, 1 mg/kg IV q8h × 2 wk	Uncomplicated native valve IE only; not acceptable for nutritionally variant streptococci
Nutritionally variant strain	Penicillin, 2-4 million units IV q4h × 4 wk, _plus_ gentamicin, 1 mg/kg IV q8h × 2 wk	For prosthetic valve IE, give 6 wk of penicillin. Nutritionally variant streptococci are often penicillin tolerant.
	Vancomycin, 15-20 mg/kg IV q8-12h × 4 wk	For penicillin allergy
Relatively Penicillin-Resistant Viridans Streptococci (MIC 0.12-<0.5 μg/mL)		
	Penicillin, 4 million units IV q4h × 4 wk, _plus_ gentamicin, 1 mg/kg IV q8h × 2 wk	
	Vancomycin, 15-20 mg/kg IV q8-12h × 4 wk	For penicillin allergy or to avoid gentamicin
Enterococci[c] and Penicillin-Resistant Viridans Streptococci (Penicillin MIC >0.5 μg/mL)		
Penicillin-susceptible, aminoglycoside-susceptible enterococci	Penicillin[d] 3-5 g IV q4h × 4-6 wk, _plus_ gentamicin, 1 mg/kg IV q8h × 4-6 wk; _or_ Ampicillin, 2 g IV q4h, _plus_ gentamicin, 1 mg/kg IV q8h × 4-6 wk	Increase duration of both drugs to 6 wk for prosthetic valve infection or for enterococcal IE with symptoms >3 mo. For older patients and those with underlying renal disease, can consider shortening the duration of gentamicin to 2 wk.
Penicillin-resistant, vancomycin-susceptible, aminoglycoside-susceptible enterococci	Vancomycin, 15-20 mg/kg IV q8-12h × 6 wk, _plus_ gentamicin, 1 mg/kg q8h × 6 wk[e]	Also for patients with penicillin allergy. This regimen is associated with enhanced risk of nephrotoxicity. Penicillin desensitization should be considered as an alternative to this regimen when possible.
Penicillin-susceptible, aminoglycoside-resistant enterococci	Ampicillin, 2 g IV q4h, _plus_ ceftriaxone, 2 g IV q12h	Useful for patients with significant underlying renal disease
Penicillin-resistant, vancomycin-resistant enterococci	No standard therapy; daptomycin, linezolid, and quinupristin-dalfopristin have been used	Consult infectious diseases specialist
HACEK Strains		
	Ceftriaxone, 2 g IV qd × 4 wk	Increase duration to 6 wk for infections involving prosthetic valves
	Ampicillin-sulbactam, 3 g IV q6h × 4 wk (if β-lactamase producing strain)[a]	Increase duration to 6 wk for infections involving prosthetic valves
Non-HACEK Gram-Negative Bacilli[f]		
Enterobacteriaceae	Extended-spectrum penicillin (e.g., piperacillin-tazobactam) or cephalosporin _plus_ aminoglycosides for susceptible strains	Treat for a minimum of 6-8 wk. Some species exhibit inducible resistance to third-generation cephalosporins. Valve surgery is often required for patients with left-sided IE caused by gram-negative bacilli, especially for prosthetic valve IE. Consultation with an infectious diseases specialist is recommended.

Continued

TABLE 27-2 Summary of Treatment Options for Endocarditis—cont'd

ORGANISM/REGIMEN[a]		COMMENTS
Non-HACEK Gram-Negative Bacilli[f]—cont'd		
Pseudomonas aeruginosa	Antipseudomonal penicillin (e.g., piperacillin) *plus* high-dose tobramycin, 8 mg/kg/day IV or IM in once-daily doses; *or* High-dose ceftazidime, cefepime, or imipenem	Goal tobramycin peak and trough concentrations of 15-20 µg/mL and ≤2 µg/mL, respectively. Treat for a minimum of 6-8 wk. Early valve surgery usually required for left-sided *Pseudomonas* IE; consultation with a specialist in infectious diseases is recommended.
Fungi[f]		
	Treatment with a parenteral antifungal agent (usually an amphotericin B–containing product) is usually recommended as initial therapy	Fungal endocarditis is usually an indication for valve replacement surgery. Long-term/lifelong suppressive therapy with oral antifungal agents is often required. Consultation with a specialist in infectious diseases is recommended.

HACEK, *Haemophilus* spp., *Aggregatibacter* spp., *Cardiobacterium hominis, Eikenella corrodens,* and *Kingella* spp.; IE, infective endocarditis; MIC, minimal inhibitory concentration.

[a]Dosages assume normal renal function. For patients with renal insufficiency, adjustments must be made for all antibiotics except nafcillin, rifampin, and ceftriaxone. Gentamicin doses should be adjusted to achieve a peak serum concentration of approximately 3 µg/mL 30 minutes after dosing and a trough gentamicin level of <1 µg/mL.

[b]Primarily relevant to left-sided IE.

[c]Enterococci must undergo antimicrobial susceptibility testing. These recommendations are for enterococci susceptible to penicillin, gentamicin, and vancomycin except as indicated.

[d]Ampicillin, 12 g/day, can be used instead of penicillin.

[e]The need to add an aminoglycoside has not been demonstrated for penicillin-resistant streptococci.

[f]Limited data exist.Modified from Baddour LM, Wilson WR, Bayer AS, et al. Infective endocarditis: diagnosis, antimicrobial therapy, and management of complications. *Circulation.* 2005;111:e394-e433.

28 Prosthetic Valve Endocarditis

Raj Palraj, Bettina M. Knoll, Larry M. Baddour, and Walter R. Wilson

DEFINITION
- Prosthetic valve endocarditis (PVE) is a potentially life-threatening infection that involves a valve prosthesis or annuloplasty ring.

EPIDEMIOLOGY
- Prosthetic valve endocarditis is an uncommon but well-recognized complication of valve replacement or repair.
- Health care–associated PVE is increasing in incidence.
- *Staphylococcus aureus* is the most common cause of PVE.

MICROBIOLOGY
- Early-onset (illness onset within 1 year of valve surgery) PVE is usually caused by microorganisms acquired perioperatively, such as *S. aureus* and coagulase-negative staphylococci (CoNS). Nosocomial gram-negative pathogens, many of which are multidrug resistant, and fungi rarely cause early-onset PVE.
- Late-onset PVE is usually caused by organisms representative of "normal microbiota" and include viridans group streptococci and enterococci.
- *S. aureus* and CoNS are also common pathogens of late-onset PVE due, in part, to an increase in frequency of health care–associated exposure in the late period.

DIAGNOSIS
- Modified Duke criteria have been used to define suspect cases of PVE.
- Blood cultures are critical in both supporting a PVE diagnosis and directing selection of antimicrobial therapy.
- Transesophageal echocardiography (TEE) is the preferred imaging modality to support a diagnosis and to identify complications such as severe valve dysfunction and perivalvular extension of infection, which may require surgical intervention.

THERAPY
- Parenteral antimicrobial therapy directed against a specific pathogen for a minimum of 6 weeks is recommended (see Table 28-1).
- TEE may need to be repeated during antimicrobial therapy to identify complications that would prompt surgical intervention.
- Early surgical intervention should be considered in complicated PVE with perivalvular extension, severe heart failure, severe valve dysfunction/dehiscence, multiple emboli, unresponsive infection, and PVE due to multidrug-resistant organisms or fungi (see Table 28-2).

PREVENTION
- Perioperative antibiotic prophylaxis, strict infection control measures, good surgical technique, and limiting the use of central venous catheters are important in preventing early-onset PVE.

TABLE 28-1 Therapy for Prosthetic Valve Endocarditis Caused by Staphylococci, Suggested by American Heart Association

REGIMEN	DOSAGE AND ROUTE	DURATION
Methicillin-Susceptible Staphylococci		
Nafcillin or oxacillin* *plus*	2 g IV q4h	≥6 wk
Rifampin[†] *plus*	300 mg PO or IV q8h	≥6 wk
Gentamicin[‡]	3 mg/kg IV/IM q24h in 2 or 3 equally divided doses	2 wk
Methicillin-Resistant Staphylococci		
Vancomycin[§] *plus*	15 mg/kg IV q12h	≥6 wk
Rifampin[†] *plus*	300 mg PO or IV q8h	≥6 wk
Gentamicin[‡]	3 mg/kg per IV/IM in 2 or 3 equally divided doses	2 wk

Dosages recommended are for patients with normal renal function.

*Penicillin G, 24 million U/24 hr IV, may be used in place of nafcillin or oxacillin if the strain is penicillin susceptible (MIC ≤0.1 µg/mL) and does not produce β-lactamase. Cefazolin 2 g IV q8h may be substituted for nafcillin or oxacillin. Cefazolin can be used in non–immediate-type allergic reaction to penicillin. Consider skin testing for patients with history of immediate-type allergy to penicillin. Vancomycin is recommended only in patients unable to tolerate penicillins and cephalosporins.

[†]It is recommended to initiate rifampin therapy only after susceptibility results are known and ideally after 2 days of effective combination therapy, in an attempt to reduce the risk of emergence of rifampin resistance.

[‡]Gentamicin should be administered in close proximity to vancomycin, nafcillin, or oxacillin to maximize synergy. Renal function and serum gentamicin concentrations should be closely monitored. Goal trough level is <1 µg/mL and peak level (1 hr postdose) is 3-4 µg/mL.

[§]Vancomycin dosage should be adjusted to a trough level of 10-15 µg/mL.

From Baddour LM, Wilson WR, Bayer AS, et al. Infective endocarditis: diagnosis, antimicrobial therapy, and management of complications: a statement for healthcare professionals from the Committee on Rheumatic Fever, Endocarditis, and Kawasaki Disease, Council on Cardiovascular Disease in the Young, and the Councils on Clinical Cardiology, Stroke, and Cardiovascular Surgery and Anesthesia, American Heart Association: endorsed by the Infectious Diseases Society of America. *Circulation.* 2005;111:e394-e434.

TABLE 28-2 Indications for Consideration of Surgical Intervention

Severe heart failure; mild-moderate heart failure unresponsive to medical therapy
Valvular dehiscence, obstruction, or leaflet perforation
Perivalvular extension of infection leading to myocardial abscess, fistula, or shunt
New severe conduction defects suggestive of perivalvular extension
Multiple (>1) systemic emboli despite appropriate antimicrobial therapy
Uncontrolled infection—persistent fever and positive blood cultures for >5 days
Fungal, *Pseudomonas* spp., or other multidrug-resistant organisms

- Maintenance of good oral hygiene is important to prevent late-onset community-acquired PVE.
- Although there has been no randomized, placebo-controlled trial to define the efficacy and safety of antibiotic prophylaxis, it is recommended for any dental procedure that involves manipulation of the gingival or periapical region of teeth or perforation of oral mucosa, as well as for procedures on the respiratory tract, infected skin, skin structures, and/or musculoskeletal tissue.

29 Infections of Nonvalvular Cardiovascular Devices

M. Rizwan Sohail, Walter R. Wilson, and Larry M. Baddour

CARDIOVASCULAR IMPLANTABLE ELECTRONIC DEVICE (CIED) INFECTIONS

- The infection rate of CIED infection is rising disproportionate to the rate of implantation.
- Most early-onset (within 6 months of implantation) CIED pocket infections are caused by device contamination at the time of implantation, whereas hematogenous seeding is a frequent source of late-onset (after 6 months of implantation) CIED lead infections.
- Hematogenous seeding of CIED leads is rare with gram-negative bacteremia from a distant source.
- Blood cultures should be obtained in all patients at initial presentation. If blood cultures are positive, then transesophageal echocardiography should be done to exclude endocarditis.
- Complete removal of the CIED system is required for eradication of infection.
- A replacement device can be implanted once blood cultures are negative for 72 hours and perhaps earlier in cases in which admission blood cultures are negative. A 2-week delay is recommended for patients with valvular endocarditis.
- All patients should receive perioperative antibiotics as primary prevention of CIED infection.

LEFT VENTRICULAR ASSIST DEVICE (LVAD) INFECTIONS

- In addition to being a bridge to transplantation, LVADs are increasingly being used as destination therapy for patients with end-stage heart failure who are not transplant candidates.
- Continuous-flow pumps are at lower risk of infection compared with devices with pulsatile flow pumps.
- Driveline exit-site infections are the most common type of LVAD-specific infections, followed by LVAD-related bacteremia and endocarditis.
- *Staphylococcus aureus* and coagulase-negative staphylococci are responsible for the majority of LVAD-specific infections.
- Most LVAD infections are treated with the infected device left in situ because device removal is not an option in most cases.
- Suppressive antibiotics are continued lifelong or until the infected LVAD is removed and cardiac transplantation is performed.
- Immobilizing the driveline at the skin exit site to prevent repeated skin trauma reduces the risk of local infections.

PROSTHETIC VASCULAR GRAFT INFECTIONS (PVGIS)

- Staphylococcal species are the predominant pathogens in PVGIs.
- Microbial seeding of a graft at the time of implantation or in the immediate postoperative period is operative in graft infections.
- Computed tomographic (CT) scanning is the best tool in the diagnostic evaluation of graft infection. CT findings of perigraft fluid accumulation, fat stranding or gas bubbles, lack of

fat plane between graft and bowel, and anastomotic aneurysms are all suggestive of graft infection.

- Surgical management of an infected graft includes complete excision of infected graft material, débridement of all infected and devitalized tissues, and revascularization of distal tissues.
- If complete excision of an infected graft is not feasible, patients should be prescribed lifelong oral suppressive antibiotics after an initial 4-week course of parenteral antimicrobial therapy.

30 Prophylaxis of Infective Endocarditis

David T. Durack

DEFINITION OF THE ISSUE

Infective endocarditis (IE) continues to cause serious morbidity and mortality; therefore, prevention of IE is a priority.

EPIDEMIOLOGY

- The incidence of IE is increasing in developing countries.
- Contributing factors include aging populations, the steadily increasing number of medical procedures, implants and prostheses, and the rising frequency of health care–associated infections, especially catheter-related bloodstream infections.

MICROBIOLOGY

- Staphylococci have superseded viridans streptococci as the predominant pathogens.
- Methicillin-sensitive, methicillin-resistant, and coagulase-negative strains of staphylococci all contribute to the increase in cases of staphylococcal IE.
- Increasing resistance to β-lactams, aminoglycosides, and vancomycin among staphylococci, streptococci, and enterococci presents new challenges for prevention and therapy of IE.

PREVENTION OF INFECTIVE ENDOCARDITIS

- Many dental, medical, and diagnostic procedures cause bacteremias, which occasionally result in IE.
- Antibiotics can prevent IE in vivo in experimental animals.
- For more than 50 years, administration of antibiotics before procedures known to cause bacteremias was recommended to prevent IE, but there is no definitive evidence that this practice is effective or cost-effective in humans. Antibiotics can cause unwanted side effects, including profound and persistent alterations of the microbiome.
- Therefore, recent guidelines sharply restrict use of antibiotic prophylaxis for IE, limiting it to patients at highest risk of an adverse outcome of IE: those with prosthetic heart valves; with cyanotic congenital heart disease (CHD); with repaired CHD with implanted prosthetic material, for the first 6 months only; with a history of previous episode(s) of IE; with valvulopathy after a heart transplant (see Table 30-1).
- For this small group of high-risk patients, the standard regimen is a single 2-g dose of amoxicillin given orally 30 to 60 minutes before the dental procedure. Alternative regimens are recommended for penicillin-allergic patients and those unable to take oral medication, and dosages are adjusted for children (see Table 30-2).
- There is no evidence that this major change in prevention guidelines has resulted in any increase in the number of cases of IE.
- Continuing surveillance of epidemiologic trends and microbial resistance, together with education of patients at risk for IE and their health care providers, is recommended.
- Prevention and prompt treatment of health care–associated infections is important, to reduce the incidence of bacteremias that can cause IE.
- Because preventive measures may fail, early diagnosis and prompt therapy of IE are important, to reduce morbidity and mortality.

TABLE 30-1 Preexisting Cardiac Conditions Associated with Highest Risk of Adverse Outcome from Infective Endocarditis

- Prosthetic cardiac valve(s) or prosthetic material inserted for cardiac valve repair
- Previous infective endocarditis
- Congenital heart disease (CHD)
  - Unrepaired cyanotic CHD, including palliative shunts and conduits
  - Completely repaired CHD with prosthetic material or device, whether placed by surgery or catheter intervention, during the first 6 months after the procedure
  - Repaired CHD with residual defects at site or adjacent to site of prosthetic patch or prosthetic device (which inhibit endothelialization)
- Cardiac transplant recipients who develop cardiac valvulopathy

Modified from Wilson W, Taubert KA, Gewitz M, et al. Prevention of infective endocarditis: guidelines from the American Heart Association: a guideline from the American Heart Association Rheumatic Fever, Endocarditis, and Kawasaki Disease Committee; Council on Cardiovascular Disease in the Young; and the Council on Clinical Cardiology; Council on Cardiovascular Surgery and Anesthesia; and the Quality of Care and Outcomes Research Interdisciplinary Working Group. *Circulation*. 2007;116:1736-1754.

TABLE 30-2 Regimens for Antibiotic Prophylaxis of Infective Endocarditis during Dental Procedures*

CLINICAL SITUATION	ANTIBIOTIC	DOSAGE FOR ADULTS[†]	DOSAGE FOR CHILDREN[†,‡]
Standard oral regimen—for most patients	Amoxicillin	2.0 g PO	50 mg/kg PO
If unable to take oral medication	Ampicillin or ceftriaxone	2.0 g IM or IV 1.0 g IM or IV	50 mg/kg IM or IV 50 mg/kg IM or IV
If allergic to penicillins	Clindamycin or azithromycin or clarithromycin	600 mg PO 500 mg PO 500 mg PO	15 mg/kg PO 15 mg/kg PO 15 mg/kg PO
If allergic to penicillins and unable to take oral medication	Clindamycin	600 mg IM or IV	20 mg/kg IM or IV

IM, intramuscular; IV, intravenous; PO, oral.
*Only for patients with highest risk of adverse outcome of infective endocarditis; see Table 30-1.
[†]Single dose, 30 to 60 minutes before procedure.
[‡]Not to exceed adult dose.
Modified from Wilson W, Taubert KA, Gewitz M, et al. Prevention of infective endocarditis: guidelines from the American Heart Association: a guideline from the American Heart Association Rheumatic Fever, Endocarditis, and Kawasaki Disease Committee; Council on Cardiovascular Disease in the Young; and the Council on Clinical Cardiology; Council on Cardiovascular Surgery and Anesthesia; and the Quality of Care and Outcomes Research Interdisciplinary Working Group. *Circulation*. 2007;116:1736-1754.

31 Myocarditis and Pericarditis

Kirk U. Knowlton, Anna Narezkina, Maria C. Savoia, and Michael N. Oxman

MYOCARDITIS

- Inflammation of the myocardium, which is clinically manifested by chest pain, arrhythmias, or congestive heart failure (CHF)

Etiologic Agents

- Most commonly associated with viral infections, particularly enteroviruses, adenoviruses, parvovirus B19, human herpesvirus 6, and dengue viruses (see Table 31-1).
- Occasionally caused by bacteria, as a result of bacteremia, direct extension from a contiguous focus, or a bacterial toxin.
- Caused by *Trypanosoma cruzi,* the cause of Chagas' disease, which is prevalent in South and Central America.

Diagnosis

- In the setting of clinical suspicion, elevations of cardiac enzymes, electrocardiographic changes (nonspecific), echocardiography, and cardiac magnetic resonance imaging are helpful.
- Evidence of coincident viral infection, either by culture or serology, is circumstantial.
- Endomyocardial biopsy can provide a definitive diagnosis, but sampling errors limit its utility.

Treatment

- Supportive care and management of CHF are essential.
- The benefit of immunosuppressive therapy is not established.
- The efficacy of intravenous immunoglobulin therapy is also not established.

PERICARDITIS

- Inflammation of the pericardium is clinically manifested by chest pain, pericardial friction rub, and pericardial effusion. These may be present individually or in combination. Monitoring for cardiac tamponade is important.

Etiologic Agents

- Enteroviruses are most common, but other viruses may sometimes be responsible (see Table 31-2).
- Bacteria rarely may cause purulent pericarditis, usually as a complication of pneumonia.
- *Mycobacterium tuberculosis* can cause pericarditis, usually as a complication of pulmonary tuberculosis. This is a major problem in Africa in association with acquired immunodeficiency syndrome.

Diagnosis

- Etiology is often undetermined in individual cases.
- Pericardiocentesis may yield an etiologic agent but is negative in the majority of patients.

TABLE 31-1   Infectious Causes of Myocarditis

Viruses	Bacteria and Rickettsiae—cont'd
Coxsackie B viruses	*Francisella tularensis*
Coxsackie A viruses	*Neisseria meningitidis*
Adenoviruses	*Salmonella*
Echoviruses	*Shigella*
Parvovirus B19	*Streptococcus pyogenes*
Nonpolio enteroviruses	*Staphylococcus aureus*
Polioviruses	*Listeria monocytogenes*
Rabies virus	*Vibrio cholerae*
Mumps virus	*Mycobacterium tuberculosis*
Rubeola (measles) virus	*Legionella pneumophila*
Influenza A and B viruses	*Mycoplasma pneumoniae*
Rubella	*Chlamydia psittaci*
Dengue viruses	*Chlamydia pneumoniae*
Chikungunya virus	*Rickettsia rickettsii*
Yellow fever virus	*Rickettsia prowazekii*
Argentine hemorrhagic fever virus (Junin virus)	*Rickettsia (Orientia) tsutsugamushi*
Bolivian hemorrhagic fever virus (Machupo virus)	*Coxiella burnetii*
Lymphocytic choriomeningitis virus	*Ehrlichia*
Lassa fever virus	*Borrelia burgdorferi*
Varicella-zoster virus	*Tropheryma whippelii*
Human cytomegalovirus	*Ureaplasma* spp.
Epstein-Barr virus	**Fungi**
Human herpesvirus 6	*Aspergillus*
Herpes simplex virus	*Candida* species
Variola virus	*Blastomyces*
Vaccinia virus	*Coccidioides immitis*
Hepatitis B virus	*Cryptococcus neoformans*
Hepatitis C virus	*Histoplasma capsulatum*
Respiratory syncytial virus	**Parasites**
Human immunodeficiency virus	*Trypanosoma cruzi*
Bacteria and Rickettsiae	*Trypanosoma gambiense*
Brucella	*Trypanosoma rhodesiense*
Campylobacter	*Trichinella spiralis*
Corynebacterium diphtheriae	*Toxoplasma gondii*
Clostridium perfringens	*Toxocara canis*

- Evidence of viral infection by detection in peripheral samples or by serology provides only circumstantial evidence of possible etiology.
- Percutaneous pericardial biopsy or pericardiotomy with biopsy and drainage increase the diagnostic yield.

Treatment

- For presumed viral or idiopathic pericarditis, analgesic treatment with nonsteroidal anti-inflammatory drugs (NSAIDs), together with bed rest, is often successful in relieving symptoms. NSAIDs are generally continued for 1 to 2 weeks, or until symptoms resolve.
- Colchicine given with NSAIDs has been found to improve rate of recovery and reduce recurrence.
- Purulent pericarditis usually requires drainage together with appropriate antibiotics.
- Tuberculous pericarditis requires appropriate antituberculous therapy; concomitant administration of corticosteroids reduces development of constrictive pericarditis and the need for repeated pericardiocentesis.

TABLE 31-2 Infectious Causes of Pericarditis

Viruses

Coxsackie A viruses
Coxsackie B viruses
Echoviruses
Adenoviruses
Mumps virus
Influenza A and B viruses
Lymphocytic choriomeningitis virus
Lassa fever virus
Varicella-zoster virus
Human cytomegalovirus
Epstein-Barr virus
Herpes simplex virus
Variola (smallpox) virus
Vaccinia virus
Hepatitis B virus
Human immunodeficiency virus

Bacteria and Rickettsia

Streptococcus pneumoniae
Other streptococcal species
Staphylococcus aureus
Neisseria meningitidis
Neisseria gonorrhoeae
Haemophilus influenzae
Salmonella
Yersinia
Francisella tularensis
Pseudomonas

Bacteria and Rickettsia—cont'd

Campylobacter
Brucella
Listeria monocytogenes
Nocardia
Actinomyces
Other anaerobic bacteria
Corynebacterium diphtheriae
Mycobacterium tuberculosis
Nontuberculous mycobacteria
Legionella pneumophila
Mycoplasma pneumoniae
Coxiella burnetii
Chlamydia
Borrelia burgdorferi

Fungi

Aspergillus
Candida species
Blastomyces
Coccidioides immitis
Cryptococcus neoformans
Histoplasma capsulatum

Parasites

Entamoeba histolytica
Toxoplasma gondii
Toxocara canis
Schistosoma

32 Mediastinitis

Trevor C. Van Schooneveld and Mark E. Rupp

DEFINITION
- Mediastinitis is an infection involving the structures of the mediastinum (see Fig. 32-1).

EPIDEMIOLOGY
- Acute mediastinitis usually occurs via one of three routes: esophageal perforation, extension of a head and neck infection (descending necrotizing mediastinitis), and post–cardiac surgery (see Table 32-1).
- Post–cardiac surgery mediastinitis occurs in 1% to 2% of cardiac surgery cases, and important risk factors for mediastinitis include obesity, diabetes, *Staphylococcus aureus* colonization, use of bilateral internal thoracic arteries, need for reexploration, and receipt of multiple blood products.
- Chronic/fibrosing mediastinitis is usually due to an excessive immune reaction to histoplasma antigens in mediastinal lymph nodes, which results in fibrosis and narrowing of mediastinal structures.

MICROBIOLOGY
- Oral flora, including streptococci, gram-negative bacilli, and anaerobes predominate in mediastinitis due to esophageal perforation and descending head and neck infections.
- Poststernotomy mediastinitis is most frequently due to gram-positive cocci, especially staphylococci, whereas gram-negative bacilli and candida are less common.

DIAGNOSIS
- Esophageal rupture is usually manifested by chest pain, shortness of breath, and odynophagia.
- Signs of the initiating head and neck infection (swelling, pain, erythema) predominate in descending necrotizing mediastinitis.
- Post–cardiac surgery mediastinitis findings may range from subtle to fulminant but usually present within 2 weeks of surgery. Fever, wound drainage, cellulitis, and chest pain are usually present.
- Laboratory findings often include leukocytosis and a rising procalcitonin in postmedian sternotomy patients.
- Fibrosing mediastinitis manifestations include cough, dyspnea, chest pain, and exercise intolerance but depend on the structures being occluded.
- Computed tomography is the preferred diagnostic imaging for all forms of mediastinitis.

THERAPY
- Broad-spectrum antimicrobials targeted to expected pathogens are essential.
- Aggressive surgical intervention is essential in all forms of mediastinitis with débridement of any infected or necrotic tissues.
- Early esophageal perforation may occasionally be managed with stenting, but most cases require urgent surgical repair.
- Post–cardiac surgery mediastinitis requires sternal and mediastinal débridement.

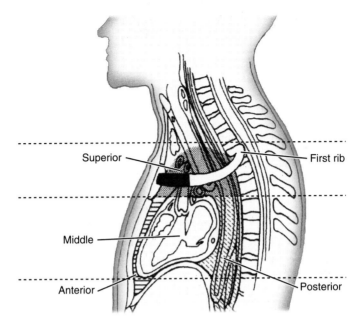

Superior
First rib

Middle

Anterior
Posterior

FIGURE 32-1 **Anatomic boundaries and divisions of the mediastinum.**

TABLE 32-1   Causes of Acute Mediastinitis

Esophageal Perforation
Iatrogenic

Esophagogastroduodenoscopy, esophageal dilation, esophageal variceal sclerotherapy, nasogastric tube, Sengstaken-Blakemore tube, endotracheal intubation, esophageal surgery including endoscopic resection, paraesophageal surgery, transesophageal echocardiography, anterior stabilization of cervical vertebral bodies, catheter ablation of atrial fibrillation

Swallowed Foreign Bodies

Bones, coins, can pull-tabs, drug-filled condoms, swords, ballpoint pens, button batteries

Trauma

Penetrating—gunshot wound, knife wound
Blunt—steering wheel injury, seatbelt injury, cardiopulmonary resuscitation, whiplash injury, barotrauma

Spontaneous or Other

Emesis, cricoid pressure during anesthesia induction, heavy lifting, defecation, parturition, carcinoma, ingestion of caustic or corrosive liquids

Head and Neck Infections

Odontogenic, Ludwig's angina, pharyngitis, tonsillitis, parotitis, epiglottitis, Lemierre syndrome

Infection Originating at Another Site

Pneumonia; pleural space infection or empyema; subphrenic abscess; pancreatitis; cellulitis or soft tissue infection of the chest wall; osteomyelitis of sternum, clavicle, ribs, or vertebrae; hematogenous spread from distant foci
Lymph nodes—necrosis and hemorrhage (anthrax) or caseous necrosis (tuberculosis)

Cardiothoracic Surgery (Median Sternotomy)

Coronary artery bypass grafting, cardiac valve replacement, repair of congenital heart defect, heart transplantation, heart-lung transplantation, cardiac assist devices, extracorporeal membrane oxygenation (ECMO), other types of cardiothoracic surgery

- Multiple surgical techniques can be utilized for surgical treatment of poststernotomy mediastinitis with increasing use of vacuum-assisted closure and soft tissue flaps for reconstruction.
- The role, if any, for antifungal therapy in fibrosing mediastinitis is not established.
- In fibrosing mediastinitis, stenoses of vessels and other structures are often successfully managed by either surgical bypass or stenting.

PREVENTION

- Prevention of post–cardiac surgery is a major focus of quality measures and guidelines.
- Key factors associated with decreased post–cardiac surgery infection rates include appropriate antimicrobial prophylaxis (administration within 1 hour before surgery and for no longer than 24 to 48 hours and use of the appropriate agent), control of postoperative blood glucose, and use of nasal mupirocin in patients colonized with *S. aureus*.

33 Acute Meningitis

Allan R. Tunkel, Diederik van de Beek, and W. Michael Scheld

DEFINITION

- Meningitis, or inflammation of the meninges, is identified by an abnormal number of white blood cells in cerebrospinal fluid (CSF). Acute meningitis is clinically defined as a syndrome characterized by the onset of meningeal symptoms over the course of hours to up to several days.

EPIDEMIOLOGY

- Estimates from the Centers for Disease Control and Prevention (CDC) indicate that 10 to 15 million symptomatic enteroviral infections occur annually in the United States, which includes 30,000 to 75,000 cases of meningitis.
- In a surveillance study among residents in eight surveillance areas representing 17.4 million persons from 1998 to 2007, the impact of the heptavalent pneumococcal conjugate vaccine was appreciated, in which the incidence of bacterial meningitis caused by vaccine serotypes decreased from 0.61 cases/100,000 population in 1998 to 1999 to 0.05 cases/100,000 population in 2006 to 2007.
- In patients 16 years old or older, the relative frequency of isolation of meningeal pathogens in patients with community-acquired bacterial meningitis is somewhat different than in infants and children, with most cases caused by *Streptococcus pneumoniae*, *Neisseria meningitidis*, and *Listeria monocytogenes*.

MICROBIOLOGY

- Enteroviruses, currently the leading recognizable cause of aseptic meningitis syndrome, account for 85% to 95% of all cases in which a pathogen is identified.
- DNA of herpes simplex virus (HSV) has been detected in the CSF of published cases of Mollaret's meningitis (now termed *recurrent benign lymphocytic meningitis*), almost all being HSV-2.
- A profound reduction has been seen in the incidence of invasive infections (including bacterial meningitis) caused by *Haemophilus influenzae* type b in the United States and Western Europe; this decrease in infection is attributed, in part, to the widespread use of conjugate vaccines against *H. influenzae* type b that have been licensed for routine use in all children beginning at 2 months of age.
- From 1998 to 2007, a total of 2262 cases of meningococcal disease were reported to the Active Bacterial Core surveillance sites, with an annual incidence of 0.53 cases/100,000 population; the incidence decreased from 0.92 cases/100,000 population in 1998 to 0.33 cases/100,000 population in 2007 before the introduction of the quadrivalent meningococcal conjugate vaccine.
- Patients with pneumococcal meningitis often have contiguous or distant foci of pneumococcal infection, such as pneumonia, otitis media, mastoiditis, sinusitis, and endocarditis; serious infection may be observed in patients with various underlying conditions (e.g., splenectomy or asplenic states, multiple myeloma, hypogammaglobulinemia, alcoholism, malnutrition, chronic liver or renal disease, malignancy, and diabetes mellitus).

- Outbreaks of *Listeria* infection have been associated with the consumption of contaminated coleslaw, raw vegetables, milk, and cheese, with sporadic cases traced to contaminated turkey franks, alfalfa tablets, cantaloupe, diced celery, hog head cheese (a meat jelly made from hog heads and feet), and processed meats, thus pointing to the intestinal tract as the usual portal of entry.
- Group B streptococcus is a common cause of meningitis in neonates, with 52% of all cases in the United States reported during the first month of life.
- Aerobic gram-negative bacilli (e.g., *Klebsiella* spp., *Escherichia coli*, *Serratia marcescens*, *Pseudomonas aeruginosa*, *Acinetobacter* spp., *Salmonella* spp.) have become increasingly important as etiologic agents in patients with bacterial meningitis; these agents may be isolated from the CSF of patients after head trauma or neurosurgical procedures and may also be found in neonates, older adults, immunosuppressed patients, and patients with gram-negative sepsis.

DIAGNOSIS

- Nucleic acid amplification tests, such as polymerase chain reaction (PCR) assay, are the most promising alternatives to viral culture for the diagnosis of enteroviral meningitis.
- CSF culture is the gold standard in diagnosis of bacterial meningitis and is positive in 80% to 90% of patients of community-acquired disease if CSF is obtained before the start of antimicrobial therapy.
- Broad-based bacterial PCR can be used to detect the most common microorganisms of bacterial meningitis in only one test and has adequate sensitivity and excellent specificity; these tests can be done within 2 hours in most industrialized countries, but they are scarce in resource-poor countries.
- The diagnostic accuracy of CSF lactate is better than that of the CSF white blood cell count, glucose, and protein in the differentiation of bacterial from aseptic meningitis, with sensitivities of 93% and 97% and specificities of 96% and 94%, respectively.

THERAPY

- The initial management of a patient with presumed bacterial meningitis includes performance of a lumbar puncture to determine whether the CSF formula is consistent with that diagnosis.
- If purulent meningitis is present, institution of antimicrobial therapy should be based on the results of Gram staining; however, if no etiologic agent can be identified by this means or if performance of the lumbar puncture is delayed, institution of empirical antimicrobial therapy should be based on the patient's age and underlying disease status.
- Certain patients with bacterial meningitis should also be treated with adjunctive dexamethasone. In a Cochrane Database Systematic review of 24 studies involving 4041 participants, adjunctive dexamethasone did not reduce overall mortality but there was a trend to lower mortality in adults; corticosteroids were associated with lower rates of severe hearing loss, any hearing loss, and neurologic sequelae, although these benefits were only seen in studies from high-income countries.
- Penicillin can never be recommended as empirical therapy in patients with suspected pneumococcal meningitis; as an empirical regimen, the combination of vancomycin plus a third-generation cephalosporin (either cefotaxime or ceftriaxone) is recommended.
- Empirical treatment of gram-negative meningitis could begin with ceftazidime, cefepime, or meropenem. If the organism is later found to be resistant to these cephalosporins and the carbapenems, colistin (usually formulated as colistimethate sodium) or polymyxin B should be substituted for meropenem and may also need to be administered by the intraventricular or intrathecal route.

PREVENTION

- Chemoprophylaxis is also necessary for close contacts of patients with invasive meningococcal disease; the CDC currently recommends the administration of rifampin, ciprofloxacin, or ceftriaxone, which are all 90% to 95% effective at eradicating nasopharyngeal carriage, although cases of ciprofloxacin-resistant *N. meningitidis* have been reported in North Dakota and Minnesota, leading the CDC to no longer recommend ciprofloxacin for meningococcal chemoprophylaxis in selected counties of these states.

- Vaccination to prevent infection with specific meningeal pathogens is a very useful measure for decreasing the incidence of bacterial meningitis.
- For *H. influenzae* type b, the availability of conjugate vaccines has decreased the number of cases of *H. influenzae* type b meningitis more than 90%.
- The first meningococcal conjugate vaccine (meningococcal polysaccharide-diphtheria toxoid conjugate vaccine containing serogroups A, C, W135, and Y polysaccharides) was licensed for use in the United States for routine vaccination of all persons aged 11 to 18 years with one dose; in updated guidelines, a booster dose is now recommended at age 16 years and a two-dose primary series is administered 2 months apart for persons aged 2 through 54 years with persistent complement component deficiency or functional or anatomic asplenia and for adolescents with human immunodeficiency virus infection; other persons who are at risk for meningococcal disease (e.g., microbiologists or travelers to an epidemic or highly endemic country) should receive a single dose.
- The Advisory Committee on Immunization Practices now recommends use of the 13-valent pneumococcal conjugate vaccine to prevent pneumococcal disease in infants and young children aged younger than 6 years; this vaccine has activity against the serotypes that were present in the heptavalent vaccine (4, 6B, 9V, 14, 18C, 19F, and 23F) along with six additional serotypes (1, 3, 5, 6A, 7F, and 19A).

34 Chronic Meningitis

John E. Bennett

DEFINITION

- Chronic meningitis, defined here as at least 4 weeks of symptoms with signs of inflammation in the cerebrospinal fluid, must be distinguished from recurrent aseptic meningitis, chronic myeloradiculitis, and chronic encephalitis.

ETIOLOGY

- Major causes are fungal infections, tuberculosis, syphilis, and malignancy (see Table 34-1)

DIAGNOSIS

- Major diagnostic tools are gadolinium-enhanced magnetic resonance imaging and cerebrospinal fluid studies (see Table 34-2). Surgical biopsy has a low yield.
- Polymerase chain reaction assay has taken on an increasing role, including its use in the diagnosis of Whipple's disease, chronic enteroviral meningitis, lymphoma, toxoplasmosis, and tuberculosis.

THERAPY

- Empirical therapy for suspected tuberculous meningitis is often done because of disease severity, but addition of prednisone may cause deterioration of unsuspected fungal meningitis. Worsening of infection may not be detected initially because corticosteroids can temporarily improve hypoglycorrhachia, fever, and cerebral edema on T2-weighted magnetic resonance images. The same issue arises with corticosteroid treatment of suspected sarcoid or autoimmune meningitis. It is only when subsequent, potentially irreversible deterioration occurs despite corticosteroids that an infectious cause is found. The benefit of corticosteroids in empirical regimens is usually outweighed by the harm.

TABLE 34-1 Differential Diagnosis of Chronic Meningitis

Mycoses

Cryptococcus (cryptococcosis)
Coccidioides (coccidioidomycosis)
Histoplasma (histoplasmosis)
Candida (candidiasis)
Sporothrix (sporotrichosis [rare])
Blastomyces (blastomycosis [rare])
Other molds (rare): *Scedosporium, Aspergillus, Cladophialophora* and other dark-walled molds

Bacteria

Mycobacterium tuberculosis (tuberculosis)
Treponema pallidum (syphilis)
Borrelia burgdorferi (Lyme disease)
Tropheryma whipplei (Whipple's disease)
Actinomyces (actinomycosis [parameningeal, rare])
Nocardia (nocardiosis [with brain abscess])
Brucella (brucellosis [rare])

Parasites

Acanthamoeba (acanthamebiasis)
Taenia solium (cysticercosis)
Angiostrongylus cantonensis (angiostrongyliasis)

Viruses

Echovirus (meningoencephalitis)

Postneurosurgical Causes

Infected cerebrospinal fluid shunt
Infected prosthetic material

Tumors

Diffuse gliomatosis
Metastatic meningeal malignancy, including lymphomatous meningitis

Other Causes

Sarcoidosis
Vogt-Koyanagi-Harada syndrome
Behçet's syndrome
IgG4-related hypertrophic pachymeningitis

TABLE 34-2 Diagnostic Tests for Chronic Meningitis

Cerebrospinal Fluid Tests

Glucose, blood, protein, and cell count and differential (including eosinophils)
India ink on centrifuged sediment
Fungal culture of 3 to 5 mL of cerebrospinal fluid
Cytopathology for malignant cells, including polymerase chain reaction assay or flow cytometry for
    monoclonal B cells
Periodic acid–Schiff stain of cytopathologic specimen for Whipple's disease
Venereal Disease Research Laboratory test (VDRL) for syphilis
Cryptococcal antigen
Histoplasma antigen
Aspergillus galactomannan antigen
Complement fixation for antibody to *Coccidioides* species
MTB Direct (Gen-Probe, San Diego, CA)
Polymerase chain reaction assay for tuberculosis, Whipple's disease, enterovirus infection, toxoplasmosis,
    lymphoma
Culture for enterovirus, *Acanthamoeba*

Serum Tests

Rapid plasma reagin (RPR) test or antitreponemal antibody test
Antibody to *Coccidioides, Histoplasma, Toxoplasma, Brucella*
Histoplasma antigen

35 Encephalitis

J. David Beckham and Kenneth L. Tyler

DEFINITION
- Encephalitis is an inflammatory process involving the brain parenchyma associated with clinical or laboratory evidence of neurologic dysfunction.

EPIDEMIOLOGY
- It occurs most frequently in infants younger than 1 year of age and in elderly patients older than the age of 65 with intermediate incidence in individuals between these age extremes.

MICROBIOLOGY
- Up to 60% of encephalitis cases result from an unidentified etiologic agent.
- Viruses, bacteria, and autoimmune inflammation cause the majority of known encephalitis cases.

DIAGNOSIS
- A compatible febrile syndrome with evidence of central nervous system impairment exists (see Table 35-1).
- Standard cerebral spinal fluid (CSF) analysis and neuroimaging with magnetic resonance imaging are preferred.
- Specific CSF or serum studies for defined etiologies of encephalitis, or both, are warranted (see Table 35-2).

THERAPY
- Early, empirical use of high-dose acyclovir is warranted to treat possible herpes simplex encephalitis pending diagnostic studies.
- Antiviral therapy is indicated for the treatment of other herpes viruses that cause encephalitis.
- Empirical antiviral therapy is recommended for suspected encephalitis associated with influenza.
- There is currently no therapy of known benefit for patients with encephalitis due to arboviruses.

PREVENTION
- Routine vaccination for common pathogens and vaccination for Japanese encephalitis virus in selected travelers may prevent some cases of encephalitis.
- Procedures to decrease exposure to mosquito bites may decrease the risk for arbovirus-related cases of encephalitis.

TABLE 35-1 Comparison of Encephalitis and Encephalopathy

	ENCEPHALITIS	ENCEPHALOPATHY
Clinical Features		
Fever	Common	Uncommon
Headache	Common	Uncommon
Depressed mental status	May fluctuate	Steady decline in mental status
Focal neurologic signs	Common	Uncommon
Seizures	Common	Uncommon
Types of seizures	Generalized or focal	Generalized
Laboratory Results		
Complete blood count	Leukocytosis common	Leukocytosis uncommon
Cerebrospinal fluid	Pleocytosis common	Pleocytosis uncommon
Electroencephalogram	Diffuse slowing and occasional focal abnormalities or periodic patterns	Diffuse slowing
Magnetic resonance imaging	May have focal abnormalities	No focal abnormalities

Modified from Davis LE. Diagnosis and treatment of acute encephalitis. *Neurologist.* 2000;6:145-159.

TABLE 35-2 Other Important and Emerging Causes of Viral Encephalitis

VIRAL ETIOLOGY	EPIDEMIOLOGY	CLINICAL FEATURES	DIAGNOSIS	TREATMENT
Adenovirus	Children and immunocompromised patients	Associated pneumonia	PCR or culture of brain biopsy specimen or CSF	Supportive
Chikungunya virus	Epidemic setting; India and Southeast Asia; mosquito vector	Febrile syndrome with rash and arthralgias	CSF and serum IgM and PCR	Supportive
Hendra virus	Australia; fruit bat reservoir; humans infected by secretions of bats	Fever, drowsiness, seizures, and coma associated with a flulike prodrome	Contact Special Pathogens Branch at CDC	Supportive
HIV	Worldwide epidemic; recent high-risk behavior	Fever, headache-associated acute retroviral syndrome; commonly associated with HIV dementia	HIV serology testing and HIV quantitative PCR of CSF; MRI may reveal T2 or FLAIR hyperintense lesions in periventricular regions and centrum semiovale	Combination antiretroviral therapy
Influenza	Fall and winter seasonal predilection; worldwide distribution; rare complication in children	Associated febrile syndrome, myalgias, respiratory prodrome; may be associated with bilateral thalamic necrosis	Viral culture, antigen detection, and PCR in respiratory secretions	Oseltamivir (C-III); poor outcomes
Japanese encephalitis	Mosquito vector, swine and bird reservoirs; most common cause of epidemic viral encephalitis throughout Southeast Asia and Australia	Seizures and parkinsonian features common; acute flaccid paralysis; case-fatality rate of 20%-30%	Serum IgM or acute/convalescent IgG; CSF IgM or antigen; MRI can show T2 and FLAIR hyperintense lesions at basal ganglia, thalami, and midbrain	Supportive; formalin-inactivated mouse brain–derived vaccine available for prevention

Continued

Part I Major Clinical Syndromes

TABLE 35-2 Other Important and Emerging Causes of Viral Encephalitis—cont'd

VIRAL ETIOLOGY	EPIDEMIOLOGY	CLINICAL FEATURES	DIAGNOSIS	TREATMENT
JC virus	Cell-mediated immunodeficiencies (AIDS) and immunomodulating therapy (natalizumab, rituximab, efalizumab)	Cognitive dysfunction, limb weakness, gait disturbance, visual loss, focal neurologic findings	CSF PCR (sensitivity 50%-70% for PML); MRI shows ≥1 nonenhancing, confluent subcortical white matter hyperintensity on T2 and FLAIR sequences	Combination antiretroviral therapy in AIDS patients or reversal of immunosuppression
Louping ill virus	Tick-borne disease; found in Ireland, Scotland, and England; associated with livestock	Usually mild febrile illness with associated confusion and stupor in some; deaths are rare	Serum IgM ELISA or a 4-fold increase in IgG antibody in paired acute and convalescent sera	Supportive
LCMV	Rodent-borne virus infects humans with exposure to infected urine, feces, saliva, or blood; severe disease in immunocompromised patients	Fever, headache, leukopenia, and thrombocytopenia; encephalitis characterized by personality changes, increased ICP, paraplegia, and cranial nerve and sensory dysfunction	CSF and serum IgM ELISA	Supportive
Me Tri virus	Mosquito-borne; Southeast Asia; transmitted among livestock	Fever, rash, seizures, lethargy, and meningismus	CSF PCR and IgM ELISA, serology	Supportive
Monkeypox	Prairie dog exposure	Vesiculopustular rash on head, extremities, palms, and soles; adenopathy; encephalitis is rare, with confusion, somnolence, and diminished reflexes	Skin biopsy, CSF, and serum IgM, serology; MRI showing T2 and FLAIR hyperintense lesions of the pons, thalamus, and subparietal cortex	Supportive care; consider cidofovir or vaccinia immune globulin (C-III)
Mumps virus	Unvaccinated	Previous parotitis followed by headaches, vomiting, seizures, altered consciousness, and sensorineural hearing loss	4-fold IgG increase in paired acute and convalescent sera, culture of saliva, CSF culture and PCR	Supportive
Murray Valley encephalitis virus	Mosquito vector; bird reservoir; Australia and New Guinea	Rapid onset in infants with case-fatality rate of 15%-30%	IgG antibody testing with 4-fold increase in paired acute and convalescent sera	Supportive
Nipah virus	Exposure to infected pigs; pteropid bat reservoir; exposure to infected bats or bat roosting sites; close contact to infected humans; South Asia	Fever, headache, altered consciousness, dizziness, vomiting, myoclonus, dystonia, areflexia, hypotonia; pneumonitis	4-fold IgG increase in paired acute and convalescent sera; CSF culture; MRI may show T2 focal hyperintensity of subcortical and deep white matter of cerebral hemispheres; contact Special Pathogens Branch at CDC	Supportive; ribavirin (C-III)

TABLE 35-2 Other Important and Emerging Causes of Viral Encephalitis—cont'd

VIRAL ETIOLOGY	EPIDEMIOLOGY	CLINICAL FEATURES	DIAGNOSIS	TREATMENT
Powassan virus	Tick vector; rodent reservoir; New England states, Canada, and Asia	Case-fatality rate of 10%-15% and focal neurologic findings in >50% of patients	Serum and CSF IgM; IgG antibody 4-fold increase in acute and convalescent paired sera	Supportive
Rift Valley fever virus	Sub-Saharan Africa, Egypt, Saudi Arabia, Yemen; mosquito vector and livestock reservoir; humans infected via exposure to infected animal secretions	1% of infected humans develop encephalitis with headache, meningismus, and altered consciousness	ELISA antigen detection or culture from serum and PCR; contact Special Pathogens Branch at CDC	Supportive
Rocio virus	Cause of epidemic encephalitis in Brazil; mosquito vector	Fever, headache, confusion, motor impairment, and cerebellar syndrome; sequelae include ataxia, dysphagia, incontinence, and memory problems	4-fold IgG increase in acute and convalescent sera	Supportive
Rubella virus	Unvaccinated adults	Rash followed by headache, dizziness, behavioral changes, and seizures	CSF IgM; 4-fold IgG increase in paired acute and convalescent sera	Supportive
Snowshoe hare virus	Mosquito-borne; North America; children predominantly affected by encephalitis	Fever, headache, confusion, and lethargy; low mortality and rare long-term neurologic sequelae	CSF and serum IgM ELISA or 4-fold increase in IgG acute and convalescent sera	Supportive
Tick-borne encephalitis virus	Tick vector; rodent reservoir; unpasteurized milk; Eastern Russia, central Europe, Far East	Acute encephalitis; acute flaccid paralysis	Serum IgM or 4-fold increase in IgG antibody in paired acute and convalescent sera	Supportive
Toscana virus	Sandfly vector; infection during summer months in Mediterranean countries	Fever, headache, meningismus, and meningoencephalitis with coma, lethargy, hydrocephalus, and hepatosplenomegaly	CSF PCR; serum and CSF IgM; 4-fold increase in IgG acute and convalescent sera	Supportive
Vaccinia	Most cases are postinfectious; rare event after vaccination	Abrupt encephalopathy with focal neurologic signs 2-30 days postvaccination	CSF PCR or IgM	Supportive; corticosteroids if postvaccination (C-III); consider cidofovir or vaccinia immune globulin

AIDS, acquired immunodeficiency syndrome; CDC, Centers for Disease Control and Prevention; CSF, cerebrospinal fluid; ELISA, enzyme-linked immunosorbent assay; FLAIR, fluid-attenuated inversion recovery; HIV, human immunodeficiency virus; ICP, intracranial pressure; LCMV, lymphocytic choriomeningitis virus; MRI, magnetic resonance imaging; PCR, polymerase chain reaction; PML, progressive multifocal leukoencephalopathy.
Modified from Tunkel AR, Glaser CA, Bloch KC, et al. The management of encephalitis: clinical practice guidelines by the Infectious Disease Society of America. *Clin Infect Dis.* 2008;47:303-327.

36 Brain Abscess

Allan R. Tunkel

DEFINITION
- Brain abscess is a focal, intracerebral infection that begins as a localized area of cerebritis and develops into a collection of pus surrounded by a well-vascularized capsule.

EPIDEMIOLOGY
- Before the advent of human immunodeficiency virus (HIV) infection, brain abscess accounted for 1500 to 2500 cases treated in the United States each year; the incidence was estimated at 0.3 to 1.3 cases per 100,000 people per year.
- In most pediatric and adult series, a male predominance exists (a ratio of 2:1 to 3:1) with a median age of 30 to 40 years, although the age distribution varies depending on the predisposing condition leading to the formation of brain abscess.
- The incidence of brain abscess is also affected by the general health of the population. In one study of 973 patients from one tertiary hospital in South Africa from 1983 to 2002, the incidence declined during the study period as a result of improvements in socioeconomic standards and availability of health care services.
- The incidence of otogenic abscesses has decreased, whereas the incidence of post-traumatic and postoperative brain abscesses has increased.

MICROBIOLOGY
- Streptococci (aerobic, anaerobic, and microaerophilic) are the bacteria most commonly (70% of cases) cultured from patients with bacterial brain abscess, and they are frequently isolated in mixed infections (30% to 60% of cases).
- *Staphylococcus aureus* accounts for 10% to 20% of isolates, usually in patients with cranial trauma or infective endocarditis, and it is often isolated in pure culture; cases caused by community-associated methicillin-resistant *S. aureus* strains have been reported.
- The attention to proper culture techniques has increased the isolation of anaerobes from brain abscesses with *Bacteroides* and *Prevotella* spp., isolated in 20% to 40% of patients, often in mixed culture.
- Enteric gram-negative bacilli (e.g., *Proteus* spp., *Escherichia coli*, *Klebsiella* spp., and *Pseudomonas* spp.) are isolated in 23% to 33% of patients, often in patients with otitic foci of infection, with septicemia, who have had neurosurgical procedures, or who are immunocompromised.
- Nocardial brain abscess may occur as an isolated central nervous system (CNS) lesion or as part of a disseminated infection in association with pulmonary or cutaneous disease.
- The incidence of fungal brain abscess has increased as a result of the prevalent administration of immunosuppressive agents, broad-spectrum antimicrobial therapy, and corticosteroids.

DIAGNOSIS
- Magnetic resonance imaging (MRI) has been extensively evaluated in the diagnosis of brain abscess and is the first imaging choice in the evaluation of a patient suspected to have this disorder.

TABLE 36-1 Empirical Antimicrobial Therapy for Bacterial Brain Abscess

PREDISPOSING CONDITION	ANTIMICROBIAL REGIMEN
Otitis media or mastoiditis	Metronidazole + third-generation cephalosporin*
Sinusitis (frontoethmoid or sphenoid)	Metronidazole + third-generation cephalosporin*†
Dental infection	Penicillin + metronidazole
Penetrating trauma or postneurosurgical	Vancomycin + third- or fourth-generation cephalosporin*‡
Lung abscess, empyema, bronchiectasis	Penicillin + metronidazole + sulfonamide§
Bacterial endocarditis	Vancomycin‖
Congenital heart disease	Third-generation cephalosporin*
Unknown	Vancomycin + metronidazole + third- or fourth-generation cephalosporin*‡

*Cefotaxime or ceftriaxone; the fourth-generation cephalosporin cefepime may also be used.
†Add vancomycin when infection caused by methicillin-resistant *Staphylococcus aureus* is suspected.
‡Use ceftazidime or cefepime as the cephalosporin if *Pseudomonas aeruginosa* is suspected.
§Trimethoprim-sulfamethoxazole; include if a *Nocardia* spp. is suspected.
‖Additional agents should be added based upon other likely microbiologic etiologies.

- The combined use of proton MR spectroscopy, diffusion-weighted imaging, and diffusion tensor imaging has been shown to improve the specificity of diagnosis of focal ring-enhancing lesions and differentiating brain abscess from other cystic lesions of the brain, including tumors.
- A major advance in the use of computed tomography (CT) in patients with suspected brain abscess is the ability to perform stereotactic CT-guided aspiration to facilitate microbiologic diagnosis and to guide antimicrobial therapy; at the time of aspiration, specimens should be sent for Gram stain, routine aerobic and anaerobic cultures, and cultures for mycobacteria and fungi.

THERAPY

- When abscess material has been obtained for microbiologic and histopathologic studies, empirical antimicrobial therapy should be initiated on the basis of the patient's predisposing conditions and the presumed pathogenesis of abscess formation (see Table 36-1).
- In HIV-infected patients with CNS mass lesions, the initial approach to management is different because of the high likelihood of the diagnosis of toxoplasmic encephalitis.
- Antimicrobial therapy with high-dose intravenous agents has traditionally been administered for 6 to 8 weeks in patients with bacterial brain abscesses.
- Most patients with bacterial brain abscess require surgical management for optimal therapy.
- The combination of surgical aspiration or removal of all abscesses larger than 2.5 cm in diameter, a 6-week or longer course of intravenous antimicrobial therapy, and response on follow-up neuroimaging should result in a cure rate of more than 90%.

37 Subdural Empyema, Epidural Abscess, and Suppurative Intracranial Thrombophlebitis

Allan R. Tunkel

DEFINITION
- Subdural empyema refers to a collection of pus between the dura and arachnoid.
- Epidural abscess is a localized collection of pus between the dura mater and overlying skull or vertebral column.
- Suppurative intracranial thrombophlebitis includes dural venous sinus thrombosis and suppuration.

EPIDEMIOLOGY
- The most common conditions predisposing to cranial subdural empyema are otorhinologic infections, especially of the paranasal sinuses, which are affected in 40% to 80% of cases. Spinal subdural empyema originates hematogenously.
- About 0.2 to 2/10,000 hospitalized patients have spinal epidural abscess, with most cases usually secondary to extension from vertebral osteomyelitis.
- Suppurative intracranial thrombophlebitis may occur after infection of the paranasal sinuses, middle ear, mastoid, face, or oropharynx.

MICROBIOLOGY
- A number of bacterial species have been isolated in patients with cranial subdural empyema, including aerobic streptococci, staphylococci, aerobic gram-negative bacilli, and anaerobic streptococci and other anaerobes.
- *Staphylococcus aureus* is the most common etiologic agent in patients with spinal epidural abscess.
- The likely infecting pathogens in patients with suppurative intracranial thrombophlebitis depend on the pathogenesis of infection.

DIAGNOSIS
- Magnetic resonance imaging (MRI), with gadolinium enhancement, is the diagnostic procedure of choice in patients with subdural empyema and epidural abscess.
- The noninvasive diagnostic procedure of choice in patients with suppurative intracranial thrombophlebitis is MRI and magnetic resonance venography; computed tomography venography is done in patients unable to undergo MRI.

THERAPY
- Subdural empyema is a medical and surgical emergency. The goals of surgery are to achieve adequate decompression of the brain and completely evacuate the empyema; based on retrospective outcome data, craniotomy is the surgical procedure of choice.
- The principles of therapy for spinal epidural abscess are prompt laminectomy and surgical decompression in patients with neurologic dysfunction, drainage of the abscess, and long-term antimicrobial therapy. Antimicrobial therapy alone can be considered in patients with localized pain and radicular symptoms without long-tract findings, but frequent neurologic

examinations and serial MRI studies should be performed to demonstrate resolution of the abscess.

- Empirical antimicrobial therapy for suppurative intracranial thrombophlebitis is usually vancomycin, metronidazole, and a third- or fourth-generation cephalosporin; anticoagulation should also be used in patients with septic cavernous sinus thrombosis unless there are contraindications.

38 Cerebrospinal Fluid Shunt and Drain Infections

Adarsh Bhimraj, James M. Drake, and Allan R. Tunkel

DEFINITION

- Ventriculoperitoneal (VP) shunt infections can be either superficial, involving the skin and soft tissue adjacent to the shunt valve or reservoir, or it can be a deeper infection, involving the cerebral ventricles, proximally or the peritoneum distally.
- Cerebrospinal fluid (CSF) drain infections can be tunnel infections, catheter exit site infections, or ventriculitis.

EPIDEMIOLOGY

- The case incidence of CSF shunt infection (i.e., the occurrence of infection in any given patient) has ranged from 5% to 41%, although usually it is 4% to 17%.
- The operative incidence (i.e., the occurrence of infection per procedure) has ranged from 2.8% to 14%, although usually it is less than 4%.
- In patients with CSF drains, the incidence of ventriculitis has ranged from zero to 22%.

MICROBIOLOGY

- Staphylococcal species account for the majority of isolates in patients with CSF shunt infections, with *Staphylococcus epidermidis* most frequently isolated (47% to 64% of infections), followed by *Staphylococcus aureus* (12% to 29% of infections).
- The most common isolated gram-negative species are *Escherichia coli, Klebsiella, Proteus,* and *Pseudomonas;* cases of *Acinetobacter* meningitis have also been reported in patients with VP shunts.
- In recent years, an increasing prevalence of diphtheroids (including *Propionibacterium acnes*) has been found in CSF shunt infections.

DIAGNOSIS

- The diagnosis is established by either direct culture of the CSF obtained by shunt aspiration or by culture of the proximal shunt components if the shunt is explanted.
- CSF culture from the shunt, reservoir, or drain is the most important test to establish the diagnosis of infection.
- In patients with lumbar drains or externalized ventricular drains, definite infection is defined as a positive CSF culture (obtained from the ventricular or lumbar catheter) associated with CSF pleocytosis.

THERAPY

- The principles of antimicrobial therapy for CSF shunt infections are generally the same as those for acute bacterial meningitis; the agent selected must penetrate the central nervous system, attain adequate CSF concentrations, and have bactericidal activity against the infecting pathogen.
- Empirical therapy with intravenous vancomycin plus either cefepime, ceftazidime, or meropenem is appropriate.

- Optimal therapy of an infected CSF shunt is an initial intravenous antimicrobial, followed by removal of all components of the infected shunt, insertion of a fresh ventricular catheter, and a period of external drainage. Later, the drain is removed and a new shunt is placed.
- Direct instillation of antimicrobial agents into the lateral ventricle or, in the case of lumbar shunts, into the lumbar thecal sac may be necessary in patients with shunt infections that are difficult to eradicate with intravenous antimicrobial therapy and shunt removal or when the patient is unable to undergo shunt replacement.

PREVENTION

- There is evidence to support the use of periprocedural prophylactic antimicrobial administration for patients undergoing CSF shunt insertion and placement of external ventricular drains.
- Use of antimicrobial-impregnated CSF shunts and CSF drains appears to be safe and effective in prevention of ventriculitis, although prospective, randomized controlled trials are needed to firmly confirm their benefits.
- Use of a standardized protocol and reducing variation by adherence to a common protocol are effective at reducing CSF shunt infection rates.

39 Cellulitis, Necrotizing Fasciitis, and Subcutaneous Tissue Infections

Mark S. Pasternack and Morton N. Swartz*

DEFINITION

- Skin and soft tissue infections are characterized by location, depth of infection, etiologic agent, and clinical setting and may result from either primary cutaneous inoculation or, less commonly, hematogenous seeding.
- *Impetigo* is a superficial crusting and at times bullous infection of the skin; localized progression into the dermis leads to ecthyma.
- *Folliculitis* is a localized infection of hair follicles, which can extend into subcutaneous tissue, resulting in furuncles. These, in turn, may coalesce, leading to carbuncle formation.
- *Erysipelas* is a rapidly progressive infection of the superficial dermis, with sharp erythematous borders; *cellulitis* reflects deeper dermal involvement.
- Necrotizing skin and soft tissue infections, including *necrotizing fasciitis,* are rare life-threatening infections, occur in a variety of clinical settings, and require prompt diagnosis and surgical intervention.

EPIDEMIOLOGY

- Significant skin and soft tissue infection may occur throughout the age spectrum. Minor local trauma as the initial pathogenic event is a common feature of these processes. Although invasive infections may occur in previously healthy individuals, a variety of systemic risk factors predisposes individuals to these infections.

MICROBIOLOGY

- Hemolytic streptococci and *Staphylococcus aureus,* including methicillin-resistant *S. aureus* (MRSA), are the most common causes of superficial cutaneous infection.
- Mixed infection of facultative gram-negative bacilli, anaerobes, and gram-positive organisms most frequently cause necrotizing infection, but group A streptococci, clostridia, and *Vibrio* species can also cause necrotizing fasciitis.
- A broad differential diagnosis most be considered in confronting infections in immunocompromised patients.

DIAGNOSIS

- Most cutaneous infections are not associated with bacteremia, and diagnosis and empirical therapy are based on physical findings and clinical setting.
- In compromised hosts, tissue biopsy for microbiologic and histologic study is critical to plan definitive therapy.

---

*Morton N. Swartz, a long-time contributor to chapters in previous editions of *Principles and Practice of Infectious Diseases,* died on September 9, 2013.

THERAPY

- Oral therapy targeted against gram-positive pathogens is appropriate for mild disease, with close follow-up and revision of therapy for inadequate response. Parenteral therapy targeted more broadly against gram-positive organisms, including *S. aureus* and MRSA, gram-negative pathogens, and anaerobes is required in many settings of severe infection, particularly in compromised hosts.
- Necrotizing infections require urgent surgical débridement.
- Infections associated with toxic shock syndrome are treated with protein-synthesis inhibitors such as clindamycin and with intravenous immune globulin to neutralize streptococcal toxins.

PREVENTION

- Good hygienic practices and attention to early therapy for superficial processes such as dermatophyte infection reduce the risk for cutaneous and soft tissue infection.
- Individuals with recurrent cellulitis may benefit from chronic antibiotic suppression.

40 Myositis and Myonecrosis

*Mark S. Pasternack and Morton N. Swartz**

DEFINITION

- Myositis is an inflammatory and generally necrotizing process primarily due to hematogenous seeding of muscle with subsequent bacterial invasion. Direct inoculation of muscle as the result of penetrating trauma is also an important mechanism of infection (associated with clostridial myonecrosis). More generalized muscle inflammation may also accompany a variety of acute and chronic viral and parasitic disorders.

EPIDEMIOLOGY

- Pyomyositis occurs across the age spectrum in temperate regions and may occur in previously healthy as well as immunocompromised individuals; in warm climates, infections in children predominate (i.e., tropical pyomyositis). Clostridial myonecrosis most commonly complicates penetrating trauma (e.g., vehicular accidents, war, natural disasters), especially in resource-limited settings.

MICROBIOLOGY

- *Staphylococcus aureus* is the classic cause of pyomyositis, but similar illnesses have been associated with a wide variety of bacterial pathogens, particularly in compromised hosts. *Clostridium perfringens* myonecrosis complicates penetrating trauma, but nontraumatic clostridial myonecrosis may develop after hematogenous dissemination of more aerotolerant species (e.g., *C. septicum, C. sordellii*). Group A streptococci can also cause severe myonecrotic infection, which is a true medical emergency. Acute generalized muscle inflammation occurs after influenza and dengue virus infections, but a wide variety of viral pathogens have sporadically led to significant muscle injury and even severe rhabdomyolysis.

DIAGNOSIS

- Consideration of these uncommon processes is the first step toward the proper diagnosis, because the focal progressive pain of pyomyositis mimics a variety of disorders. Blood cultures and (percutaneous) drainage based on the findings of cross-sectional imaging confirm the diagnosis and guide therapy. Pyomyositis may accompany toxic shock, and investigation of a focal process responsible for fulminant systemic illness is essential. Gas production in muscle and soft tissue in the setting of a rapidly progressive illness occurs in clostridial myonecrosis and related infections; this is a surgical emergency and exploration for débridement of nonviable tissue and appropriate cultures is critical.

THERAPY

- Ideally, after expedited imaging and drainage, empirical broad-spectrum antibacterial therapy effective against *S. aureus* (including methicillin-resistant *S. aureus*) and

---

*Morton N. Swartz, a long-time contributor to chapters in previous editions of *Principles and Practice of Infectious Diseases,* died on September 9, 2013.

gram-negative bacilli as well as anaerobes should be administered. The findings of associated toxic shock mandate the addition of a protein synthesis inhibitor (e.g., clindamycin) and possibly intravenous immunoglobulin therapy. Narrow-spectrum therapy is appropriate after identification and sensitivity testing of the isolated pathogen. Patients presenting with the clinical findings of gas gangrene (clostridial myonecrosis) require immediate high-dose penicillin and clindamycin and urgent surgical exploration.

PREVENTION

- Because most episodes of pyomyositis develop after transient bacteremia, prevention is not practical. Prompt débridement of devitalized tissue after penetrating injury is highly effective at preventing clostridial myonecrosis.

41 Lymphadenitis and Lymphangitis

Mark S. Pasternack and Morton N. Swartz*

DEFINITION: LYMPHADENITIS

- Acute (suppurative) or chronic (often granulomatous) inflammation of the lymph nodes

EPIDEMIOLOGY

- Suppurative lymphadenitis most common among young children; granulomatous lymphadenitis may occur in individuals of all ages.

MICROBIOLOGY (SEE TABLE 41-1)

- Suppurative lymphadenitis primarily due to *Staphylococcus aureus* (methicillin sensitive and methicillin resistant) and group A streptococci in normal hosts; a variety of pathogens may cause suppurative lymphadenitis in immunocompromised individuals.
- Granulomatous lymphadenitis is due primarily to nontuberculous mycobacteria in healthy children. *Mycobacterium tuberculosis* is the most important etiology in older patients but may be due to a variety of pathogens in compromised hosts.

DIAGNOSIS

- Needle aspiration, incisional biopsy, or excisional biopsy, depending on the tempo and severity of the illness and possible immunodeficiency

THERAPY

- Drainage of established abscesses and conventional antimicrobial therapy against gram-positive pathogens for acute suppurative lymphadenitis
- Targeted therapy based on microbiologic/histopathologic investigation for chronic granulomatous lymphadenitis

PREVENTION

- Early therapy of primary superficial infections and early therapy of acute adenitis episodes may reduce the risk of suppuration and need for surgical drainage.

DEFINITION: LYMPHANGITIS

- Lymphangitis is an inflammation of lymphatic channels, usually in subcutaneous tissues. It is caused by an acute process of bacterial origin or as a chronic process of mycotic, mycobacterial, or filarial etiology (see Table 41-2).

---

*Morton Swartz, a long-term contributor to previous editions of *Principles and Practice of Infectious Diseases,* died on September 9, 2013.

TABLE 41-1 Forms of Lymphadenitis

DISEASE	INFECTING ORGANISM	REGIONAL	REGIONAL WITH SUPPURATION (OR CASEATION)	INGUINAL BUBO FORMATION	ULCEROGLANDULAR	OCULOGLANDULAR	GENERAL
Bacterial							
Pyogenic	Group A or B streptococci, Staphylococcus aureus	+	+				
Scarlet fever	Group A streptococci	+	+				+
Diphtheria	Corynebacterium diphtheriae	+					
Fusospirochetal angina	Prevotella melaninogenica, peptostreptococci, etc.	+					
Scrofula	Mycobacterium tuberculosis	+	+				
	Mycobacterium scrofulaceum	+	+				
	Mycobacterium avium-intracellulare	+	+				
Miliary tuberculosis	M. tuberculosis	+					+
Brucellosis	Brucella	+					+
Leptospirosis	Leptospira	+					+
Syphilis	Treponema pallidum	+					+
Chancroid	Haemophilus ducreyi	+					
Plague	Yersinia pestis	+	+	+			
Tularemia	Francisella tularensis	+	+	+	+	+	
Rat-bite fever	Streptobacillus moniliformis	+					
	Spirillum minus	+			+		
Anthrax	Bacillus anthracis	+	+		+		
Listeriosis	Listeria monocytogenes	+					
Melioidosis	Burkholderia pseudomallei	+	+	+			
Glanders	Burkholderia mallei	+	+	+			
Cat-scratch disease	Bartonella henselae	+	+	±	±	+	
Typhoid fever	Salmonella typhi	+					
Mycotic							
Histoplasmosis	Histoplasma capsulatum	+					
	H. capsulatum var. duboisii	+					
Coccidioidomycosis	Coccidioides immitis	+					
Paracoccidioidomycosis	Paracoccidioides brasiliensis	+					
Cryptococcosis	Cryptococcus neoformans	+	+				
Rickettsiae							
Boutonneuse fever, etc.	Rickettsia conorii	+					
Scrub typhus	Rickettsia tsutsugamushi	+					
Rickettsialpox	Rickettsia akari	+					
Chlamydial							
Lymphogranuloma venereum	Chlamydia trachomatis	+	+	+			

Continued

TABLE 41-1 Forms of Lymphadenitis—cont'd

DISEASE	INFECTING ORGANISM	REGIONAL	REGIONAL WITH SUPPURATION (OR CASEATION)	INGUINAL BUBO FORMATION	ULCEROGLANDULAR	OCULOGLANDULAR	GENERAL
Viral							
Measles	Measles virus						+
Rubella	Rubella virus						+
Infectious mononucleosis	Epstein-Barr virus						+
Cytomegalovirus mononucleosis	Cytomegalovirus						+
Dengue fever	Dengue virus						+
West Nile fever	West Nile virus						+
Lassa fever	Lassa fever virus						+
Oropharyngeal herpes infection	Herpes simplex virus type 1	+	±				+
Genital herpes infection	Herpes simplex virus type 2	+					
Primary HHV-6 infection	Human herpesvirus 6	+					
Primary HHV-7 infection	Human herpesvirus 7	+					
Cowpox	Cowpox virus	+	±				
Pharyngoconjunctival fever	Adenovirus (types 3 and 7)	+	+				
Epidemic keratoconjunctivitis	Adenovirus (types 8 and 19)	+					
AIDS, AIDS-related complex	Human immunodeficiency virus						+
Protozoan							
Kala azar	Leishmania donovani						+
African trypanosomiasis	Trypanosoma brucei				+		+
Chagas' disease	Trypanosoma cruzi					+	+
Toxoplasmosis	Toxoplasma gondii	+				+	+
Helminthic							
Filariasis	Wuchereria bancrofti	+					+
	Brugia malayi	+					+
Loiasis	Loa loa			+			
Onchocerciasis	Onchocerca volvulus			+			

AIDS, acquired immunodeficiency syndrome; HHV, human herpesvirus; +, present; ±, rare.

TABLE 41-2 Causes of Lymphangitis

CLINICAL FORM	ETIOLOGIC AGENT	RELATIVE FREQUENCY AS CAUSE OF LYMPHANGITIS
Acute	Group A streptococci	Common
	Staphylococcus aureus	Occasional
	Pasteurella multocida	Occasional
	Streptobacillus moniliformis (rat-bite fever)	Rare
	Wuchereria bancrofti; Brugia malayi (filariasis)	Rare (only in immigrants from endemic areas)
Chronic	Sporothrix schenckii (sporotrichosis)	Occasional
	Mycobacterium marinum (swimming pool granuloma)	Occasional
	Mycobacterium kansasii	Rare
	Nocardia brasiliensis	Rare
	W. bancrofti; B. malayi	Rare (only in immigrants from endemic areas)
	Nocardia asteroides	Very rare
	Mycobacterium chelonae	Very rare
	S. aureus (botryomycosis)	Very rare
	Leishmania brasiliensis or Leishmania mexicana	Very rare
	Francisella tularensis	Very rare

42 Esophagitis

Paul S. Graman

DEFINITION
- Inflammation of the esophagus, of noninfectious or infectious etiology

EPIDEMIOLOGY
- Gastroesophageal reflux disease is the most common cause. Esophageal infections occur predominantly in patients with impaired immunity, particularly those with acquired immunodeficiency syndrome or receiving cancer chemotherapy. Immunocompetent persons are occasionally affected.

MICROBIOLOGY
- *Candida* species, herpes simplex virus (HSV), and cytomegalovirus are most common.

DIAGNOSIS
- Endoscopy and biopsy for immunohistopathology and culture, polymerase chain reaction

THERAPY (SEE TABLE 42-1)
- *Candida:* fluconazole, itraconazole, amphotericin lipid formulations, voriconazole, echinocandins
- Herpes simplex virus: acyclovir or valacyclovir, famciclovir; foscarnet for acyclovir-resistant HSV
- Cytomegalovirus: ganciclovir, valganciclovir, or foscarnet
- Aphthous ulceration (in acquired immunodeficiency syndrome): prednisone, thalidomide

PREVENTION
- Recipients of allogeneic hematologic stem cell transplants who are neutropenic commonly receive antiviral and antifungal prophylaxis.

TABLE 42-1 Treatment of Esophagitis

CAUSE	USUAL TREATMENT (ADULT DOSE)	ALTERNATIVE DRUGS
Candida	Fluconazole, 100-200 mg/day PO or IV for 14-21 days; maintenance suppressive therapy may be necessary in AIDS (fluconazole, 100-200 mg/day PO)	Itraconazole oral suspension, 100-200 mg bid PO Voriconazole, 200 mg bid PO* Amphotericin B, 0.3-0.7 mg/kg/day IV for 7 days Caspofungin, 50 mg/day IV after 70-mg loading dose* Micafungin, 150 mg/day IV Anidulafungin, 100 mg on day 1, then 50 mg/day IV
Herpes simplex virus	Acyclovir, 5 mg/kg IV q8h for 7-14 days or 400 mg 5 times daily PO for 14-21 days Or valacyclovir, 1 g PO tid for 14-21 days†; maintenance suppressive therapy may be necessary in AIDS	Famciclovir, 500 mg bid PO for 14-21 days (not for acyclovir-resistant infection) Foscarnet, 90 mg/kg q12h IV for 7-14 days (used for acyclovir-resistant infection)
Cytomegalovirus	Ganciclovir, 5 mg/kg IV q12h for 14-21 days; maintenance suppressive therapy usually is necessary in AIDS (ganciclovir, 5 mg/kg/day IV 7 days/wk or 6 mg/kg/day IV 5 days/wk)	Foscarnet, 90 mg/kg q12h IV for 14-21 days; suppression with foscarnet, 90-120 mg/kg/day IV Valganciclovir, 900 mg bid PO for treatment, and 900 mg qd for maintenance/suppression†
Aphthous ulceration (in AIDS)	Prednisone, 40 mg/day PO for 14 days, then taper	Thalidomide, 200 mg/day PO†

AIDS, acquired immunodeficiency syndrome.
*Amphotericin, echinocandins, and voriconazole are indicated for severe or refractory esophageal candidiasis.
†Not approved by the U.S. Food and Drug Administration for this indication.

43 Nausea, Vomiting, and Noninflammatory Diarrhea

David A. Bobak and Richard L. Guerrant

DEFINITION

- A disease group consisting of acute and chronic forms of gastroenteritis occurs in both pediatric and adult patients, and these diseases have the unifying characteristic of being predominantly noninflammatory in nature.

EPIDEMIOLOGY

- Noninflammatory gastroenteritides are among the most common infections of humans. As a group, they are second in incidence only to viral upper respiratory infections.
- Most cases of these diseases are not tracked or reported but are estimated to affect tens of millions of people worldwide each year.
- There are baseline endemic and seasonal rates as well as epidemic outbreaks of most forms of these infections.
- The rates of infection as well as etiologic agents vary according to age, climate, and geography. In addition, there are differences in these parameters observed for place of acquisition (e.g., community- vs. health care facility–acquired infections).

MICROBIOLOGY

- Viruses, including members of the rotavirus, norovirus, adenovirus, and astrovirus genera, are the cause of most cases of noninflammatory gastroenteritis.
- Among the bacterial causes of this syndrome, certain pathogenic strains of *Escherichia coli* and some serotypes of cholera and noncholera *Vibrio* are particularly noteworthy.
- Certain protozoan types of parasites can cause a predominantly noninflammatory type of gastroenteritis and include members of the *Giardia*, *Cryptosporidium*, *Cystoisospora*, and *Cyclospora* genera.
- Although many of the etiologic agents are similar, there are also some important differences between the endemic and epidemic causes of noninflammatory gastroenteritis in developing, newly industrialized, and developed countries. Newborn nursery–associated and nosocomial outbreaks of this syndrome have differences from those cases acquired in the community.
- The number of potential infectious agents is much greater in immunocompromised compared with immunocompetent hosts.

DIAGNOSIS

- The typical clinical syndrome consists of varying degrees of nausea, vomiting, and watery diarrhea, often in combination with fever, myalgias, and arthralgias.
- Most cases of this syndrome are self-limited, and no specific etiology is identified.
- In certain instances, such as epidemic, nosocomial, and foodborne cases, an etiologic agent can be identified by either culture or molecular diagnostic assay.

THERAPY

- Adequate replacement of fluids and electrolytes remains the mainstay of all forms of gastro-enteritis, including the noninflammatory gastroenteritides discussed in this chapter.
- In most cases of noninflammatory gastroenteritis, specific antimicrobial therapy is not used. However, in more severe or specific forms of this infection, specific antiviral, antibacterial, or antiparasitic treatment may be beneficial.

PREVENTION

- Adequate sanitation for the local water supply and food processing and distribution systems helps to prevent many forms of endemic, community-acquired noninflammatory gastroenteritis.
- Although there has been tremendous interest in developing effective vaccination or immu-nization schemes for many of these infectious agents, only vaccines for rotavirus are currently available for general use.

44 Bacterial Inflammatory Enteritides

Aldo A. M. Lima, Cirle A. Warren, and Richard L. Guerrant

DEFINITION

- Acute and chronic inflammatory enteritides are caused by several specific infectious agents.

EPIDEMIOLOGY

- Acute dysenteric syndromes are influenced by the unusually low inoculum required for infection by organisms such as shigellae.
- The bacterial enteric pathogens most associated with illnesses in children younger than 5 years in the United States are nontyphoid *Salmonella*, followed by *Campylobacter*, *Yersinia enterocolitica*, and *Escherichia coli* O157.
- Venereal exposure, particularly among men who have sex with men, may implicate gonococci, herpes simplex virus, *Chlamydia trachomatis*, or *Treponema pallidum* as a cause of proctitis, or *Campylobacter*, *Shigella*, *C. trachomatis* (lymphogranuloma venereum serotypes), or *Clostridium difficile* as a cause of colitis.
- A history of antibiotic intake and/or recent admission to a health care facility would strongly suggest *C. difficile* infection.

MICROBIOLOGY

- Genomic studies of *Shigella* species have indicated that *Shigella* and enteroinvasive *E. coli* are derived from multiple origins of *E. coli* and form a single pathovar.
- The cause of a recent outbreak of bloody diarrhea and severe hemolytic-uremic syndrome, unlike prior enterohemorrhagic *E. coli* strains that had exhibited enteropathogenic *E. coli* traits of attachment and effacement, was a Shiga toxin–producing enteroaggregative *E. coli* strain.
- *Campylobacter* spp. have a small genome (1.6 to 2.0 Mb) and can cause intestinal and systemic infections.
- The primary virulence factors that are known to cause clinical disease in *C. difficile* infection are the two large toxins: *C. difficile* toxin (Tcd)A, or toxin A (308 kDa), and TcdB, or toxin B (270 kDa).
- *Vibrio parahaemolyticus* has been recognized since 1950 in Japan and is a cause of seafood poisoning.
- *Salmonella* flagellin is regulated by the *fliC* gene, which is the major ligand for the Toll-like receptor 5, nucleotide oligomerization domain–like receptors, and ICE protease-activating factor (Ipaf) protein.

DIAGNOSIS

- Any of the above microorganisms may cause an acute dysentery syndrome with blood and pus in the stool.
- Examination for leukocytes or for fecal lactoferrin may suggest intestinal inflammation, even if blood is not present in the stool on gross examination.

- Recent approaches using a laboratory-developed TaqMan Array Card for simultaneous detection of several enteropathogens hold promise, with high accuracy, sensitivity, and specificity as well as being potentially suited for surveillance or clinical purposes.

THERAPY AND PREVENTION

- Because there are many etiologic agents, the treatment and prevention rely on each specific cause of acute and chronic inflammatory enteritides

45 Enteric Fever and Other Causes of Fever and Abdominal Symptoms

Jason B. Harris and Edward T. Ryan

DEFINITION
- Enteric fever is a nonspecific febrile illness caused by typhoidal *Salmonella;* the diagnosis should be considered in any patient with otherwise unexplained prolonged fever.
- The term *typhoidal fever* is sometimes used more broadly to refer to a syndrome of persistent high-grade fevers, often with no localizing features.

EPIDEMIOLOGY
- Tens of millions of cases of enteric fever occur each year, largely in impoverished areas of Asia and Africa.
- Enteric fever is fecally/orally transmitted, with contaminated municipal water supplies being commonly involved in transmission.
- Multidrug-resistant strains of the major causative agents of enteric fever (*Salmonella enterica* serotype Typhi and Paratyphi A) are now common worldwide.

CLINICAL MANIFESTATIONS
- Common life-threatening complications of enteric fever include intestinal hemorrhage, perforation, encephalopathy, and shock.
- Untreated, patients with enteric fever may be febrile for 3 to 4 weeks or longer, with mortality rates exceeding 10%, and prolonged asthenia and fatigue are common among survivors.
- Chronic biliary carriage of typhoidal *Salmonella* may occur after resolution of the acute illness.

DIAGNOSIS
- Current diagnostic tests for enteric fever are imperfect: blood cultures are 30% to 70% sensitive, bone marrow cultures are more sensitive but are impractical, serologic assays lack both sensitivity and specificity, especially in enteric fever endemic areas, and nucleic acid amplification assays with sensitivity are not available.

THERAPY
- Given the morbidity of typhoid fever, the risk of complications, and the lack of optimal diagnostic tests, the initiation of antibiotics for treating individuals with suspected enteric fever may be based on a presumptive diagnosis, particularly in resource-limited settings.
- The most commonly used agents for treating individuals with enteric fever are fluoroquinolones, azithromycin, and cefixime or ceftriaxone. Chloramphenicol, trimethoprim-sulfamethoxazole, and amoxicillin may be used to treat patients with susceptible strains.
- An oral-attenuated typhoid vaccine and injectable polysaccharide vaccine are internationally commercially available and provide 50% to 75% protection for 5 and 2 years, respectively. Injectable typhoid conjugate vaccines are in late-stage development. No vaccine effective against paratyphoid A is currently commercially available.

46 Foodborne Disease

Rajal K. Mody and Patricia M. Griffin

DEFINITION

- Foodborne diseases are illnesses that are acquired through ingestion of food contaminated with pathogenic microorganisms, bacterial and nonbacterial toxins, or other substances.

EPIDEMIOLOGY

- An estimated 48 million foodborne illnesses caused by pathogens or their toxins are acquired annually in the United States.
- Many agents that cause foodborne infection can also be acquired in other ways, including ingestion of contaminated drinking or recreational water, through contact with animals or their environment, and from one person to another directly or through fomites.
- Some foodborne diseases can lead to long-term sequelae, such as impaired kidney function after Shiga toxin–producing *Escherichia coli* infection, Guillain-Barré syndrome after *Campylobacter* infection, and reactive arthritis and irritable bowel syndrome after a variety of infections.
- Groups at higher risk of acquiring or experiencing more severe foodborne disease include infants, young children, pregnant women, older adults, and immunocompromised persons.
- A foodborne disease outbreak should be considered when an acute illness, especially with gastrointestinal or neurologic manifestations, affects two or more people who shared a meal. However, most foodborne diseases do not occur in the context of an outbreak.

MICROBIOLOGY

- Many pathogens, including bacteria, viruses, and parasites, can cause foodborne disease.
- Some illnesses are caused by ingestion of chemicals (e.g., heavy metals, mushroom toxins) or preformed microbial toxins (e.g., staphylococcal toxin, botulinum toxin).

DIAGNOSIS

- Detection of pathogens has mostly relied on isolating bacterial pathogens in culture, by visualizing parasites by microscopy, and by enzyme-linked immunosorbent assays.
- Newer molecular tests pose opportunities and challenges to both clinical practice and public health surveillance.
- Many intoxications must be diagnosed based on clinical suspicion alone.

THERAPY

- Therapy for most foodborne diseases is supportive; replacing fluid and electrolyte losses is important in diarrheal illnesses.
- Antimicrobial agents are used to treat parasitic infections and selected bacterial infections.
- Resistance to antimicrobial agents complicates treatment and can increase the likelihood of clinically apparent infection.

PREVENTION

- To reduce contamination, food producers identify points where the risk of contamination can be controlled and use production systems that decrease the hazards.
- Outbreak investigation is important to identify food safety gaps that may be present anywhere in the food production chain, from the farm to the table.
- Individuals can reduce their risk of illness by adhering to safe food handling practices.

47 Tropical Sprue: Enteropathy

Christine A. Wanke

DEFINITION
- Syndrome of diarrhea, malabsorption of at least two distinct nutrients, abnormal duodenal histopathology, and weight loss.

EPIDEMIOLOGY
- Most frequent in Asia and the Caribbean islands, more frequent in adults than children; occurs in long-term travelers to endemic regions.

MICROBIOLOGY
- No single agent associated with causality, small bowel overgrowth common.

DIAGNOSIS
- Appropriate clinical syndrome (persistent diarrhea, malabsorption of at least two distinct nutrients, weight loss) with consistent small bowel series or upper endoscopy. Response to folate and tetracycline ultimately confirms diagnosis.

THERAPY
- Removal from area of risk, treatment with folate and tetracycline.

PREVENTION
- Good hygiene practices.

48 Infectious Arthritis of Native Joints

Christopher A. Ohl and Derek Forster

DEFINITION

- Infectious arthritis is an infection of one or more joints that can be caused by bacteria, viruses, fungi, and parasites.

CLINICAL CATEGORIES

Acute Bacterial Arthritis

- Overall incidence in native joints is 2 to 10/100,000 per year, increased in rheumatoid arthritis.
- Infection can be acquired from hematogenous dissemination, direct joint inoculation, or a contiguous focus. Most infections are monarticular; 10% to 20% are polyarticular. The knee is most often involved.
- Microbiology
  - Gram-positive organisms, including *Staphylococcus aureus* and *Streptococcus* spp. predominate.
  - Gram-negative bacilli in 5% to 20% are mainly in neonates, the elderly, intravenous drug users, and immunocompromised.
  - Prevalence rates of gonococcal arthritis have markedly decreased. There are two syndromes of joint involvement: monarticular arthritis and disseminated gonorrhea with febrile tenosynovitis and skin lesions.

Viral Arthritis

- It may occur sporadically or in community outbreaks that may be small (e.g., parvovirus B19) or explosive (e.g., chikungunya virus).
- It is caused by infection of the joint space or by immune-mediated inflammation.
- It is usually an acute polyarticular arthritis that occurs simultaneously with other systemic symptoms of viral infection.
- Causes include parvovirus B19, rubella (which may follow immunization), hepatitis B, hepatitis C, and alphaviruses, including chikungunya virus, Ross River virus, and o'nyong-nyong virus.
- It may occasionally cause prolonged or chronic arthritis after acute infection.

CLINICAL EVALUATION

- Bacterial arthritis is an emergency and should be considered in any patient with acute monoarticular or polyarticular arthritis.
- The most useful demographic risk factors are presence or absence of recent joint surgery, rheumatoid arthritis, advanced age, concomitant skin infection, or diabetes mellitus.
- The most helpful laboratory parameters are the synovial fluid leukocyte count and differential, and examination for crystals to rule out gout or pseudogout.
- Diagnostic imaging should include plain film radiography. For prolonged or atypical symptoms, or for deep joints, computed tomography or magnetic resonance imaging is recommended.

TABLE 48-1 Recommended Empirical Therapy for Adult Native Joint Bacterial Arthritis

GRAM STAIN	PREFERRED ANTIBIOTIC[a]	ALTERNATIVE ANTIBIOTIC
Gram-positive cocci	Vancomycin, 15-20 mg/kg (ABW) daily every 8-12 hr[b]	Daptomycin, 6-8 mg/kg daily[c] or linezolid, 600 mg IV or PO every 12 hr[c]
Gram-negative cocci[d]	Ceftriaxone, 1 g every 24 hr	Cefotaxime, 1 g every 8 hr[e]
Gram-negative rods[f]	Ceftazidime, 2 g every 8 hr or Cefepime, 2 g every 8 hr or Piperacillin-tazobactam, 4.5 g every 6 hr	Aztreonam, 2 g every 8 hr or Fluoroquinolone[g] or Carbapenem[h,i]
Gram-stain negative[f]	Vancomycin plus Ceftazidime or Cefepime	Daptomycin[c] or linezolid[c] plus Piperacillin-tazobactam or Aztreonam or Fluoroquinolone[g] or Carbapenem[h,i]

ABW, actual body weight; IgE, immunoglobulin E; IV, intravenous; PO, by mouth.
[a]Unless noted otherwise, dosages are IV for persons with normal renal function.
[b]Therapeutic monitoring should target a serum trough of 15-20 mg/L.
[c]For patients allergic to, or intolerant of, vancomycin.
[d]Equivocal gram-negative morphology should be considered as gram-negative rods.
[e]Gram-negative cocci with epidemiology or history suggestive of gonococcal infection should be initially treated per Centers for Disease Control and Prevention Sexually Transmitted Disease Guidelines. Alternative therapies have not been suggested for patients with a history of a Stevens-Johnson syndrome or severe IgE-mediated allergy to β-lactam antibiotics. Possible empirical options for penicillin-allergic patients, pending culture sensitivities, include azithromycin, ciprofloxacin, tobramycin, gentamicin, and spectinomycin (not available in United States).
[f]For patients with risk factors for resistant gram-negative pathogens (significant health care exposure, immunosuppression, or history of extended-spectrum β-lactamase gram-negative infection or colonization), drug selection should consider regional or local antibiograms.
[g]Ciprofloxacin, 400 mg IV every 8 hr or 750 mg PO every 12 hr or levofloxacin, 750 mg IV or PO every 24 hr.
[h]Doripenem, 500 mg every 8 hr; imipenem, 500 mg every 6 hr; or meropenem, 1 g every 8 hr.
[i]Usually reserved for patients with risk factors for resistant gram-negative pathogens (significant health care exposure, immunosuppression, or history of extended-spectrum β-lactamase gram-negative infection or colonization).

- Identification of the infecting organism on synovial fluid Gram stain and culture remains the definitive diagnostic test. The polymerase chain reaction (PCR) assay continues to show promise.

THERAPY
Acute Bacterial Arthritis
- Joint drainage by repeat aspiration, arthroscopy, or arthrotomy is required.
- Empirical selection should be based on synovial fluid Gram stain (see Table 48-1).
- Intravenous therapy, in some instances with an oral transition, is usually prescribed for a total of 2 to 4 weeks.

Chronic Infectious Arthritis
- It is usually monarticular, involving the large peripheral joints.
- It is relatively uncommon compared with acute bacterial arthritis but is increasingly seen in immunocompromised or chronically ill hosts. Etiology includes *Mycobacterium tuberculosis* and nontuberculosis mycobacteria. Fungal causes include *Candida*, dimorphic fungi (e.g., *Blastomyces, Coccidioides, Histoplasma,* and *Sporothrix*), *Cryptococcus,* and *Aspergillus,* among others.
- Therapy of *M. tuberculosis* arthritis is similar to pulmonary tuberculosis.
- Many fungal arthritides are difficult to treat and result in chronic joint disability. Treatment varies by infecting organism. Experience using the azoles (including new triazoles) and the echinocandins is growing, and in many cases, these drugs are replacing amphotericin.
- Except for *Cryptococcus* and perhaps *Sporothrix,* fungal arthritis requires surgical drainage and débridement.

SEPTIC BURSITIS

- It predominantly involves the prepatellar, olecranon, and trochanteric bursa.
- It can be caused by direct inoculation, contiguous infection, or less commonly, from a hematogenous source.
- More than 80% of cases are due to *Staphylococcus aureus*.
- Diagnosis is made from the clinical presentation and by aspirating the bursa for fluid analysis, Gram stain, and culture.
- Treatment includes antibiotics (usually 14 to 21 days) and daily aspiration of the bursa until sterile fluid is obtained. Except for severe cases, oral antistaphylococcal agents that have activity against community-acquired methicillin-resistant *S. aureus* (CA-MRSA) are recommended pending culture and sensitivity. For moderate-to-severe cases or patients with immunosuppression, intravenous antibiotics should be selected.

49 Osteomyelitis

Elie F. Berbari, James M. Steckelberg, and Douglas R. Osmon

CLASSIFICATION

- Osteomyelitis can develop as the result of contiguous spread from adjacent soft tissues and joints, hematogenous seeding, or direct inoculation of microorganisms into the bone as a result of trauma or surgery.
- The Cierny and Mader classification is based on the affected portion of the bone, the physiologic status of the host, and the local environment.
- The Lew and Waldvogel classification is based on the duration of illness (acute versus chronic), the mechanism of infection (hematogenous vs. contiguous), and the presence of vascular insufficiency.

GENERAL PRINCIPLES

- The diagnosis of osteomyelitis is suspected on clinical grounds. Confirmation usually entails a combination of radiologic, microbiologic, and pathologic tests.
- Cross-sectional imaging modalities, such as computed tomography or magnetic resonance imaging (MRI), are considered standard of care in the diagnosis of osteomyelitis.
- Repeated swab cultures of the same organism from draining wounds and sinus tracts may be of diagnostic benefit, although failure to recover the true pathogen is common, except for *Staphylococcus aureus*.
- Bone biopsy or needle aspiration is best for organism identification.
- Therapy is typically a combination of complete surgical débridement and 4 to 6 weeks of antimicrobial therapy (see Table 49-1).

OSTEOMYELITIS AFTER A CONTAMINATED OPEN FRACTURE

- Contaminated open fractures can lead to the development of osteomyelitis of the fractured bone, typically at the fracture site in 3% to 25% of cases.
- Staphylococci and aerobic gram-negative bacilli are the two most common groups of microorganisms in this setting.
- The hallmark of osteomyelitis after open fracture is nonunion of the fracture site or poor wound healing after wound closure or soft tissue coverage.
- Management of open contaminated fractures entails early aggressive wound irrigation and débridement, administration of parenteral and local antimicrobials, fracture fixation, and soft tissue coverage of exposed bone.

VERTEBRAL OSTEOMYELITIS AND SPONDYLODISKITIS

- The origin is hematogenous in most native cases; it may also occur postoperatively or postprocedurally.
- *S. aureus*, coagulase-negative staphylococci, *Mycobacterium tuberculosis,* and *Brucella* spp. are the most common microorganisms encountered in vertebral osteomyelitis.
- MRI of the spine is highly accurate in the diagnosis of vertebral osteomyelitis.
- Image-guided aspiration and biopsy is highly specific but lacks sensitivity.
- Most cases can be treated with a 6-week course of parenteral antimicrobial therapy without surgery.

TABLE 49-1 Antimicrobial Therapy of Chronic Osteomyelitis in Adults for Selected Microorganisms

MICROORGANISMS	FIRST CHOICE*	ALTERNATIVE CHOICE*
Staphylococci		
Oxacillin sensitive	Nafcillin sodium or oxacillin sodium, 1.5-2 g IV q4h for 4-6 wk, or cefazolin, 1-2 g IV q8h for 4-6 wk	Vancomycin, 15 mg/kg IV q12h for 4-6 wk; some add rifampin, 600 mg PO qd, to nafcillin/oxacillin
Oxacillin resistant (MRSA)	Vancomycin,[†] 15 mg/kg IV q12h for 4-6 wk or Daptomycin 6 mg/kg IV q24h	Linezolid, 600 mg PO/IV q12h for 6 wk, or levofloxacin,[†] 500-750 mg PO/IV daily, plus rifampin, 600-900 mg/day PO for 6 wk if susceptible to both drugs
Penicillin-sensitive streptococci	Aqueous crystalline penicillin G, 20 × 10⁶ U/24 hr IV either continuously or in six equally divided daily doses for 4-6 wk, or ceftriaxone, 1-2 g IV or IM q24h for 4-6 wk or cefazolin, 1-2 g IV q8h for 4-6 wk	Vancomycin, 15 mg/kg IV q12h for 4-6 wk
Enterococci or streptococci with MIC ≥0.5 µg/mL, or Abiotrophia or Granulicatella spp.	Aqueous crystalline penicillin G, 20 × 10⁶ U/24 hr IV either continuously or in six equally divided daily doses for 4-6 wk, or ampicillin sodium, 12 g/24 hr IV either continuously or in 6 equally divided daily doses; the addition of gentamicin sulfate, 1 mg/kg IV or IM q8h for 1-2 wk is optional	Vancomycin,[†] 15 mg/kg IV q12h for 4-6 wk; the addition of gentamicin sulfate, 1 mg/kg IV or IM q8h for 1-2 wk is optional
Enterobacteriaceae	Ceftriaxone, 1-2 g IV q24h for 4-6 wk, or ertapenem 1 g IV q24h	Ciprofloxacin,[†] 500-750 mg PO q12h for 4-6 wk, or levofloxacin 500-750 mg PO q24h
Pseudomonas aeruginosa	Cefepime, 2 g IV q12h, meropenem, 1 g IV q8h or imipenem, 500 mg IV q6h for 4-6 wk	Ciprofloxacin,[†] 750 mg PO q12h for 4-6 wk, or ceftazidime, 2 g IV q8h

MIC, minimal inhibitory concentration; MRSA, methicillin-resistant *Staphylococcus aureus*.
*Antimicrobial selection should be based on in vitro sensitivity data.
[†]Should be avoided, if possible, in pediatric patients and in osteomyelitis associated with fractures.

OSTEOMYELITIS IN PATIENTS WITH DIABETES MELLITUS OR VASCULAR INSUFFICIENCY
- Patients typically have osteomyelitis contiguous to an ulcer of the lower extremity.
- The sensitivity of exposed bone or a probe-to-bone test was 60%, and the specificity was 91%.
- This category of osteomyelitis is often polymicrobial.
- Therapy requires a combination of broad-spectrum antimicrobial regimen and surgical débridement.

ACUTE HEMATOGENOUS OSTEOMYELITIS
- Acute hematogenous osteomyelitis of long bones occurs mainly in prepubertal children, elderly patients, intravenous drug abusers, and patients with indwelling central catheters.
- The most common recovered microorganism is S. aureus.
- Acute hematogenous osteomyelitis of long bones in prepubertal children is typically treated with a 2- to 3-week course of antimicrobial therapy.

50 Orthopedic Implant–Associated Infections

Werner Zimmerli and Parham Sendi

PERIPROSTHETIC JOINT INFECTION (PJI)
Diagnosis
- Determination that a prosthetic joint is infected depends on recovery of an organism from a joint aspirate or surgically obtained material from the joint, although inflammation, wound dehiscence, a draining sinus tract, joint effusion, and loosening of the prosthesis can point toward this diagnosis.

Microbiology
- Most frequent microorganisms: *Staphylococcus aureus,* coagulase-negative staphylococci and streptococci
- *Propionibacterium acnes:* Most important microorganism in periprosthetic shoulder infection
- Microorganisms establish a biofilm on the surface of the implant

Pathogenesis
- Foreign devices are covered by host proteins (e.g., fibronectin) after implantation favoring bacterial adherence.
- Minimal infecting dose is greater than 10,000-fold lower in the presence than absence of an implant.
- Granulocyte function around the implant is impaired (activation and degranulation).

Clinical Manifestations
- Acute exogenous PJI: Local signs of inflammation (wound dehiscence, secretion, erythema)
- Acute hematogenous PJI: New-onset pain at any time after implantation, initially without local signs of infection, new-onset articular effusion
- Chronic PJI: Pain because of early loosening, local inflammation, sinus tract, chronic articular effusion

Treatment
- Cornerstone of successful treatment is early diagnosis.
- Cure is only possible with adequate surgery combined with long-term antibiotic therapy.
- A treatment algorithm (see Fig. 50-1) allows choosing the most appropriate surgical intervention: Débridement with retention, one-stage exchange, two-stage exchange, removal without replacement, or suppressive therapy.
- Guidelines: www.idsociety.org/Organ_System/#Skeletal%20%28Bones%20&%20Joints%29

INTERNAL FIXATION–ASSOCIATED INFECTION
Diagnosis
- Diagnosis of infection associated with implanted devices used to stabilize bone fractures, such as pins and rods, requires culture of the device, usually following surgical removal. Pain,

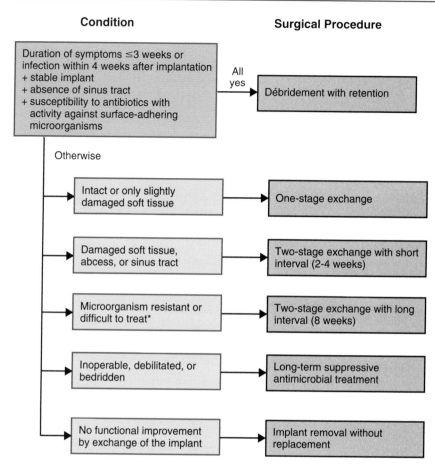

Condition   **Surgical Procedure**

FIGURE 50-1   Surgical treatment algorithm for prosthetic joint infections. *Difficult-to-treat microorganisms include microorganisms resistant to antibiotics with good oral bioavailability, rifampin-resistant staphylococci, enterococci, and quinolone-resistant gram-negative bacilli and fungi. (Modified from Trampuz A, Zimmerli W. Prosthetic joint infections: update in diagnosis and treatment. *Swiss Med Wkly.* 2005;135:243-251.)

inflammation, wound dehiscence, or loosening of the fixation device often indicates infection.

Microbiology

- Microbiology is comparable with that of PJI. Staphylococci are the most important pathogens.
- In open fractures with environmental exposure and preemptive therapy, consider selection of β-lactam–resistant gram-negative bacilli such as *Enterobacter* spp., nonfermenters.

Pathogenesis

- The exogenous route plays a more important role than the hematogenous.
- Infection may also occur via an adjacent focus (contiguous).

Clinical Manifestations

- Acute early postoperative infections: Wound healing disturbances, discharge, erythema
- Acute symptoms after an uneventful postoperative period: Systemic infection signs are dominating, pain is the most important local sign. Other local features are absent in the beginning and become apparent in the course of disease.
- Acute symptoms may also be due to reactivation of chronic post-traumatic osteomyelitis that has been silent for many years: Pain without prominent systemic inflammatory signs.
- Chronic symptoms: Sinus tract, pain, implant loosening.

Treatment

- Bone fractures are less susceptible to infection if stabilized.
- In acute infections: Retain implant with débridement and antimicrobial therapy, until fracture is consolidated.
- In delayed infections, implant must be removed after healing of bone fracture.

51 Genital Skin and Mucous Membrane Lesions

Michael H. Augenbraun

DEFINITION

- Infectious genital skin and mucous membrane lesions cover a wide spectrum of pathologic etiologies and clinical manifestations, mostly presenting as inflammatory reactions or defects in the epithelium of the genital tract in men and women.

EPIDEMIOLOGY

- Infectious genital skin and mucous membrane lesions are seen globally without seasonality.
- These lesions occur primarily among individuals who are sexually active.
- Incubation periods may vary according to etiology, that is, human papillomavirus potentially weeks, months, or years after exposure; primary syphilis weeks to months; herpes simplex outbreaks years.
- Disease may be modified in populations that are immunocompromised.
- Some conditions are currently being seen more frequently in men who have sex with men (early-stage syphilis, lymphogranuloma venereum [LGV]).

MICROBIOLOGY

- Bacteria: *Treponema pallidum* (spirochete), *Haemophilus ducreyi* (gram-negative diplococcus), *Chlamydia trachomatis* L serovars (obligate intracellular pathogen), *Klebsiella granulomatis*/donovanosis (gram-negative rod)
- Viruses: Herpes simplex virus, molluscum contagiosum virus, human papillomavirus
- Fungi: *Candida albicans*

DIAGNOSIS

- Clinical assessment alone may be misleading.
- Laboratory examination using microscopy and serologic testing is often helpful.
- Gram staining and light microscopy help to identify *H. ducreyi* and *Candida*.
- Darkfield microscopy is used to identify *Treponema pallidum*.
- Serology helps to diagnose *T. pallidum* and herpes simplex virus.
- Cell culture is used to diagnose herpes simplex virus.
- Nucleic acid amplification tests are used to identify *C. trachomatis*.

THERAPY

- Therapy is best chosen based on the likely or specific etiologic agent.
- Syphilis is treated with penicillin and tetracyclines.
- Herpes simplex virus infection is treated with acyclovir, valacyclovir, and famciclovir.
- *C. trachomatis* causing LGV should be treated with tetracyclines.

PREVENTION

- Safe sex
- Partner contact tracing
- Preemptive treatment based on contact and risk

52 Urethritis

Michael H. Augenbraun and William M. McCormack

DEFINITION

- Urethritis is an inflammatory condition involving the male urethra usually caused by sexually transmitted infectious pathogens.

EPIDEMIOLOGY

- Urethritis occurs worldwide.

MICROBIOLOGY

- Common etiologic agents include *Chlamydia trachomatis, Neisseria gonorrhoeae, Trichomonas vaginalis,* and *Mycoplasma genitalium.*

DIAGNOSIS

- Light microscopy of urethral discharge can be helpful. The presence of polymorphonuclear leukocytes is highly suggestive of inflammation. Gram stain of this material that reveals intracellular gram-negative diplococci suggests *Neisseria gonorrhoeae,* which can also be cultured using standard agar-based techniques. Nucleic acid amplification techniques are preferred for diagnosing the other etiologic agents of this condition (see Table 52-1).

THERAPY

- Treatment is directed toward the known or suspected pathogen. Infection with *Neisseria gonorrhoeae* is generally treated with third-generation cephalosporins, but resistance is an emerging concern. Infection with *Chlamydia trachomatis* responds to azalides and tetracyclines.

PREVENTION

- Condom use or abstaining from high-risk sexual activity reduces the risk for urethritis.

TABLE 52-1 Evaluation of Men Who Have Urethral Symptoms	
DIAGNOSTIC STUDIES	**COMMENTS**
Gram-stained urethral smear	
Examination of first-void urine specimen for leukocytes	
Endourethral cultures or nonculture tests	
Neisseria gonorrhoeae	Culture and NAATs are equally appropriate. Culture can provide option for susceptibility testing.
Chlamydia trachomatis	NAATs preferred
Trichomonas vaginalis	Culture or NAATs
Mycoplasma genitalium	No currently available commercial test

NAATs, nucleic acid amplification tests.

53 Vulvovaginitis and Cervicitis

William M. McCormack and Michael H. Augenbraun

DEFINITION

- Vulvovaginitis and cervicitis include infectious and noninfectious conditions involving the vulva, vagina, and cervix.

EPIDEMIOLOGY

- Trichomoniasis is a sexually transmitted condition.
- Bacterial vaginosis and vulvovaginal candidiasis are not classic sexually transmitted diseases but seldom occur in sexually inexperienced women.
- Vulvitis and desquamative inflammatory vaginitis are not sexually transmitted.
- Cervicitis may be sexually transmitted or idiopathic.

MICROBIOLOGY

- Trichomoniasis is caused by *Trichomonas vaginalis*.
- Candidiasis is caused by *Candida albicans* and other fungal species.
- Bacterial vaginosis is associated with a complex bacterial microbiota.
- Infectious cervicitis is usually caused by *Neisseria gonorrhoeae, Mycoplasma genitalium,* or *Chlamydia trachomatis.*

DIAGNOSIS

- Trichomoniasis and cervical infections due to *N. gonorrhoeae, M. genitalium,* and *C. trachomatis* can be diagnosed by identifying the causative organisms with use of culture or non-culture methods of which nucleic acid amplification testing is the most accurate.
- Bacterial vaginosis is diagnosed using clinical criteria, including vaginal pH, odor produced when potassium hydroxide is added to vaginal fluid, and detection of "clue cells" when vaginal fluid is examined microscopically.
- Vulvovaginal candidiasis is diagnosed clinically and by the identification of *C. albicans* or other fungal species in cultures of vaginal fluid.
- Desquamative inflammatory vaginitis is diagnosed by the clinical appearance of the vagina and the identification of leukocytes and parabasal cells in wet preparations of vaginal fluid.

THERAPY

- Trichomoniasis is treated with the oral administration of metronidazole or tinidazole.
- Bacterial vaginosis is treated with a 7-day course of oral metronidazole or with preparations for intravaginal use that contain metronidazole or clindamycin.
- Vulvovaginal candidiasis is treated with oral fluconazole or with preparations for vaginal use that contain nystatin, miconazole, or other antifungal agents.
- Desquamative inflammatory vaginitis is best treated with intravaginal clindamycin.
- Intravaginal administration of boric acid or corticosteroids provides symptomatic relief.

PREVENTION

- Judicious choice of sexual partners and regular use of condoms is preventative.

54 Infections of the Female Pelvis

David E. Soper

DEFINITION

- An acute inflammation of the epithelium and/or soft tissue of the pelvic organs

MICROBIOLOGY

- Microorganisms found in the endocervix and vagina
- Bacterial vaginosis microorganisms, predominantly anaerobes
- Group B *Streptococcus* and *Escherichia coli*
- Sexually transmitted microorganisms, such as *Neisseria gonorrhoeae* and *Chlamydia trachomatis*

DIAGNOSIS

- Clinical diagnosis based on fever, erythema, and tenderness in the postoperative setting
- Clinical diagnosis based on risk assessment for sexually transmitted disease and an evaluation for lower genital tract inflammation in the case of pelvic inflammatory disease

THERAPY FOR POSTOPERATIVE INFECTIONS

- Broad-spectrum antibiotic therapy
- Include coverage of penicillinase-producing anaerobes
- Use antibiotic regimens effective in an anaerobic environment

THERAPY FOR PELVIC INFLAMMATORY DISEASE

- Be aware of the emerging resistance of *N. gonorrhoeae* to quinolones, azithromycin, and, to some degree, cephalosporins
- Treat concurrently for bacterial vaginosis if the diagnosis is made concurrently

PREVENTION

- Preoperative antibiotic prophylaxis
- Screening for sexually transmitted microorganisms

55 Prostatitis, Epididymitis, and Orchitis

Catherine C. McGowan and John Krieger

DEFINITION AND CLASSIFICATION

- For the National Institutes of Health classification of prostatitis syndromes, see Table 55-1.
- Acute bacterial prostatitis is associated with lower urinary tract infection and sepsis.
- Chronic bacterial prostatitis is associated with recurrent lower urinary tract infections caused by the same bacterial clade.
- Chronic prostatitis/chronic pelvic pain syndrome (CP/CPPS) occurs in absence of uropathogenic bacteria.
- Acute epididymitis and orchitis are usually due to infectious agents or local trauma.

EPIDEMIOLOGY

- Prostatitis represents the most common urologic diagnosis in healthy young men. Fifty percent of men may experience symptoms in their lifetimes. Prevalence is 2% to 16%.
- Nearly 90% of men evaluated for genitourinary symptoms have CP/CPPS.
- Sexually transmitted epididymitis is most common in young men. Men with bacterial epididymitis may have underlying urologic pathology or recent genitourinary tract manipulation.
- Isolated orchitis is rare.

MICROBIOLOGY

- Gram-negative Enterobacteriaceae cause most episodes of bacterial prostatitis. Enterococci account for a small percentage.
- Etiology of epididymitis and orchitis reflects patient age. *Chlamydia trachomatis* and *Neisseria gonorrhoeae* predominate in young men, and coliform or *Pseudomonas* species predominate in older men.
- Most orchitis is caused by viral infections.

DIAGNOSIS

- Careful history, physical examination, urinalysis, and urine culture are essential.
- The lower urinary tract localization test (see Table 55-2) is the gold standard.
- Epididymitis and orchitis should be evaluated with a urethral swab for *C. trachomatis* and *N. gonorrhoeae*. A urethral smear for Gram stain and midstream urine culture is useful for establishing other etiologies.

THERAPY

- Fluoroquinolones are preferred oral treatment. Quinolone resistance is increasingly common, especially after genitourinary tract instrumentation.
- Septic patients should receive empirical broad-spectrum parenteral therapy.
- Combinations of antibiotics, α-blockers, anti-inflammatory agents, and pain management therapies represent the most effective treatment for CP/CPPS.
- Combination therapy with intramuscular ceftriaxone plus either azithromycin or doxycycline is recommended for *N. gonorrhoeae* infections.

TABLE 55-1 Classification of Prostatitis Syndromes on the Basis of Lower Urinary Tract Localization Studies

CONDITION	BACTERIURIA[a]	INFECTION LOCALIZED TO PROSTATE	INFLAMMATORY RESPONSE[b]	ABNORMAL RECTAL EXAMINATION OF PROSTATE[c]	SYSTEMIC ILLNESS[d]
Acute bacterial prostatitis	+	+	+	+	+
Chronic bacterial prostatitis	+	+	+	−	−
Chronic prostatitis/chronic pelvic pain syndrome					−
Inflammatory subtype[e]	−	−	+	−	−
Noninflammatory subtype[f]	−	−	−	−	−
Asymptomatic inflammatory prostatitis	−	−	+	±	−

[a]Documented with an identical organism that is shown to localize to a prostatic focus when the midstream urine culture is negative.
[b]In expressed prostatic secretions, semen, postmassage urine, or prostate tissue.
[c]Abnormal findings include exquisite tenderness and swelling that may be associated with signs of lower urinary tract obstruction.
[d]Systemic findings frequently include fever and rigors and may include signs of bacteremia.
[e]Formerly termed *nonbacterial prostatitis*.
[f]Formerly termed *prostatodynia*.
From Krieger JN, Nyberg L Jr, Nickel JC. NIH consensus definition and classification of prostatitis. *JAMA*. 1999;282:236-237.

TABLE 55-2 Lower Urinary Tract Localization Using Sequential Urine Cultures*

SPECIMEN	SYMBOL	DESCRIPTION
Voided bladder 1	VB_1	Initial 5-10 mL of urinary stream
Voided bladder 2	VB_2	Midstream specimen
Expressed prostatic secretions	EPS	Secretions expressed from prostate by digital massage
Voided bladder 3	VB_3	First 5-10 mL of urinary stream immediately after prostatic massage

*Unequivocal diagnosis of bacterial prostatitis requires that the colony count in the VB_3 specimen greatly exceed the count in the VB_1 specimen, preferably by at least 10-fold. Many patients who have chronic bacterial prostatitis harbor only small numbers of bacteria in the prostate. In these patients, direct culture of prostatic secretions is particularly useful. Microscopic examination of the EPS is useful for identifying white blood cells and oval fat bodies—large lipid-laden macrophages characteristic of the prostatic inflammatory response.
From Stamey T. *Pathogenesis and Treatment of Urinary Tract Infections*. Baltimore: Williams & Wilkins; 1980.

56 Microbial Conjunctivitis

Scott D. Barnes, Nalin M. Kumar,
Deborah Pavan-Langston, and Dimitri T. Azar

DEFINITION

- Microbial conjunctivitis involves inflammation of the thin lining of the inner eyelid and front of the eyeball, caused by bacteria, viruses, fungi, or parasites.

EPIDEMIOLOGY

- Conjunctivitis affects males and females of all ages.
- Bacterial conjunctivitis is more prevalent in children; viral conjunctivitis is more prevalent in adults.
- Risk factors include contact lens wear, contaminated ocular medications, exposure to an infected person, vaginal versus cesarean delivery, and visits to camps and swimming pools.

MICROBIOLOGY

- Common causes of bacterial conjunctivitis include *Staphylococcus aureus, Streptococcus pneumoniae, Haemophilus* species, *Moraxella, Corynebacterium diphtheriae, Neisseria* species, and enteric gram-negative rods.
- The most common cause of viral conjunctivitis is infection with adenovirus, but other viral causes include herpes simplex virus (HSV), picornavirus, and herpes zoster virus.
- Neonatal conjunctivitis is commonly due to transmission from the mother during childbirth of sexually transmitted bacteria, including *Chlamydia trachomatis* and *Neisseria gonorrhoeae*.

DIAGNOSIS

- Symptoms of conjunctivitis include itching, increased ocular secretions, swelling of the conjunctiva and/or eyelids, pink color in the white of the eyes, and light sensitivity.
- Clinical presentation of acute bacterial conjunctivitis involves rapid onset of unilateral lid edema, conjunctival injection, a mucopurulent discharge, and involvement of the second eye within 1 to 2 days. Itching is uncommon. Unlike viral and chlamydial conjunctivitis, there is no preauricular lymphadenopathy.
- Clinical presentation of viral conjunctivitis is acute, unilateral conjunctivitis with involvement of the second eye occurring often within 1 week. It is associated with a watery to mucous discharge and enlargement of preauricular lymph nodes.
- Routine laboratory evaluation is not usually required except in the first month of life where cultures and smears for bacterial, chlamydial, and herpetic causes need to be performed.
- If bacterial conjunctivitis is suspected, conjunctival scraping for identification of bacterial species by further analysis is recommended for guidance of appropriate antibiotic therapy.
- Viral conjunctivitis can often be diagnosed from signs (e.g., common cold); symptoms (e.g., watery, rather than mucus, discharge); and patient history (e.g., work environment such as if person is a veterinarian or poultry worker). Laboratory tests are not usually necessary.

THERAPY

- Acute bacterial conjunctivitis is treated with a broad-spectrum topical agent such as sulfacetamide, trimethoprim-polymyxin, or a fluoroquinolone (ciprofloxacin, levofloxacin, or moxifloxacin) as eyedrops, usually every 3 hours when awake for 7 to 10 days. Topical azithromycin has been shown to be effective in treating bacterial conjunctivitis with a 3-day course.
- Viral conjunctivitis spontaneously resolves within days to weeks, usually without adverse sequelae to the conjunctiva, but associated keratitis may have long-term sequelae. HSV conjunctivitis in newborns should be treated with intravenous acyclovir.
- Adult inclusion conjunctivitis involves systemic treatment for 3 weeks with tetracycline, doxycycline, or erythromycin, with the caution to avoid tetracycline in children younger than age 8 and in pregnant or lactating women. The use of oral azithromycin has also been found to be effective.
- For hyperacute bacterial conjunctivitis, the prevalence of penicillin-resistant organisms has made ceftriaxone the treatment of choice.
- When treating neonatal chlamydial conjunctivitis, if erythromycin or tetracycline ointment is applied to the conjunctival surface within 1 hour after delivery, the chance of developing chlamydial conjunctivitis is reportedly almost zero. Two weeks of oral erythromycin therapy is given to the newborn with laboratory-proven chlamydial conjunctivitis; a second course may be given if adequate resolution is not achieved with the initial treatment.
- Limit spread of conjunctivitis by following good hygiene steps, including washing hands often, washing any discharge from around the eyes multiple times during the day, and using fresh washcloths, cotton balls, or tissues each time.

57 Microbial Keratitis

Scott D. Barnes, Joelle Hallak, Deborah Pavan-Langston, and Dimitri T. Azar

DEFINITION
- Microbial keratitis is a vision-threatening corneal inflammatory condition, caused by bacteria, viruses, fungi, or parasites.

EPIDEMIOLOGY
- Disease burden is higher in developing than developed countries.
- Risk factors include contact lens wear, trauma (surgical and nonsurgical), contaminated ocular medications, altered structure of the corneal surface, and contributing systemic diseases.
- Contact lens use is the main cause for keratitis in the United States: poor lens storage and hygiene and overnight lens use.
- Nonsurgical ocular trauma is the main cause of keratitis in developing countries.
- Trachoma is encountered more commonly in developing countries.

MICROBIOLOGY
- Pathogens can be gram-negative organisms, such as *Pseudomonas aeruginosa.*
- Pathogens can be gram-positive organisms, such as *Staphylococcus* and *Streptococcus* spp.
- Viral pathogens include herpes simplex virus, varicella-zoster virus, adenovirus.
- Recent outbreaks of microbial keratitis in contact lens wearers have involved *Acanthamoeba* and *Fusarium* spp.

DIAGNOSIS
- Symptoms include severe pain and discomfort, tearing, photophobia, blepharospasm, and decreased vision.
- Clinical presentation includes conjunctival injection and discharge, decreased corneal transparency, corneal infiltrate, epithelial defect and/or stromal inflammation, corneal edema, corneal neovascularization, stromal melting, loss of vision.
- Knowing the nature of the stromal inflammation (suppurative or nonsuppurative), and its location (focal, multifocal, or diffuse) is helpful.

THERAPY
- Corneal scrapings and cultures should be performed on all suspected cases with infectious keratitis.
- Aggressive antimicrobial therapy should be initiated after scrapings and cultures of infectious keratitis.
- Fortified topical administration is the most common route of antimicrobial therapy. Subconjunctival injections, parenteral and oral routes, and antibiotic-soaked collagen shields/soft lenses are used infrequently.
- Fortified cefazolin and aminoglycoside should be used for more severe bacterial keratitis.
- Monotherapy with a fourth-generation fluoroquinolone is used for bacterial keratitis.
- Antifungal therapeutic agents include topical natamycin, amphotericin B, flucytosine, fluconazole, and itraconazole. Oral itraconazole or voriconazole have also shown favorable outcomes when added to topical therapy.

58 Endophthalmitis

Marlene L. Durand

DEFINITION

- Endophthalmitis is a bacterial or fungal infection inside the eye, involving the vitreous and/or aqueous. It is either exogenous, in which infection is introduced from the outside in, or endogenous, in which the eye is seeded from the bloodstream.

CLINICAL MANIFESTATIONS

- Decreased vision and eye pain are usually present. Hypopyon (layer of white blood cells in aqueous humor) is commonly seen. No fever or leukocytosis is present in exogenous cases and may also be absent in endogenous cases on presentation.

CATEGORIES AND MICROBIOLOGY (SEE TABLE 58-1)

- *Acute postcataract endophthalmitis.* Incidence is 0.1% to 0.2% of cataract surgeries, with onset within 1 week postoperatively in 75%. Etiology is contamination of aqueous from ocular surface flora. Gram-positive cocci cause 95% of cases, with coagulase-negative staphylococci the major pathogens (70% of all cases).
- *Chronic postcataract endophthalmitis.* Rare, this category presents as low-grade inflammation in aqueous postoperatively that persists for months. It may respond to topical corticosteroids initially but recurs as the drug dosage is tapered. The cause is *Propionibacterium acnes* in most cases.
- *Postinjection endophthalmitis.* Incidence is 0.1% after each intravitreal injection of anti–vascular endothelial growth factor agents (treatment of wet macular degeneration). Injections are typically given once monthly. Major pathogens are coagulase-negative staphylococci and streptococci (25% of cases), the latter usually causing severe endophthalmitis.
- *Bleb-related endophthalmitis.* A filtering bleb is a "bleb" of conjunctiva overlying a surgically created defect in the sclera. Endophthalmitis typically occurs suddenly, months to years postoperatively; incidence is 1.3% per patient-year. Infection is often fulminant because streptococci, including *Streptococcus pneumoniae,* and *Haemophilus influenzae* are major pathogens.
- *Post-traumatic endophthalmitis.* Incidence is 3% to 10% after penetrating eye trauma ("open globe") but may be much lower after protocol that includes 48 hours of prophylactic antibiotics. Coagulase-negative staphylococci and *Bacillus cereus* are major pathogens; *B. cereus* is most feared and causes fulminant infection.
- *Endogenous bacterial endophthalmitis.* Sources include endocarditis (*Staphylococcus aureus* and streptococci are major pathogens), intraabdominal abscess (liver abscess due to *Klebsiella pneumoniae* in East Asian nations), transient bacteremia (e.g., endoscopy, intravenous drug abuse).
- Candida *endophthalmitis.* This category is usually endogenous, and chorioretinitis, the earliest manifestation, is often asymptomatic. Chorioretinitis usually responds to systemic antifungal treatment alone, but cases with endophthalmitis (marked vitreous inflammation) also require intravitreal antifungal injection and often vitrectomy.

TABLE 58-1 Endophthalmitis Categories and the Most Common Pathogens in Each

CATEGORY	PATHOGEN
Acute postcataract	Coagulase-negative staphylococci
Chronic postcataract	*Propionibacterium acnes*
Postinjection	Viridans streptococci, coagulase-negative staphylococci
Bleb-related	Streptococci, *Haemophilus influenzae*
Post-traumatic	*Bacillus cereus*
Endogenous	*Staphylococcus aureus*, streptococci, gram-negative bacilli
Fungal	*Candida, Aspergillus, Fusarium*

- *Mold endophthalmitis.* Usually exogenous, this infection occurs after eye surgery, eye trauma, or as an extension of keratomycosis (fungal corneal infection). *Aspergillus* and *Fusarium* are the most common pathogens.

DIAGNOSIS

- Exogenous cases, and some endogenous cases, require vitreous aspirate or vitrectomy for culture (aqueous may also be cultured). Endogenous cases with positive blood cultures are usually presumed to be due to the same organism.

THERAPY

- Intravitreal antibiotics and often vitrectomy (surgical débridement of the vitreous) are required in all cases. Systemic antibiotics alone are not used to treat endophthalmitis, except in cases of *Candida* chorioretinitis.

59 Infectious Causes of Uveitis

Marlene L. Durand

DEFINITION AND CATEGORIES

- *Uveitis* means inflammation of the uvea (iris, ciliary body, choroid) or retina.
- Divided into categories by site of greatest inflammation:
  - Anterior (iritis, iridocyclitis)
  - Intermediate (pars planitis)
  - Posterior (choroiditis, retinitis, chorioretinitis)
  - Panuveitis
- Noninfectious causes of uveitis (idiopathic, autoimmune) are more common than infectious causes, but the frequency of each varies depending on category.
- Approximately 10% of anterior uveitis cases have an infectious etiology.
- Approximately 50% of posterior uveitis cases have an infectious etiology.

EPIDEMIOLOGY AND ETIOLOGY

- The most likely infectious etiologies vary by uveitis category and by location in the world (see Table 59-1).
- Infectious causes of anterior include herpes simplex virus (HSV) (90% of infectious etiologies), varicella-zoster virus (VZV), syphilis, tuberculosis (TB), and Lyme disease.
- Infectious causes of intermediate uveitis are rare and include Lyme disease.
- Infectious causes of posterior uveitis include ocular toxoplasmosis, acute retinal necrosis (HSV, VZV, sometimes cytomegalovirus [CMV]), CMV retinitis (severely immunocompromised patients), ocular *Toxocara,* syphilis, cat-scratch disease, and *Candida* endophthalmitis.
- Infectious causes of panuveitis include syphilis, TB, and *Candida* endophthalmitis.
- Other infectious etiologies of uveitis seen primarily in tropical regions or developing countries include leptospirosis (panuveitis without retinal or choroidal lesions), leprosy (anterior uveitis), *Brucella* (chronic relapsing uveitis), and Chikungunya virus (anterior uveitis, retinitis, or optic neuritis).

DIAGNOSIS

- Varies by etiology. Ocular syphilis is presumed in cases of uveitis with positive specific treponemal serology. Polymerase chain reaction of aqueous or vitreous for HSV, VZV, and CMV may be helpful in some chronic anterior uveitis cases (aqueous) and in some cases of acute retinal necrosis (vitreous higher yield than aqueous, but vitreous sampling carries more risk).

THERAPY

- Varies by etiology. Acute retinal necrosis is a medical emergency and requires antiviral treatment directed against HSV and VZV and against CMV as well in immunocompromised patients. Ocular toxoplasmosis is discussed in Chapter 280 of *Mandell, Douglas, and Bennett's Principles and Practice of Infectious Diseases,* 8th Edition. Ocular TB and ocular syphilis should be treated the same way as TB meningitis and neurosyphilis, respectively.

Part I Major Clinical Syndromes

TABLE 59-1 Classification of Uveitis and Major Infectious Etiologies in Each Category

CATEGORY	OCULAR FINDINGS	MAJOR INFECTIOUS ETIOLOGIES (%)*
Anterior (iritis, cyclitis, iridocyclitis)	WBCs in aqueous, keratic precipitates, iris nodules, synechiae	Herpes simplex (10%); syphilis (<1%); TB (<1%); Lyme disease (<1%); leprosy (<1%)
Intermediate	WBCs or *snowballs* in the vitreous, pars plana *snow bank*	Lyme disease (<1%)
Posterior (choroiditis, chorioretinitis, retinitis)	Lesions in choroid, retina, or both; vitritis in some	*Toxoplasma* (25%); CMV (12%)[†]; ARN (6%); *Toxocara* (3%); syphilis (2%); *Candida* (<1%)
Panuveitis	WBCs in aqueous and vitreous	Syphilis (6%); TB (2%); *Candida* (2%)

ARN, acute retinal necrosis; CMV, cytomegalovirus; TB, tuberculosis; WBCs, white blood cells.

*Percentage of uveitis cases in each category (not of total uveitis cases), based on 1237 cases of uveitis seen at Massachusetts Eye & Ear Infirmary, Boston, 1982-1992, by Foster's group (Rodriguez A, Calonge M, Pedoza-Seres M, et al. Referral patterns of uveitis in a tertiary eye care center. *Arch Ophthalmol.* 1996;114:593-599).

[†]Series was before use of highly active antiretroviral therapy, and rate for CMV retinitis would be lower now.

60 Periocular Infections

Marlene L. Durand

DEFINITION

- Periocular infections include infections of the eyelids, lacrimal system, and orbit.
- Eyelid infections include preseptal cellulitis, infections of the meibomian glands of the lids (hordeolum, stye), sterile inflammatory granulomatous nodule in the lid (chalazion), and marginal blepharitis (inflammation at the lid margins).
- Lacrimal system infections include dacryoadenitis (infection of the lacrimal gland), canaliculitis (infection of the canaliculi that collect tears in the medial canthus and drain into the lacrimal sac), and dacryocystitis (infection of the lacrimal sac).
- Orbital infections include orbital cellulitis, subperiosteal abscess, orbital abscess, and cavernous sinus thrombophlebitis. Acute sinusitis is the most common cause of orbital infections.

MICROBIOLOGY

- Lid infections: *Staphylococcus aureus,* streptococci
- Canaliculitis: *Actinomyces israelii,* also staphylococci, streptococci
- Dacryocystitis: *S. aureus,* streptococci; also gram-negative bacilli
- Orbital infections: *S. aureus* including methicillin-resistant *S. aureus, Streptococcus anginosus (milleri),* other streptococci (including *Streptococcus pneumoniae*), gram-negative bacilli, anaerobes. Mixed infections common.

DIAGNOSIS

- Clinical examination in lid infections, lacrimal system infections, supported by culture.
- Preseptal cellulitis must be distinguished from orbital infections (orbital cellulitis, subperiosteal and orbital abscess). Orbital infections usually have one or more of the following findings: proptosis (which may not be grossly apparent but can be measured as 2 mm or more difference in Hertel's exophthalmometer measurements), ophthalmoplegia, and vision loss. Preseptal cellulitis has none of these features—only lid edema and erythema. Computed tomography (CT) scan should be performed on any patient with orbital findings. CT should be considered in children who present with what appears to be severe preseptal cellulitis because they may have subperiosteal abscess.

THERAPY

- Varies by diagnosis
- Orbital infections are much more serious than preseptal cellulitis, and all orbital infections must be treated with intravenous antibiotics. Subperiosteal abscesses usually require surgical drainage, and orbital abscesses almost always do. Drainage of an adjacent infected sinus may be indicated.

61 | Viral Hepatitis

Jules L. Dienstag and Andrew S. Delemos

ACUTE HEPATITIS

- Acute clinical illnesses caused by the five hepatitis viruses (HAV, HBV, HCV, HDV, and HEV) are similar.
- Illness ranges from asymptomatic to fulminant.
- Asymptomatic infections are 10 to 30 times more common than symptomatic ones.

CHRONIC HEPATITIS

- Chronic hepatitis affects more than 500 million people worldwide.
- HBV, HCV, and HDV cause chronic hepatitis.
- HEV causes protracted and chronic hepatitis only in immunosuppressed patients.

INDIVIDUAL HEPATITIS VIRUSES (SEE TABLE 61-1)
Hepatitis A Virus (HAV)

- HAV is an RNA virus that is a member of the *Hepatovirus* genus.
- HAV is transmitted via the fecal-oral route.
- It typically causes an acute, self-limited illness, more often symptomatic in adults than in children.
- HAV is more severe in patients with preexisting chronic hepatitis B or C.
- Relapsing and cholestatic hepatitis may occur.
- Diagnosis is by serology (IgM anti-HAV) (see Table 61-2).
- Treatment is usually not necessary beyond supportive care.
- Prevention—highly effective HAV vaccines that have markedly reduced incidence where used are available.
- Passive immunization with immune globulin intramuscularly is effective in postexposure prophylaxis.

Hepatitis B Virus (HBV)
Virology/Epidemiology

- HBV is a double-stranded DNA virus in the *Orthohepadnavirus* genus and the *Hepadnavirus* family; 10 genotypes have been identified.
- Worldwide, 350 million people are infected chronically with HBV.
- One million deaths annually result from complications of chronic infection—cirrhosis, hepatocellular carcinoma (HCC).
- Prevalence in Asia is estimated at greater than 10%, resulting primarily from perinatal transmission, after which the likelihood of acquiring chronic infection is 90%.
- In adults, transmission of hepatitis B occurs primarily following high-risk behaviors (injection drug use, sexual activity) or after occupational exposure but resolves in greater than 95% of otherwise healthy persons.

TABLE 61-1 Hepatitis Viruses and Characteristics of Infection

CHARACTERISTIC	A	B	C	D	E
Virus family	Picornaviridae	Hepadnaviridae	Flaviviridae	Unassigned	Hepeviridae
Genus	Hepatovirus	Orthohepadnavirus	Hepacivirus	Deltavirus	Hepevirus
Nucleic acid	RNA	DNA	RNA	RNA	RNA
Incubation period (days)	15-48 (mean 30)	30-180 (mean 60-90)	15-160 (mean 50)	30-180 (mean 60-90)	14-60 (mean 40)
Mode of transmission:					
Fecal-oral	Yes	No	No	No	Yes
Sexual	Possible	Yes	Rare	Yes	No
Blood	Rare	Yes	Yes	Yes	No*
Chronic infection	No	Yes	Yes	Yes	Yes†
Cirrhosis and hepatocellular carcinoma	No	Yes	Yes	With hepatitis B	No‡

*Can be bloodborne in endemic areas.
†Acute hepatitis in normal hosts, protracted and chronic infection only in immunosuppressed patients.
‡Cirrhosis can occur after chronic infection, which is confined to immunosuppressed patients.

TABLE 61-2 Simplified Diagnostic Approach in Patients Presenting with Acute Hepatitis

DIAGNOSTIC INTERPRETATION	SEROLOGIC TESTS OF PATIENT'S SERUM			
	HBsAg	IgM Anti-HAV	IgM Anti-HBc	Anti-HCV
Acute hepatitis B	+	–	+	–
Chronic hepatitis B	+	–	–	–
Acute hepatitis A superimposed on chronic hepatitis B	+	+	–	–
Acute hepatitis A and B	+	+	+	–
Acute hepatitis A	–	+	–	–
Acute hepatitis A and B (HBsAg below detection threshold)	–	+	+	–
Acute hepatitis B (HBsAg below detection threshold)	–	–	+	–
Acute hepatitis C	–	–	–	+

HAV, hepatitis A virus; HBc, hepatitis B core; HBsAg, hepatitis B surface antigen; HCV, hepatitis C virus.
Modified from Longo D, Fauci A, Kasper D, et al. *Harrison's Principles of Internal Medicine*. 18th ed. New York: McGraw Hill; 2011.

Diagnosis
- Acute hepatitis B is a symptomatic infection typified by right upper quadrant pain, nausea, malaise, jaundice, elevated alanine aminotransferase (ALT) and aspartate aminotransferase (AST), and IgM antibody to hepatitis B core antigen.
- Different categories of chronic infection are diagnosed on the basis of serologic testing and HBV DNA level (see Table 61-3).
- Liver biopsy is not required for diagnosis but may inform treatment decisions in chronic infection.

Treatment
- Indications (see Table 61-4):
  - Hepatitis B e antigen (HBeAg)-positive or HBeAg-negative patients with ALT > 2× upper limit of normal or moderate to severe hepatitis on liver biopsy and HBV DNA > 20,000 IU/mL

TABLE 61-3 Viral and Laboratory Markers of Hepatitis B Virus Infection

DIAGNOSIS	HBsAg	Anti-HBs	IgM Anti-HBc	IgG Anti-HBc	HBeAg	Anti-HBe	ALT
Acute hepatitis	+	−	+	−	+	−	Elevated
Recovered (immune)	−	+	−	+	−	+	Normal
HBeAg-positive chronic hepatitis B	+	−	−	+	+	−	Elevated
HBeAg-negative chronic hepatitis B	+	−	−	+	−	+	Elevated (may be intermittent)
Vaccinated (immune)	−	+	−	−	−	−	Normal
Inactive carrier	+	−	−	+	−	+	Normal

ALT, alanine aminotransferase; HBc, hepatitis B core (antigen); HBe, HBeAg, hepatitis B e antigen; HBs, HBsAg, hepatitis B surface antigen; IgG, immunoglobulin G; IgM, immunoglobulin M.

TABLE 61-4 Recommendations/Guidelines of the American Association for the Study of Liver Diseases for the Treatment of Chronic Hepatitis B

HBeAg	HBV DNA (IU/mL)	ALT	TREATMENT	FIRST-LINE AGENTS
Chronic Hepatitis B without Cirrhosis				
+	$>2 \times 10^4$	$>2 \times$ ULN	Recommended	PEG IFN, ETV, TDF
+	$>2 \times 10^4$	$\leq 2 \times$ ULN	Not recommended	
−	$>2 \times 10^4$	$>2 \times$ ULN	Recommended	PEG IFN, ETV, TDF
−	$>2 \times 10^3$	1 to $>2 \times$ ULN	Histology determines*	
−	$\leq 2 \times 10^3$	Normal	Not recommended†	
Cirrhosis				
±	Detectable (PCR‡)	Normal or ↑	Recommended	Compensated: treat with ETV or TDF for HBV DNA $>2 \times 10^3$; for HBV DNA $<2 \times 10^3$, treat if ALT ↑ Decompensated§: treat with ETV or combination nucleoside/nucleotide
±	Undetectable (PCR‡)	Normal or ↑	Not recommended	§

ALT, alanine aminotransferase; ETV, entecavir; HBeAg, hepatitis B e antigen; HBV, hepatitis B virus; IU, international units; PCR, polymerase chain reaction; PEG IFN, pegylated interferon; TDF, tenofovir; ULN, upper limit of normal.
Table is updated to reflect supplanting of the less effective drugs by the best available antiviral drugs.
*If liver biopsy reveals advanced necroinflammatory activity or fibrosis, consider treatment.
†Inactive carrier.
‡$>10^2$ to 10^3 IU/mL.
§If decompensated, coordinate care with a liver transplantation center.

- HBeAg-negative patients with low-level HBV DNA but evidence of fibrosis or moderate to severe hepatitis on liver biopsy
- Cirrhosis associated with chronic HBV irrespective of HBV DNA level
- Inactive carrier (hepatitis B surface antigen [HBsAg] positive) preemptively when starting chemotherapy or other immunosuppressive therapy (including anti–tumor necrosis factor)
- Therapy (see Table 61-5):
  - Tenofovir 300 mg daily or entecavir 0.5 mg daily (1 mg dose approved for prior lamivudine resistance but not a viable alternative to adding tenofovir)

TABLE 61-5 Approved Antiviral Drugs for Chronic Hepatitis B

	IFN	PEG IFN	LAM	ADV	ETV	TBV	TDF
Dose	5 MU/day*	180 µg/wk	100 mg/day	10 mg/day	0.5 mg/day	600 mg/day	300 mg/day
Route	Subcutaneous	Subcutaneous	Oral	Oral	Oral	Oral	Oral
Duration in trials	4 mo	48 wk	48-52 wk	48 wk	48 wk	52 wk	48 wk
Tolerability	Poor	Poor	Excellent	Excellent†	Excellent	Excellent	Excellent†
HBeAg seroconversion	18%-20%	27%‡	16%-21%	12%	21%	22%	21%
$\log_{10}$ HBV DNA reduction							
HBeAg-positive	?§	4.5	5.5	3.5	6.9	6.5	6.2
HBeAg-negative	?§	4.1	4.7	3.9	5.0	5.2	4.6
HBV DNA PCR-negative							
HBeAg-positive	?	25%	44%	21%	67%	60%	76%
HBeAg-negative	?	63%	73%	64%	90%	88%	93%
ALT normalization							
HBeAg-positive	?‖	39%	75%	61%	68%	77%	68%
HBeAg-negative	?‖	38%	79%	77%	78%	74%	76%
HBsAg loss during treatment	up to 8%	3%-4%	≤1%	0%	2%	<1%	3%
Viral resistance	None	None	15%-30%	None	None	2%-5%	0%
>1 yr	None	None	5 yr: 70%	5 yr: 29%	≤1%	2 yr: 9%-22%	0%
Cost (U.S. $)	5600*	18,500	2500	6600	8700	6000	6000

ADV, adefovir; ALT, alanine aminotransferase; ETV, entecavir; HBeAg, hepatitis B e antigen; HBsAg, hepatitis B virus surface antigen; HBV, hepatitis B virus; IFN, interferon; LAM, lamivudine; PCR, polymerase chain reaction; PEG IFN, pegylated IFN; MU, million units; TBV, telbivudine; TDF, tenofovir.

Data shown are maximum reported values for up to 1 yr (48-52 wk) of treatment in registration trials. These comparisons are head to head only for PEG IFN vs. LAM, ETV vs. LAM, TBV vs. LMV, and TDF vs. ADV.

*5 MU daily to 10 MU three times a wk for 16 to 24 wk; the cost is that of a complete course, not of a yr of therapy.

†Creatinine monitoring recommended.

‡At 32% 24 wk after therapy.

§When these studies were conducted, HBV DNA was measured with insensitive hybridization assays.

‖ALT is generally normal in those with adequate serologic/virologic response; reports rarely include ALT levels at the end of treatment. In HBeAg-reactive patients, a meta-analysis showed a 23% advantage in ALT normalization (after therapy) in treated vs. untreated patients.

- 48 weeks of pegylated interferon (PEG IFN) in noncirrhotic HBeAg-positive patients also an option
- Consider stopping oral therapy in HBeAg-positive patients 6 to 12 months after HBeAg seroconversion (HBeAg-negative and anti-HBe-positive); ≥40% chance of seroconversion after 5 years of therapy
- Indefinite treatment for chronic HBeAg-negative hepatitis B; consider stopping therapy for HBsAg seroconversion

Prevention
- Universal vaccination of infants beginning at birth (≥3 intramuscular doses)
- Prenatal maternal HBsAg screening and if HBsAg positive, hepatitis B immune globulin 0.5 mL at birth along with vaccination
- Tenofovir 300 mg starting in the third trimester in women with HBV DNA >10^8 IU/mL (some authorities recommend antiviral therapy for mothers with HBV DNA >10^6 IU/mL)

Hepatitis D Virus (HDV)
- HDV is a percutaneously transmitted, circular RNA virus (genus: *Deltavirus*) that requires HBV (or other hepadnaviruses) to replicate and persist.
- Acute coinfection can occur and follows the clinical course of acute HBV infection.
- HDV superinfection results in chronic infection in patients with prior chronic hepatitis B and has clinical features similar to chronic hepatitis B infection, although with increased severity and risk of progression to cirrhosis.
- The diagnosis is made by serologic testing for antibodies to HDV or by polymerase chain reaction (PCR) for HDV RNA.
- Oral antivirals for hepatitis B are not active against HDV, but prolonged treatment with PEG IFN may benefit a proportion of patients.

Hepatitis C Virus (HCV)
Virology/Epidemiology
- HCV is a single-stranded RNA virus (genus: *Hepacivirus*) with six main genotypes (1 to 6); it exists as quasi-species because of its high mutation rate.
- HCV requires host lipid membrane assembly/secretion apparatus for replication.
- Worldwide, 185 million patients have chronic HCV, with more than 4 million residing in the United States.
- Transmission occurs predominantly through injection drug use, but other modes include blood transfusion before the availability of screening or nonsterile practices in which blood/body fluids are exchanged [note—the risk of hepatitis C is not increased in people with tattoos or in health workers].
- Chronic HCV infection develops in at least 85% of patients with acute infection and, in the absence of treatment, results in cirrhosis in approximately 20% of patients after 20 years of infection.
- The annual incidence of HCC in persons with HCV-associated cirrhosis is 1% to 4%.
- HCV is the leading indication for liver transplantation in the United States.

Diagnosis
- Symptomatic hepatitis and jaundice develop in fewer than 10% to 20% of patients with acute hepatitis C, which often portends viral clearance.
- Chronic hepatitis C tends to be asymptomatic, although patients often complain of fatigue.
- Patients with HCV-associated cirrhosis may present clinically with complications of end-stage liver disease such as variceal bleeding, hepatic encephalopathy, or ascites.
- The detection of antibody to HCV is the initial diagnostic test, but PCR testing for HCV RNA distinguishes ongoing chronic infection (commonly) from prior exposure with subsequent clearance (rare).

750 mg (two 375-mg tablets) q8h with food (not low fat)
eRVR = HCV negative weeks 4 and 12

Treatment Naïve and Previous Relapsers

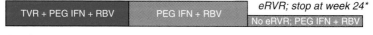

Previous Partial or Null Responders

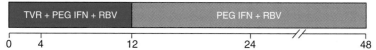

*Treatment-naïve patients with compensated cirrhosis and eRVR may benefit from continuing PEG IFN + RBV to week 48.

Time Point	Criterion	Stopping Rule
Week 4 or 12	HCV RNA >1000 IU/mL	Discontinue all therapy
Week 24	Detectable HCV RNA	Discontinue PEG IFN/RBV
Any	Discontinuation of PEG IFN/RBV for any reason	Discontinue TVR

FIGURE 61-1 **Recommended approach to treating patients with chronic hepatitis C virus (HCV), genotype 1, with telaprevir (TVR)-based therapy.** eRVR, extended rapid virologic response; IU, international units; PEG IFN, pegylated interferon; RBV, ribavirin; RNA, ribonucleic acid. As of January 2015, telaprevir is no longer recommended for treatment of hepatitis C (see Table 61-6).

Treatment

- The goal of therapy in chronic hepatitis C is to achieve a sustained virologic response (SVR), which is defined as undetectable HCV RNA 24 weeks following completion of therapy (12 weeks has been adopted as the SVR endpoint in recent clinical trials).
- **Standard of care 2011-2013:** for genotypes 2 and 3, 24 weeks of PEG IFN-α2a or -α2b and ribavirin (RBV) 800 mg daily; for genotype 1, PEG IFN, weight-based RBV, and either boceprevir (BOC) or telaprevir (TVR) (see Fig. 61-1). In prior treatment-naïve patients, treatment regimens are either 24 weeks (TVR), 28 weeks (BOC, after 4 weeks of PEG IFN/ RBV lead-in), or up to 48 weeks (with triple-drug therapy for 12 weeks and PEG IFN/RBV thereafter for TVR or BOC-based triple-drug therapy for up to week 36 and PEG IFN/RBV thereafter) and are based on HCV RNA response milestones (i.e., response-guided therapy; see Figs. 61-1 and 61-2), except in cirrhotics, in whom treatment for a full 48 weeks is recommended. In treatment-experienced patients, relapsers are treated the same way as treatment-naïve patients, while prior nonresponders are treated for up to 48 weeks (with triple-drug therapy for 12 weeks and PEG IFN/RBV thereafter for TVR or triple-drug therapy up to 44 weeks following 4 weeks of PEG IFN/RBV lead-in for BOC).
- **Standard of care 2014**
  - Treatment-naïve patients:
    - Genotype 1: sofosbuvir (SOF) 400 mg daily with PEG IFN/RBV (weight-based, 1000 to 1200 mg daily) for 12 weeks or simeprevir (SMV) 150 mg with PEG IFN/RBV for 12 weeks followed by another 12 weeks of PEG IFN/RBV; an alternative for IFN-ineligible patients is combination SOF, SMV, and RBV for 12 weeks.
    - Genotype 2: SOF 400 mg daily with RBV (weight-based, 1000 to 1200 mg daily) for 12 weeks.
    - Genotype 3: SOF 400 mg daily with RBV (weight-based, 1000 to 1200 mg daily) for 24 weeks (an alternative is SOF with PEG IFN/RBV for 12 weeks).
    - Genotypes 4 to 6: similar to genotype 1 with minor modifications (see www.hcvguidelines.org).

800 mg (four 200-mg capsules) q8h with food
Early response = HCV RNA negative at weeks 8 and 24

Treatment Naïve and Previous Relapsers

| PEG IFN + RBV | BOC + PEG IFN + RBV | *Early response; stop at week 28* |
| | BOC + PEG IFN + RBV | PEG IFN + RBV |

Previous Relapsers or Partial Responders (noncirrhotic)

| PEG IFN + RBV | BOC + PEG IFN + RBV | |
| | BOC + PEG IFN + RBV | PEG IFN + RBV |

0   4   8   12   24   28   36   48
                        Weeks

Additional recommendations:

Cirrhotics and null responders should receive lead-in and then PEG IFN/RBV + BOC for 44 weeks (no RGT).
Week 4 <1 $\log_{10}$ HCV RNA reduction: consider PEG IFN/RBV + BOC for 44 weeks after lead-in (no RGT).
EU label: fixed-duration therapy for all treatment-experienced patients: LI + 32 weeks triple + 12 weeks PR (no RGT).

Time Point	Criterion	Stopping Rule
Week 12	HCV RNA ≥100 IU/mL	Discontinue all therapy
Week 24	Detectable HCV RNA	Discontinue all therapy
Any	Discontinuation of PEG/RBV for any reason	Discontinue BOC

FIGURE 61-2 **Recommended approach to treating patients with chronic hepatitis C virus (HCV), genotype 1, with boceprevir (BOC)-based therapy.** EU, European Union; IU, international units; LI, lead-in; PEG IFN, pegylated interferon; PR, pegylated; RBV, ribavirin; RGT, response-guided therapy; RNA, ribonucleic acid. As of January 2015, boceprevir is no longer recommended for treatment of hepatitis C (see Table 61-6).

- Patients with prior PEG IFN/RBV treatment failure:
  - Genotype 1: SOF 400 mg daily, SMV 150 mg daily, and RBV (1000 to 1200 mg daily) for 12 weeks (an alternative is SOF for 12 weeks with PEG IFN/RBV for 12 to 24 weeks or SMV 150 mg for 12 weeks with PEG IFN/RBV for 48 weeks).
  - Genotype 2: SOF 400 mg daily with RBV (weight-based, 1000 to 1200 mg daily) for 12 weeks (an alternative is SOF 400 mg daily with PEG IFN/RBV [weight-based, 1000 to 1200 mg daily] for 12 weeks).
  - Genotype 3: SOF 400 mg daily with RBV (weight-based, 1000 to 1200 mg daily) for 24 weeks (an alternative is SOF 400 mg daily with PEG IFN/RBV [weight-based, 1000 to 1200 mg daily] for 12 weeks).
  - Genotypes 4 to 6: SOF 400 mg daily with PEG IFN/RBV (weight-based, 1000 to 1200 mg daily) for 12 weeks.
  - Patients with genotype 1 and prior TVR or BOC protease inhibitor failure: SOF for 12 weeks with PEG IFN/RBV for 12 to 24 weeks.
- **Standard of care: January 2015**
  - The approval of new direct-acting antivirals in October and December 2014 has led to IFN-free regimens of shorter duration and extraordinarily high efficacy, both in treatment-naïve and treatment-experienced patients (see Table 61-6).
  - Newly recommended treatment regimens:
    - Ledipasvir/sofosbuvir (Harvoni): fixed-dose daily combination for genotypes 1a, 1b, 4, and 6
    - Paritaprevir/ritonavir/ombitasvir plus dasabuvir ± ribavirin for genotypes 1a, 1b, and 4

Hepatitis E (HEV)

- HEV is an RNA virus (genus: *Hepevirus*).
- It spreads by fecally contaminated water in endemic areas.
- HEV causes acute, self-limited hepatitis, similar to HAV, in normal hosts.

TABLE 61-6 AASLD and IDSA Recommendations for HCV Treatment-Naïve Patients: January 2015

GENOTYPE	RECOMMENDATION*
1a	Daily fixed-dose combination of ledipasvir (90 mg)/sofosbuvir (400 mg) for 12 wk Daily fixed-dose combination of paritaprevir (150 mg)/ritonavir (100 mg)/ombitasvir (25 mg) plus twice-daily–dosed dasabuvir (250 mg) and weight-based RBV for 12 wk (no cirrhosis) or 24 wk (cirrhosis) Daily sofosbuvir (400 mg) plus simeprevir (150 mg) with or without weight-based RBV for 12 wk (no cirrhosis) or 24 wk (cirrhosis)
1b	Daily fixed-dose combination of ledipasvir (90 mg)/sofosbuvir (400 mg) for 12 wk Daily fixed-dose combination of paritaprevir (150 mg)/ritonavir (100 mg)/ombitasvir (25 mg) plus twice-daily–dosed dasabuvir (250 mg) for 12 wk; weight-based RBV recommended for patients with cirrhosis Daily sofosbuvir (400 mg) plus simeprevir (150 mg) for 12 wk (no cirrhosis) or 24 wk (cirrhosis)
2	Daily sofosbuvir (400 mg) and weight-based RBV for 12 wk (no cirrhosis) or 16 wk (cirrhosis)
3	Daily sofosbuvir (400 mg) and weight-based RBV for 24 wk
4	Daily fixed-dose combination of ledipasvir (90 mg)/sofosbuvir (400 mg) for 12 wk Daily fixed-dose combination of paritaprevir (150 mg)/ritonavir (100 mg)/ombitasvir (25 mg) and weight-based RBV for 12 wk Daily sofosbuvir (400 mg) and weight-based RBV for 24 wk
5	Daily sofosbuvir (400 mg) and weight-based RBV plus weekly PEG IFN for 12 wk
6	Daily ledipasvir (90 mg)/sofosbuvir (400 mg) for 12 wk

AASLD, American Association for the Study of Liver Diseases; HCV, hepatitis C virus; IDSA, Infectious Diseases Society of America; PEG IFN, pegylated interferon; RBV, ribavirin.

*Listed alphabetically—see www.hcvguidelines.org for alternative treatments, treatments in experienced patients, and special populations.

- Case fatality rates are 0.9% to 2.8% in men and 20% in pregnant women, particularly in the third trimester.
- In immunosuppressed patients, particularly solid organ transplants, HEV can cause protracted infection, chronic hepatitis, and cirrhosis.
- Diagnosis is by serologic tests (IgM antibody to HEV) or PCR in blood or stool.
- Treatment: acute hepatitis E is usually self-limited; chronic hepatitis E responds to ribavirin therapy.
- Highly effective vaccines consisting of recombinant capsid proteins have been developed for use in endemic areas. One (Hecolin) has been recently licensed in China.

62 Diagnosis of Human Immunodeficiency Virus Infection

Francesco R. Simonetti, Robin Dewar, and Frank Maldarelli

DEFINITION

- Human immunodeficiency virus (HIV) detection is the cornerstone of the medical and public health response to the HIV epidemic. HIV detection is accurate and sensitive, and precise assays have been designed for three general purposes: patient diagnosis and clinical management, epidemiologic surveillance, and donor screening for blood and tissue products.

EPIDEMIOLOGY

- By the end of 2011, more than 34 million individuals were living with HIV infection throughout the world. In the United States, the percent of individuals ever tested for HIV increased from 36% to 45% in 2000-2011, but the yearly testing rate has remained relatively stable at 9.6% to 10.4% despite the promotion of rapid testing modalities and expansion of testing resources. Although the proportion of people with HIV aware of their status is about 80% in the United States, the United Nations estimates that only 30% of infected individuals worldwide are aware of their status.

MICROBIOLOGY

- The genetic diversity of HIV-1 during early infection period is limited, and it is likely that the majority of individuals are infected with a single variant, with slow, predictable accumulation in genetic diversity reflecting both the intrinsic mutation rate of HIV-1 and strong selection pressure, likely including immune responses. At present, useful tools to detect HIV infection in vivo include viral components (HIV RNA and p24 antigen) and humoral responses (detected by enzyme-linked immunosorbent assay–, Western blot–, and immunofluorescence-based studies).

DIAGNOSIS

- Diagnosis proceeds from history, physical examination, and laboratory studies. Laboratory detection of HIV is a two-step sequential process using a highly sensitive *screening* test followed by a highly specific *confirmatory* assay (see Table 62-1).
- A variety of formats are available, and rapid tests are now U.S. Food and Drug Administration approved for HIV screening and confirmation (see Table 62-2). In many circumstances, it is now possible to screen and confirm HIV infection using rapid tests without having patients return for results.
- HIV testing is undergoing expansion in the United States; Centers for Disease Control and Prevention (CDC) recommendations for opt-out testing for all individuals from 15 to 65 years have been adopted by the U.S. Preventive Services Task Force, and the cost for opt-out testing will be substantially underwritten through the Affordable Care Act.
- In 2014, the CDC issued updated recommendations for the diagnosis of HIV infection (see Table 62-1). Initial tests are fourth-generation antigen/antibody combination assays, and confirmatory tests are HIV-1/HIV-2 antibody differentiation assays, followed by an HIV-1 nucleic acid test if needed.

TABLE 62-1   CDC-Recommended Laboratory HIV Testing Algorithm for Serum or Plasma Specimens*

Step 1: HIV-1/2 antigen/antibody combination immunoassay. If positive, proceed to Step 2.[†]
Step 2: HIV-1/HIV-2 antibody differentiation immunoassay. If negative or indeterminate for HIV-1 and negative for HIV-2, proceed to Step 3.[‡]
Step 3: HIV-1 nucleic acid test (NAT). Positive NAT indicates acute HIV-1 infection.[§]

*This algorithm, starting with the HIV-1/2 antigen/antibody combination immunoassay, should also be used after a reactive result from any rapid HIV test.
[†]No further testing is required for specimens that are nonreactive on the initial immunoassay.
[‡]Reactive results on the initial antigen/antibody combination immunoassay and the HIV-1/HIV-2 antibody differentiation immunoassay should be interpreted as positive for HIV-1 antibodies, HIV-2 antibodies, or, in the case where both HIV-1 and HIV-2 test results are reactive on the antibody differentiation assay, HIV antibodies, undifferentiated.
[§]A negative HIV-1 NAT result and nonreactive or indeterminate HIV-1/HIV-2 antibody differentiation immunoassay result indicates a false-positive result on the initial immunoassay.
CDC, Centers for Disease Control and Prevention; HIV, human immunodeficiency virus.

TABLE 62-2   FDA-Approved Formats for HIV Testing

Source for HIV Testing	FDA-APPROVED TESTING MODALITY*					
	ELISA	Rapid EIA	Western Blot	IFA	p24 Antigen Capture	HIV-1 TMA/HPA
Whole blood	X	X				
Dried blood	X					
Plasma	X	X	X	X	X	X
Serum	X	X	X	X	X	
Oral fluid	X	X	X			
Urine	X		X			
Mini-pools (donor screen)	X					X
Cadaveric serum	X					X

EIA, enzyme immunoassay; ELISA, enzyme-linked immunosorbent assay; FDA, U.S. Food and Drug Administration; HIV, human immunodeficiency virus; IFA, indirect immunofluorescence assay; TMA/HPA, transcription-mediated amplification/hybridization protection assay.
*Names and manufacturers of individual testing kits are available at www.fda.gov.

- No assay or test strategy is perfect, and familiarity with assay limitations is essential to ensure accurate identification of HIV infection.

THERAPY

- HIV diagnosis is essential to introduce specific antiretroviral therapy for treatment of disease and now as part of preexposure prophylaxis strategies.
- Screening tests are necessary, but not sufficient, to introduce therapy for HIV infection, and confirmation of HIV infection is essential before introduction of antiretroviral therapy.
- A nonreactive HIV screening test result has been useful in identifying patients at high risk of HIV infection who may undergo preexposure prophylaxis. Regimens for preexposure prophylaxis are distinct from and less potent than routine combination antiretroviral therapy, and it is essential to evaluate patients carefully for HIV infection.
- Specific guidelines are available for testing for treatment and prophylaxis purposes.

PREVENTION

- Preexposure prophylaxis represents a strategy to treat high-risk individuals with antiretroviral therapy to prevent HIV infection. Careful evaluation to rule out HIV infection is necessary.

General Clinical Manifestations of Human Immunodeficiency Virus Infection (Including Acute Retroviral Syndrome and Oral, Cutaneous, Renal, Ocular, Metabolic, and Cardiac Diseases)

Timothy R. Sterling and Richard E. Chaisson

ACUTE RETROVIRAL SYNDROME

- This syndrome is the initial manifestation of human immunodeficiency virus (HIV) infection.
- One half to two thirds of patients present with an acute "mononucleosis-like" illness (see Table 63-1), often with a truncal exanthem.
- Symptoms generally resolve within 10 to 15 days.

PERSISTENT GENERALIZED LYMPHADENOPATHY

- This disorder occurs in 50% to 70% of HIV-infected individuals and usually affects the cervical, submandibular, occipital, and axillary regions.
- In patients treated with antiretroviral therapy, previously involuted nodes may enlarge.

METABOLIC AND ENDOCRINE ABNORMALITIES

- Hypogonadism, constitutional wasting, lipid abnormalities, insulin resistance, and lipodystrophy have been reported.

ORAL DISEASE

- Oral candidiasis, oral hairy leukoplakia, gingivitis, and periodontitis may occur.

CUTANEOUS DISEASE

- Dermatologic consequences include cutaneous infections (herpes simplex virus, varicella-zoster virus, molluscum contagiosum, scabies, bacillary angiomatosis, and Kaposi sarcoma).

RENAL DISEASE

- Multiple causes of renal disease may afflict patients with HIV infection, as well as a specific HIV-related nephropathy, which includes proteinuria, mildly elevated serum creatinine concentration, reflecting glomerular injury, mesangial proliferation, and tubular degeneration.

CARDIAC DISEASE

- Accelerated atherosclerosis with myocardial infarction is seen in HIV-infected patients who have been treated with antiretroviral therapy and appears to be associated with elevations in proinflammatory cytokines and prothrombotic markers.
- Myocarditis and pericarditis are also found.

IMMUNE RECONSTITUTION SYNDROMES

- Immune reconstitution syndromes are seen after antiretroviral therapy and can involve *Mycobacterium tuberculosis*, *Mycobacterium avium* complex, cytomegalovirus, hepatitis B and C, and other opportunistic infections.

TABLE 63-1 Symptoms and Signs of the Acute Retroviral Syndrome in 209 Patients

SYMPTOM OR SIGN	NO. WITH FINDING	FREQUENCY (%)
Fever	200	96
Adenopathy	154	74
Pharyngitis	146	70
Rash	146	70
Myalgia or arthralgia	112	54
Thrombocytopenia	94	45
Leukopenia	80	38
Diarrhea	67	32
Headache	66	32
Nausea, vomiting	56	27
Elevated aminotransferase levels*	38	21
Hepatosplenomegaly	30	14
Thrush	24	12
Neuropathy	13	6
Encephalopathy	12	6

*Based on 178 subjects.
Modified from Niu MT, Stein DS, Schnittman SM. Primary human immunodeficiency virus type 1 infection: review of pathogenesis and early treatment intervention in human and animal retrovirus infections. *J Infect Dis.* 1993;168:1490-1501.

64 Pulmonary Manifestations of Human Immunodeficiency Virus Infection

Paul E. Sax and Kevin L. Ard

EPIDEMIOLOGY

- Human immunodeficiency virus (HIV) infection increases the risk of infectious and noninfectious respiratory conditions.
- Most complications occur in those not receiving antiretroviral therapy (ART).
- Effective ART has reduced, but not eliminated, the excess risk of pulmonary infections such as *Pneumocystis jirovecii* pneumonia (PCP) and to a lesser extent bacterial pneumonia.
- Noninfectious conditions, such as chronic obstructive pulmonary disease and lung cancer, are assuming greater importance as HIV-infected individuals live longer.

APPROACH TO THE PATIENT

- The differential diagnosis is influenced by the stage of immunosuppression, ART, prophylaxis for opportunistic infections, and the local epidemiology of conditions such as tuberculosis and endemic fungal infections.
- Lower CD4 cell counts increase the risk of all pulmonary infections, including those that also occur at higher CD4 cell counts.
- Findings on chest radiography can help guide the differential diagnosis (see Table 64-1).

PNEUMOCYSTIS JIROVECII PNEUMONIA

- Most cases of PCP occur at CD4 cell counts of fewer than 200 cells/mm^3 in patients not receiving ART.
- Patients with PCP typically report cough and fever of at least several weeks' duration.
- Radiographic findings include diffuse interstitial infiltrates most commonly, but cavities, pneumothoraces, pleural effusions, and normal radiographs can occur.
- Diagnosis relies on identification of the organism in respiratory secretions, often through induced sputum or bronchoalveolar lavage, which is more sensitive.
- Serum $(1{\rightarrow}3)$-β-D-glucan is also highly sensitive for the diagnosis of PCP.

BACTERIAL PNEUMONIA

- *Streptococcus pneumoniae* and *Haemophilus influenzae* are the most commonly isolated pathogens.
- With worsening immunosuppression, pneumonias due to *Staphylococcus aureus*, *Pseudomonas aeruginosa* (especially in the setting of neutropenia), *Nocardia* spp., and *Rhodococcus equi* can occur.

MYCOBACTERIAL PNEUMONIA

- The features of *Mycobacterium tuberculosis* pulmonary infection vary based on the degree of immunosuppression.
- HIV-infected patients with respiratory symptoms who are from tuberculosis-endemic areas or have other risk factors for tuberculosis, who have a positive test for latent tuberculosis without a history of prophylactic therapy, or who have a personal history of tuberculosis

TABLE 64-1 Radiographic Appearance of Pulmonary Diseases in Human Immunodeficiency Virus Infection

Diffuse Interstitial Infiltrates	Cavitary Disease
Pneumocystis jirovecii	Pyogenic bacterial pneumonia from *Pseudomonas*
Mycobacterium tuberculosis, especially with advanced human immunodeficiency virus disease	*aeruginosa, Staphylococcus aureus,* Enterobacteriaceae
Histoplasma capsulatum	*M. tuberculosis*
Coccidioides spp.	*C. neoformans*
Cryptococcus neoformans	*R. equi*
Toxoplasma gondii	*Aspergillus* spp.
Cytomegalovirus	*Nocardia* spp.
Influenza	*Mycobacterium avium* complex
Lymphocytic interstitial pneumonitis	*P. jirovecii*
Abacavir hypersensitivity	**Nodules or Masses**
Focal Consolidation	*M. tuberculosis*
Pyogenic bacterial pneumonia from *Streptococcus pneumoniae, Haemophilus influenzae*	*C. neoformans*
M. tuberculosis	*Aspergillus* spp.
Legionella spp.	*H. capsulatum*
Rhodococcus equi	*Nocardia* spp.
Hilar Adenopathy	Non-Hodgkin's lymphoma
	Kaposi sarcoma
M. tuberculosis	Lung cancer
H. capsulatum	**Normal Radiograph**
Coccidioides spp.	*P. jirovecii*
Non-Hodgkin's or Hodgkin's lymphoma	*M. tuberculosis*
Mycobacterium avium complex	

without documentation of appropriate treatment should be placed in negative air pressure rooms until the diagnosis of pulmonary tuberculosis is excluded.
- Sputum nucleic acid amplification tests can hasten diagnosis, particularly in smear-negative cases.

FUNGAL PNEUMONIA
- Fungal pneumonia tends to occur with CD4 cell count fewer than 100 cells/mm^3, often as a component of disseminated fungal infection (cryptococcosis, histoplasmosis, coccidioidomycosis, blastomycosis).
- Histoplasmosis and coccidioidomycosis are important causes of pneumonia in those who have resided in or traveled to endemic areas; *Blastomyces* rarely causes pulmonary infection in patients with HIV.
- Pulmonary aspergillosis is usually in severely immunocompromised individuals with neutropenia or corticosteroid use.

VIRAL PNEUMONIA
- During the influenza season, influenza is the most common diagnosis in HIV-infected patients with fever and respiratory symptoms, although adenovirus, respiratory syncytial virus, and parainfluenza virus can cause a similar presentation.

NONINFECTIOUS RESPIRATORY DISORDERS
- Pulmonary Kaposi sarcoma usually occurs with cutaneous or mucosal disease.
- Pulmonary lymphoma causes nodules, masses, or pleural effusions and is usually diagnosed via video-assisted thorascopic surgery (VATS).
- Lymphocytic interstitial pneumonitis, a rare cause of interstitial infiltrates, is typically diagnosed on biopsy. It primarily occurs in children but may develop in adults, particularly those with higher CD4 counts than are seen with many opportunistic infections.

65 Gastrointestinal, Hepatobiliary, and Pancreatic Manifestations of Human Immunodeficiency Virus Infection

Charles Haines and Mark S. Sulkowski

DEFINITION

- Gastrointestinal and hepatobiliary diseases are a common cause of morbidity in persons with human immunodeficiency virus (HIV) infection and often result from both host factors and exposures.

DISORDERS OF THE ESOPHAGUS

- Disorders of the esophagus typically manifest as dysphagia or odynophagia and affect up to one third of patients with acquired immunodeficiency syndrome (AIDS).
- Infectious causes include *Candida*, cytomegalovirus (CMV), herpes simplex virus, varicella-zoster virus, mycobacteria, *Histoplasma,* and *Pneumocystis jirovecii.*
- Noninfectious causes include reflux esophagitis and pill esophagitis.
- Malignant causes include esophageal carcinoma, lymphoma, and Kaposi sarcoma.
- Presumptive diagnoses can often be made with a careful history and physical examination.
- Upper endoscopy with biopsy of lesions is highly sensitive in many cases.

DISORDERS OF THE STOMACH

- Gastric disorders can result from opportunistic infections but more commonly are not related to HIV-induced immunosuppression.
- *Helicobacter pylori,* CMV, and Kaposi sarcoma are common causes of gastric disorders.
- Upper endoscopy and gastric biopsies are often needed for definitive diagnosis.

DISORDERS OF THE LIVER

- Because of shared modes of transmission, hepatitis caused by acute or chronic infection with hepatitis B and C viruses is common.
- Newly available directly acting antivirals against hepatitis C virus (HCV) are recommended for treatment of patients coinfected with HIV and HCV.
- Drug-induced liver injury has been observed with some antiretroviral agents and other drugs used in persons with HIV infection.

DISORDERS OF THE BILIARY TREE, GALLBLADDER, AND PANCREAS

- Acalculous cholecystitis and cholangitis are found primarily in advanced AIDS and may involve the pancreas.
- CMV, *Cryptosporidium,* and microsporidia are most commonly implicated.
- AIDS-related acalculous cholecystitis and cholangitis are rare in settings where antiretroviral therapy (ART) is widely used, and non–AIDS-related gallbladder and biliary diseases may be more common in such settings.
- Endoscopic retrograde cholangiopancreatography can be used for both diagnosis and treatment.
- Didanosine and systemic pentamidine can cause pancreatitis.

TABLE 65-1 Causes of Lower Gastrointestinal Tract Disease in Patients with Human Immunodeficiency Virus

Causes of Enterocolitis

Bacteria

Campylobacter jejuni and other spp.
Salmonella spp.
Shigella flexneri
Aeromonas hydrophila
Plesiomonas shigelloides
Yersinia enterocolitica
Vibrio spp.
Mycobacterium avium complex
Mycobacterium tuberculosis
Escherichia coli (enterotoxigenic, enteroadherent)
Bacterial overgrowth
Clostridium difficile (toxin)

Parasites

Cryptosporidium parvum
Microsporidia (Enterocytozoon bieneusi, Septata intestinalis)
Cystoisospora belli
Entamoeba histolytica
Giardia lamblia
Cyclospora cayetanensis

Viruses

Cytomegalovirus
Adenovirus
Calicivirus
Astrovirus
Picobirnavirus
Human immunodeficiency virus

Fungi

Histoplasma capsulatum

Causes of Proctitis

Bacteria

Chlamydia trachomatis
Neisseria gonorrhoeae
Treponema pallidum

Viruses

Herpes simplex
Cytomegalovirus

- Pancreatic infections with mycobacteria, *Cryptococcus, Toxoplasma gondii, P. jirovecii,* and CMV have been described, often in disseminated disease.

DISORDERS OF THE SMALL AND LARGE INTESTINE

- Causes of enterocolitis include bacterial, protozoal, and viral pathogens (see Table 65-1).
- *Clostridium difficile* is the most common cause of diarrhea in HIV-infected patients.
- CMV, *Cryptosporidium,* and *Mycobacterium avium* complex infections are more common in the setting of severe immunocompromise.
- HIV-associated enteropathy causes culture-negative diarrhea and may improve with ART. Human papillomavirus (HPV) and high-grade anal dysplasia are elevated in HIV, but the utility of anal HPV screening is not clear.

Chapter 65 Gastrointestinal, Hepatobiliary, and Pancreatic Manifestations of Human Immunodeficiency Virus Infection

66 Neurologic Diseases Caused by Human Immunodeficiency Virus Type 1 and Opportunistic Infections

Omar K. Siddiqi and Igor J. Koralnik

DEFINITION

- Human immunodeficiency virus (HIV) and associated infections can adversely affect any aspect of the central and peripheral nervous system.

EPIDEMIOLOGY

- Ten percent of HIV-positive patients initially present with neurologic disease.
- Thirty to fifty percent of HIV-positive patients have neurologic complications.
- Eighty percent of HIV-positive patients have nervous system involvement at autopsy.

COGNITIVE MANIFESTATIONS

- HIV-associated neurocognitive disorder occurs in 15% of patients with AIDS and can be the first manifestation of disease in 3% to 10% of patients.

CENTRAL NERVOUS SYSTEM (CNS) MASS LESIONS

- Toxoplasmosis is the most frequent cerebral mass lesion. Incidence depends on the seropositivity of the population. Empirical treatment with pyrimethamine and sulfadiazine is useful when clinical and radiologic findings are consistent with the diagnosis.
- Primary CNS lymphoma is the most common HIV-associated brain malignancy and is associated with Epstein-Barr virus infection.
- Progressive multifocal leukoencephalopathy is caused by JC polyomavirus, which induces lytic infection of oligodendrocytes causing multifocal CNS demyelination.

SPINAL CORD

- Vacuolar myelopathy is present at autopsy in 17% to 46% of patients with acquired immunodeficiency syndrome.
- Presenting symptoms are gait disturbance, weakness, sensory changes, and urinary dysfunction.
- Diagnosis is one of exclusion.
- Etiology is unclear.

PERIPHERAL NERVOUS SYSTEM

- HIV-associated distal sensory polyneuropathy is the most common peripheral neuropathy seen in HIV. Symmetrical paresthesia, numbness, and painful dysesthesia of the lower extremities can occur.
- Nucleoside neuropathy is associated with nucleoside analogue reverse-transcriptase inhibitors zalcitabine, didanosine, and stavudine.
- Clinical and electrophysiologic manifestations are indistinguishable from DSNP. Symptoms can improve upon discontinuation of offending medication.

67 Pediatric Human Immunodeficiency Virus Infection

Geoffrey A. Weinberg and George K. Siberry

EPIDEMIOLOGY

- A remarkable decline in U.S. pediatric human immunodeficiency virus (HIV) infection has occurred as a result of both the majority of currently infected children surviving into young adulthood and the tremendous success in interrupting new mother-to-child transmission (MTCT). Such success may be achieved globally wherever effective HIV screening and therapy for pregnant women is accomplished.
- A small influx of HIV-infected immigrants, refugees, and adoptees, as well as uncommon domestic MTCT, will continue to contribute to a minor but definite presence of pediatric HIV infection in the United States.
- An alarming increase in adolescent acquisition of HIV infection is occurring among young men who have sex with men, especially African-American and Hispanic men.

ELIMINATION OF NEW PEDIATRIC HIV INFECTION IN THE UNITED STATES

- Prevention of pediatric HIV infection critically depends on prevention of HIV MTCT, which in turn depends on primary prevention of HIV infection in women, universal HIV testing of pregnant women to identify those who are HIV infected, and appropriate antiretroviral therapy in HIV-infected women and their infants.
- Each episode of perinatal HIV infection in the United States should be viewed as a sentinel public health event indicating a woman whose HIV infection was either undiagnosed before or during pregnancy or a woman with a known diagnosis who did not receive adequate prenatal care including appropriate interventions to prevent MTCT.
- Prevention of adolescent HIV infection involves similar strategies to those used for adults (safer sex, avoidance of intravenous or injection drug use) but with special attention to the adolescent's unique developmental and biopsychosocial challenges. Additional challenges may be posed by interrupted health insurance, homelessness, and stigma among young men who have sex with men.

THERAPY FOR AGING HIV-INFECTED YOUTH

- Disclosure of the diagnosis of perinatal HIV infection to the aging child requires discussion and planning and is a process that may take place over months to years based on several factors, including the developmental level of the child and the parent's or caretaker's readiness to disclose. Disclosure is best accomplished by early adolescence to more fully engage youth in their own care, preferably before the age of sexual debut.
- Adherence with medical care may suffer during adolescence because of issues revolving around psychosocial developmental, confidentiality, peer pressure, and socioeconomic factors. This contributes to the substantial presence of antiretroviral resistance of HIV strains in aging adolescents.

- Transition from the pediatric care model to the adult care model is a multifaceted process that requires time and planning to keep the aging adolescent successfully engaged in care.
- Complications of long-standing perinatal HIV infection and its therapy among maturing youth include impaired growth and bone mineral accrual, possibly increased cardiovascular risk factors, increased incidence of behavioral and psychiatric disorders, and increased risk for cervical dysplasia and preterm birth among young women.

68 Antiretroviral Therapy for Human Immunodeficiency Virus Infection

Athe M. N. Tsibris and Martin S. Hirsch

DEFINITION

- Treatment of human immunodeficiency virus (HIV) infection uses a combination of at least three drugs to arrest virus replication and disease progression.

THERAPY CHOICES

- Antiretroviral therapy targets and inhibits HIV-specific enzymes.
  - Nucleoside and nucleotide reverse-transcriptase inhibitors (see Table 68-1)
  - Non-nucleoside reverse-transcriptase inhibitors (see Table 68-2)
  - Protease inhibitors (see Table 68-3)
  - Integrase inhibitor (see Table 68-4)
- CCR5 antagonists are the only drug class to target a host protein.
  - Entry inhibitors (see Table 68-4)

THERAPY STRATEGIES

- Preferred regimens will use two nucleoside reverse-transcriptase inhibitors in combination with either a non-nucleoside reverse-transcriptase inhibitor, a protease inhibitor, or an integrase strand transfer inhibitor.

THERAPY GOALS

- The goal of antiretroviral therapy, in all patients, is durable suppression of virus load to levels undetectable in commercial assays.

Part I Major Clinical Syndromes

TABLE 68-1 Approved Nucleoside and Nucleotide Reverse-Transcriptase Inhibitors

AGENT	TRADE NAME	ORAL BIOAVAILABILITY (%)	SERUM HALF-LIFE (hr)	INTRACELLULAR HALF-LIFE OF TRIPHOSPHATE (hr)	ELIMINATION	ADULT DOSE	DOSAGE FORMS
Zidovudine	Retrovir	64	1.1	3-4	Hepatic glucuronidation Renal excretion	300 mg PO q12h or 200 mg PO q8h 2 mg/kg IV loading dose, followed by 1 mg/kg/hr until umbilical cord is clamped	300-mg tablets 100-mg capsules 50-mg/5 mL syrup 10-mg/mL solution for IV infusion
Didanosine	Videx Videx EC	40 fasted	1.5	25-40	Cellular metabolism	≥60 kg: 400 mg PO qd 25 kg < weight < 60 kg: 250 mg PO qd	125-, 200-, 250-, and 400-mg capsules 2- and 4-g powder packets (makes 10-mg/mL solution)
Stavudine	Zerit	86	1.1	3	Renal excretion	≥60 kg: capsules or solution, 40 mg PO q12h; <60 kg: capsules or solution, 30 mg PO q12h	15-, 20-, 30-, and 40-mg capsules 1-mg/mL oral solution
Lamivudine	Epivir	86	2.5	12-18	Renal excretion	300 mg PO qd or 150 mg PO q12h	150- and 300-mg tablets 10-mg/mL solution
Abacavir	Ziagen	83	1.5	3.3	Hepatic glucuronidation and carboxylation	600 mg PO qd or 300 mg PO q12h	300-mg tablets 20-mg/mL solution
Tenofovir	Viread	39 with meal	12-14	>11*	Renal excretion	300 mg PO qd	150-, 200-, 250-, and 300-mg tablet Oral powder 40 mg/g
Emtricitabine	Emtriva	93	8-10	>24	Renal excretion	200 mg PO qd solution, 240 mg PO qd	200-mg capsules 10-mg/mL solution
Zidovudine + lamivudine	Combivir†					One tablet PO q12h	300-mg zidovudine/150-mg lamivudine tablets

TABLE 68-1   Approved Nucleoside and Nucleotide Reverse-Transcriptase Inhibitors—cont'd

AGENT	TRADE NAME	ORAL BIOAVAILABILITY (%)	SERUM HALF-LIFE (hr)	INTRACELLULAR HALF-LIFE OF TRIPHOSPHATE (hr)	ELIMINATION	ADULT DOSE	DOSAGE FORMS
Abacavir + lamivudine	Epzicom[†] Kivexa					One tablet PO qd	Abacavir 600-mg/ lamivudine 300-mg tablet
Tenofovir + emtricitabine	Truvada[†]					One tablet PO qd	Tenofovir 300-mg/ emtricitabine 200-mg tablet
Zidovudine + lamivudine + abacavir	Trizivir[†]					One tablet PO q12h	300-mg zidovudine/ 150-mg lamivudine/300-mg abacavir tablets
Tenofovir + emtricitabine + efavirenz	Atripla[†]					One tablet PO qd on an empty stomach	Tenofovir 300-mg/ emtricitabine 200-mg/efavirenz 600-mg tablet
Tenofovir + emtricitabine + rilpivirine	Complera Eviplera[†]					One tablet PO qd with a meal	Tenofovir 300-mg/ emtricitabine 200-mg/rilpivirine 27.5-mg tablet
Tenofovir + emtricitabine + elvitegravir + cobicistat	Stribild[†]					One tablet PO qd with food	Tenofovir 300-mg/ emtricitabine 200-mg/elvitegravir 150-mg/cobicistat 150-mg tablet
Abacavir + lamivudine + dolutegravir	Triumeq[†]					One tablet PO qd with or without food	Abacavir 600-mg/ lamivudine 300-mg/ dolutegravir 50-mg tablet

*Diphosphate form in activated cells.
[†]Pharmacokinetic properties are similar to those of the component drugs used separately.

TABLE 68-2　Approved Non-Nucleoside Reverse-Transcriptase Inhibitors

AGENT	TRADE NAME	ORAL BIOAVAILABILITY (%)	SERUM HALF-LIFE (hr)	ELIMINATION	ADULT DOSE	DOSAGE FORMS
Nevirapine	Viramune	>90	45 after first dose 25-30 after 2 wk	Hepatic cytochrome P-450, CYP3A4 and CYP2B6	200 mg PO qd for 14 days, then, if no rash develops, 200 mg PO q12h or 400 mg XR PO qd	200-mg tablets 50 mg/5-mL solution
Delavirdine	Rescriptor	85	5.8	Hepatic cytochrome P-450, CYP3A4	400 mg PO q8h	100- and 200-mg tablets
Efavirenz	Sustiva Stocrin	40-45	40-55	Hepatic cytochrome P-450, CYP2B6, and CYP3A4	600 mg PO qd	50- and 200-mg capsules 600-mg tablet
Etravirine	Intelence	Unknown	41 ± 20	Hepatic cytochrome P-450, CYP3A4, 2C9, and 2C19	200 mg PO q12h after meals	25-, 100-, and 200-mg tablets
Rilpivirine	Edurant	Unknown	50	Hepatic cytochrome P-450, CYP3A	25 mg PO qd with a meal	25-mg tablet

TABLE 68-3　Approved Protease Inhibitors

AGENT	TRADE NAME	ORAL BIOAVAILABILITY (%)	SERUM HALF-LIFE (hr)	ELIMINATION	ADULT DOSE*	DOSAGE FORMS
Saquinavir	Invirase	4	1-2	Hepatic and intestinal cytochrome P-450, CYP3A4	1000 mg PO q12h with ritonavir 100 mg PO q12h	200-mg capsules 500-mg tablets
Ritonavir	Norvir	70	3-5	Hepatic cytochrome P-450, CYP3A4, and 2D6	300 mg PO q12h with escalation over 6-9 days to 600 mg PO q12h; rarely used as single agent	100-mg capsules and tablets 80 mg/mL solution
Indinavir	Crixivan	60-65	1.8	Hepatic cytochrome P-450, CYP3A4	800 mg PO q8h Drink $\geq$1.5L of water daily	200- and 400-mg capsules

TABLE 68-3 Approved Protease Inhibitors—cont'd

AGENT	TRADE NAME	ORAL BIOAVAILABILITY (%)	SERUM HALF-LIFE (hr)	ELIMINATION	ADULT DOSE*	DOSAGE FORMS
Nelfinavir	Viracept	70-80	3.5-5	Hepatic cytochrome P-450, CYP2C19, CYP3A4, and CYP2D6	1250 mg PO q12h or 750 mg PO q8h	250- and 625-mg tablets 50-mg/g powder
Fosamprenavir	Lexiva Telzir	—	7-11	Hepatic cytochrome P-450, CYP3A4 Biliary excretion	Treatment-naïve: 1400 mg PO q12h without food, or 1400 mg PO qd with ritonavir 200 mg PO qd, or 1400 mg PO qd with ritonavir 100 mg PO qd, or 700 mg PO q12h with ritonavir 100 mg PO q12h PI-experienced: 700 mg PO q12h with ritonavir 100 mg PO q12h	700-mg tablets 50-mg/mL suspension
Lopinavir + ritonavir	Kaletra	—	5-6	Hepatic cytochrome P-450, CYP3A4	Two tablets PO q12h	Lopinavir/ ritonavir 100-mg/ 25-mg and 200-mg/50-mg tablets Lopinavir/ ritonavir 80-mg/ 20-mg per mL solution
Atazanavir	Reyataz	—	7	Hepatic cytochrome P-450, CYP3A4	Treatment-naïve: 400 mg PO qd with food or 300 mg PO qd with ritonavir 100 mg PO qd with food. Treatment-experienced or with tenofovir: 300 mg PO qd with ritonavir 100 mg PO qd	100-, 150-, 200-, and 300-mg capsules
Tipranavir	Aptivus	—	5-6	Hepatic cytochrome P-450, CYP3A4	500 mg PO q12h with ritonavir 200 mg PO q12h	250-mg capsules 100-mg/mL solution
Darunavir	Prezista	—	15 (with ritonavir)	Hepatic cytochrome P-450, CYP3A4	Treatment-naïve: 800 mg PO qd with ritonavir 100 mg qd and with food. Treatment-experienced: 800 mg PO qd with ritonavir 100 mg PO qd and with food, or 600 mg PO q12h with ritonavir 100 mg PO q12h and with food	75-, 150-, 400-, 600-, and 800-mg tablets 100-mg/mL suspension

PI, protease inhibitor.
*Consult product monograph for appropriate dose when low-dose ritonavir is used for pharmacokinetic enhancement.

Part I Major Clinical Syndromes

TABLE 68-4	Approved Entry Inhibitors and Integrase Inhibitor					
AGENT	TRADE NAME	BIOAVAILABILITY (%)	SERUM HALF-LIFE (hr)	ELIMINATION	ADULT DOSE*	AVAILABILITY
Enfuvirtide	Fuzeon	84	3.8	Catabolism to constituent amino acids	90 mg SC q12h	108-mg single-use vials, for reconstitution with 1.1 mL sterile water
Maraviroc	Selzentry Celsentri	33	14-18	Hepatic cytochrome P-450, CYP3A	300 mg PO q12h	150- and 300-mg tablets
Raltegravir	Isentress	Not established	9	UGT1A1-mediated glucuronidation	400 mg PO q12h	400-mg tablet Chewable 25- and 100-mg tablets
Dolutegravir	Tivicay	Not established	14	UGT1A1-mediated glucuronidation Hepatic cytochrome P-450, CYP3A	Treatment- or INSTI-naïve: 50 mg PO qd INSTI-experienced or when co-administered with UGT1A/CYP3A inducers: 50 mg PO bid	50-mg tablet

INSTI, integrase strand transfer inhibitor.
*Elvitegravir is not available as a single drug.

Management of Opportunistic Infections Associated with Human Immunodeficiency Virus Infection

Henry Masur

DEFINITION

- Acquired immunodeficiency syndrome (AIDS)-related opportunistic infections are defined as those infections that occur with increased frequency or severity in patients with human immunodeficiency virus (HIV) infection or AIDS.

EPIDEMIOLOGY

- The incidence of HIV-related opportunistic infections depends on the degree of immunosuppression and environmental exposure.
- The occurrence of specific infections in some cases is due to primary infection; in other cases, disease is the result of reactivation of latent infection.

MICROBIOLOGY

- The constellation of infections that characterize AIDS is unique: *Pneumocystis* pneumonia, *Toxoplasma* encephalitis, cytomegaloviral retinitis, pneumococcal pneumonia, disseminated *Mycobacterium avium* complex, cryptosporidiosis, cryptococcal meningitis, and *Mycobacterium tuberculosis* infection. The occurrence of these infections individually or in a cluster should prompt consideration of underlying HIV infection/AIDS in any patient without a clear predisposing immunodeficiency.
- The organisms that cause HIV-related opportunistic infections include bacteria, fungi, viruses, and protozoa. Some are transmitted person to person, whereas others are present in certain environmental niches.

DIAGNOSIS

- Given the broad range of pathogens that can cause infectious syndromes in patients with HIV infection/AIDS, and the potential toxicities of therapeutic agents, specific microbiologic diagnoses should be established when possible. AIDS-related opportunistic infections are diagnosed by a wide variety of techniques, including bacterial and fungal and viral culture, serum or body fluid antigen assays or polymerase chain reaction assays, colorimetric and immunofluorescent stain of secretions or tissue, and histology.

THERAPY

- There are specific agents that can successfully treat most HIV-related opportunistic infections (see Table 69-1). Prognosis depends on the severity of the acute illness as well as prognosis for comorbidities and availability of effective and well-tolerated therapies. For some HIV-related opportunistic infections, such as cryptosporidiosis, microsporidiosis, and JC virus encephalitis, there is no effective specific therapy; clinical response depends on improving immune response by initiating effective antiretroviral therapy.

PREVENTION

- Because patients with HIV infection have an extraordinarily high rate of opportunistic infections, and because these opportunistic infections characteristically recur unless patients either are reconstituted with antiretroviral therapy (ART) or administered chemoprophylaxis, both ART and chemoprophylaxis are both important preventive strategies (see Table 69-2). For some infections such as *Pneumocystis* pneumonia, *Toxoplasma* encephalitis, and disseminated *Mycobacterium avium* complex, primary prevention is effective, safe, and well tolerated and should be part of standard patient management. Immunization is also an important part of routine infection prevention strategy.

• Recommendations for discontinuing or restarting prophylactic medications are available.

TABLE 69-1 Treatment of AIDS-Associated Opportunistic Infections

OPPORTUNISTIC INFECTION	PREFERRED THERAPY	ALTERNATIVE THERAPY	OTHER COMMENTS
Pneumocystis pneumonia (PCP)	Patients who develop PCP despite TMP-SMX prophylaxis can usually be treated with standard doses of TMP-SMX. Duration of PCP treatment: 21 days		Indications for adjunctive corticosteroids: PaO$_2$ <70 mm Hg at room air, *or* Alveolar-arterial O$_2$ gradient >35 mm Hg Prednisone doses (beginning as early as possible and within 72 hr of PCP therapy):
	For moderate-to-severe PCP: TMP-SMX: (TMP 15-20 mg and SMX 75-100 mg)/day IV given q6h or q8h; may switch to PO after clinical improvement	For moderate-to-severe PCP: Pentamidine 4 mg/kg IV daily infused over ≥60 min; can reduce dose to 3 mg/kg IV daily because of toxicities, *or* Primaquine 30 mg (base) PO daily + clindamycin 600 mg q6h IV, *or* 900 mg IV q8h, *or* clindamycin 300 mg PO q6h, *or* 450 mg PO q8h	Days 1-5: 40 mg PO bid Days 6-10: 40 mg PO daily Days 11-21: 20 mg PO daily IV methylprednisolone can be administered as 75% of prednisone dose. Benefit of corticosteroid if started after 72 hr of treatment is unknown, but some clinicians will use it for moderate-to-severe PCP.
	For mild-to-moderate PCP: TMP-SMX: (TMP 15-20 mg and SMX 75-100 mg)/kg/day, given PO in three divided doses, *or* TMP-SMX: (160 mg/800 mg or DS) 2 tablets PO tid	For mild-to-moderate PCP: Dapsone 100 mg PO daily + TMP 5 mg/kg PO tid, *or* Primaquine 30 mg (base) PO daily + clindamycin 300 mg PO q6h, *or* 450 mg PO q8h, *or* Atovaquone 750 mg PO bid with food	Whenever possible, patients should be tested for G6PD before use of dapsone or primaquine. Alternative therapy should be used in patients found to have G6PD deficiency. Patients who are receiving pyrimethamine-sulfadiazine for treatment or suppression of toxoplasmosis do not require additional PCP prophylaxis.
	Secondary prophylaxis, after completion of PCP treatment: TMP-SMX DS: 1 tablet PO daily *or* TMP-SMX (80 mg/400 mg or SS): 1 tablet PO daily	Secondary prophylaxis, after completion of PCP treatment: TMP-SMX DS: 1 tablet PO three times a week, *or* Dapsone 100 mg PO daily, *or* Dapsone 50 mg PO daily + pyrimethamine 50 mg + leucovorin 25 mg PO weekly, *or* Dapsone 200 mg + pyrimethamine 75 mg + leucovorin 25 mg PO weekly, *or* Aerosolized pentamidine 300 mg monthly via Respirgard II nebulizer, *or* Atovaquone 1500 mg PO daily, *or* Atovaquone 1500 mg + pyrimethamine 25 mg + leucovorin 10 mg PO daily	If TMP-SMX is discontinued because of a mild adverse reaction, reinstitution should be considered after the reaction resolves. The dose can be increased gradually (desensitization), reduced, or the frequency modified. TMP-SMX should be permanently discontinued in patients with possible or definite Stevens-Johnson syndrome or toxic epidermal necrosis.

TABLE 69-1 Treatment of AIDS-Associated Opportunistic Infections—cont'd

OPPORTUNISTIC INFECTION	PREFERRED THERAPY	ALTERNATIVE THERAPY	OTHER COMMENTS
Toxoplasma gondii encephalitis	Treatment of acute infection: Pyrimethamine 200 mg PO 1 time, followed by weight-based therapy: If <60 kg, pyrimethamine 50 mg PO once daily + sulfadiazine 1000 mg PO q6h + leucovorin 10-25 mg PO once daily If ≥60 kg, pyrimethamine 75 mg PO once daily + sulfadiazine 1500 mg PO q6h + leucovorin 10-25 mg PO once daily Leucovorin dose can be increased to 50 mg daily or bid. Duration for acute therapy: At least 6 wk; longer duration if clinical or radiologic disease is extensive or response is incomplete at 6 wk Chronic maintenance therapy: Pyrimethamine 25-50 mg PO daily + sulfadiazine 2000-4000 mg PO daily (in two to four divided doses) + leucovorin 10-25 mg PO daily	Treatment of acute infection: Pyrimethamine (leucovorin)* + clindamycin 600 mg IV or PO q6h, *or* TMP-SMX (TMP 5 mg/kg and SMX 25 mg/kg) IV or PO bid, *or* Atovaquone 1500 mg PO bid with food + pyrimethamine (leucovorin), *or* Atovaquone 1500 mg PO bid with food + sulfadiazine 1000-1500 mg PO q6h (weight-based dosing, as in preferred therapy), *or* Atovaquone 1500 mg PO bid with food, *or* Pyrimethamine (leucovorin)* + azithromycin 900-1200 mg PO daily Chronic maintenance therapy: Clindamycin 600 mg PO q8h + (pyrimethamine 25-50 mg + leucovorin 10-25 mg) PO daily, *or* TMP-SMX DS 1 tablet bid, *or* Atovaquone 750-1500 mg PO bid + (pyrimethamine 25 mg + leucovorin 10 mg) PO daily, *or* Atovaquone 750-1500 mg PO bid + sulfadiazine 2000-4000 mg PO daily (in two to four divided doses), *or* Atovaquone 750-1500 mg PO bid with food	Adjunctive corticosteroids (e.g., dexamethasone) should only be administered when clinically indicated to treat mass effect associated with focal lesions or associated edema; discontinue as soon as clinically feasible. Anticonvulsants should be administered to patients with a history of seizures and continued through acute treatment but should not be used as seizure prophylaxis. If clindamycin is used in place of sulfadiazine, additional therapy must be added to prevent PCP.

Continued

Part I Major Clinical Syndromes

TABLE 69-1 Treatment of AIDS-Associated Opportunistic Infections—cont'd

OPPORTUNISTIC INFECTION	PREFERRED THERAPY	ALTERNATIVE THERAPY	OTHER COMMENTS
Mycobacterium tuberculosis disease	After collecting specimen for culture and molecular diagnostic tests, empirical TB treatment should be started in individuals with clinical and radiographic presentation suggestive of TB. *Initial phase (2 mo, given daily, 5-7 times/wk by DOT):* INH + [RIF or RFB] + PZA + EMB *Continuation phase:* INH + (RIF or RFB) daily (5-7 times/wk) or three times a week *Total duration of therapy (for drug-susceptible TB):* Pulmonary TB: 6 mo Pulmonary TB and culture positive after 2 mo of TB treatment: 9 mo Extrapulmonary TB with CNS infection: 9-12 mo Extrapulmonary TB with bone or joint involvement: 6 to 9 mo Extrapulmonary TB in other sites: 6 mo Total duration of therapy should be based on number of doses received, not on calendar time.	Treatment of drug-resistant TB Resistant to INH: (RIF or RFB) + EMB + PZA + (moxifloxacin or levofloxacin) for 2 mo; followed by (RIF or RFB) + EMB + (moxifloxacin or levofloxacin) for 7 mo *Resistant to rifamycins ± other drugs:* Regimen and duration of treatment should be individualized based on resistance pattern, clinical and microbiologic responses, and in close consultation with experienced specialists.	Adjunctive corticosteroid improves survival for TB meningitis and pericarditis. RIF is *not* recommended for patients receiving HIV PI because of its induction of PI metabolism. RFB is a less potent CYP3A4 inducer than RIF and is preferred in patients receiving PIs. Once-weekly rifapentine can result in development of rifamycin resistance in HIV-infected patients and is *not* recommended. Therapeutic drug monitoring should be considered in patients receiving rifamycin and interacting ART. Paradoxical IRIS that is not severe can be treated with NSAIDs without a change in TB or HIV therapy. For severe IRIS reaction, consider prednisone and taper over 4 wk based on clinical symptoms. For example: *If receiving RIF:* prednisone 1.5 mg/kg/day for 2 wk, then 0.75 mg/kg/day for 2 wk *If receiving RFB:* prednisone 1.0 mg/kg/day for 2 wk, then 0.5 mg/kg/day for 2 wk A more gradual tapering schedule over a few months may be necessary for some patients.
Disseminated *Mycobacterium avium* complex (MAC) disease	At least two drugs as initial therapy with: Clarithromycin 500 mg PO bid + ethambutol 15 mg/kg PO daily, *or* Azithromycin 500-600 mg + ethambutol 15 mg/kg PO daily if drug interaction or intolerance precludes the use of clarithromycin *Duration:* At least 12 mo of therapy, can discontinue if no signs and symptoms of MAC disease and sustained (>6 mo) CD4 count >100 cells/mm³ in response to ART	Addition of a third or fourth drug should be considered for patients with advanced immunosuppression (CD4 counts <50 cells/mm³), high mycobacterial loads (>2 log CFU/mL of blood), or in the absence of effective ART. Third or fourth drug options may include: RFB 300 mg PO daily (dosage adjustment may be necessary based on drug interactions), Amikacin 10-15 mg/kg IV daily or streptomycin 1 g IV or IM daily, *or* Moxifloxacin 400 mg PO daily or levofloxacin 500 mg PO daily	Testing of susceptibility to clarithromycin and azithromycin is recommended. NSAIDs can be used for patients who experience moderate to severe symptoms attributed to IRIS. If IRIS symptoms persist, short-term (4-8 wk) systemic corticosteroids (equivalent to 20-40 mg prednisone) can be used.

TABLE 69-1 Treatment of AIDS-Associated Opportunistic Infections—cont'd

OPPORTUNISTIC INFECTION	PREFERRED THERAPY	ALTERNATIVE THERAPY	OTHER COMMENTS
Bacterial respiratory diseases *(with focus on pneumonia)*	Empirical antibiotic therapy should be initiated promptly for patients presenting with clinical and radiographic evidence consistent with bacterial pneumonia. The recommendations listed are suggested empirical therapy. The regimen should be modified as needed once microbiologic results are available.		Fluoroquinolones should be used with caution in patients in whom TB is suspected but is not being treated. Empirical therapy with a macrolide alone is not routinely recommended, because of increasing pneumococcal resistance. Patients receiving a macrolide for MAC prophylaxis should not receive macrolide monotherapy for empirical treatment of bacterial pneumonia. For patients begun on IV antibiotic therapy, switching to PO should be considered when they are clinically improved and able to tolerate oral medications. Chemoprophylaxis can be considered for patients with frequent recurrences of serious bacterial pneumonia. Clinicians should be cautious about using antibiotics to prevent recurrences because of the potential for developing drug resistance and drug toxicities.
	Empirical outpatient therapy: A PO β-lactam + a PO macrolide (azithromycin or clarithromycin) Preferred β-lactams: High-dose amoxicillin or amoxicillin/clavulanate Alternative β-lactams: Cefpodoxime or cefuroxime, or For penicillin-allergic patients: Levofloxacin 750 mg PO once daily, or moxifloxacin 400 mg PO once daily Duration: 7-10 days (a minimum of 5 days). Patients should be afebrile for 48-72 hr and clinically stable before stopping antibiotics.	Empirical outpatient therapy: A PO β-lactam + PO doxycycline Preferred β-lactams: High-dose amoxicillin or amoxicillin-clavulanate Alternative β-lactams: Cefpodoxime or cefuroxime	
	Empirical therapy for non-ICU hospitalized patients: An IV β-lactam + a macrolide (azithromycin or clarithromycin) Preferred β-lactams: ceftriaxone, cefotaxime, or ampicillin-sulbactam For penicillin-allergic patients: Levofloxacin, 750 mg IV once daily, or moxifloxacin, 400 mg IV once daily	Empirical therapy for non-ICU hospitalized patients: An IV β-lactam + doxycycline	
	Empirical therapy for ICU patients: An IV β-lactam + IV azithromycin, or An IV β-lactam + (levofloxacin 750 mg IV once daily or moxifloxacin 400 mg IV once daily) Preferred β-lactams: Ceftriaxone, cefotaxime, or ampicillin-sulbactam	Empirical therapy for ICU patients: For penicillin-allergic patients: Aztreonam IV + (levofloxacin 750 mg IV once daily or moxifloxacin 400 mg IV once daily)	

Continued

TABLE 69-1 Treatment of AIDS-Associated Opportunistic Infections—cont'd

OPPORTUNISTIC INFECTION	PREFERRED THERAPY	ALTERNATIVE THERAPY	OTHER COMMENTS
	Empirical therapy for patients at risk for _Pseudomonas_ pneumonia: An IV antipneumococcal, antipseudomonal β-lactam + (ciprofloxacin 400 mg IV q8-12h or levofloxacin 750 mg IV once daily) _Preferred β-lactams:_ Piperacillin-tazobactam, cefepime, imipenem, or meropenem	Empirical therapy for patients at risk for _Pseudomonas_ pneumonia: An IV antipneumococcal, antipseudomonal β-lactam + an aminoglycoside + azithromycin, or Above β-lactam + an aminoglycoside + (levofloxacin 750 mg IV once daily or moxifloxacin 400 mg IV once daily), or _For penicillin-allergic patients:_ Replace the β-lactam with aztreonam	
	Empirical therapy for patients at risk for methicillin-resistant Staphylococcus aureus pneumonia: Add vancomycin IV or linezolid (IV or PO) to the baseline regimen. Addition of clindamycin to vancomycin (but not to linezolid) can be considered for severe necrotizing pneumonia to minimize bacterial toxin production.		
Salmonellosis	Ciprofloxacin 500-750 mg PO (or 400 mg IV) q12h, if susceptible Duration of therapy: _For gastroenteritis without bacteremia:_ If CD4 count ≥ 200 cells/ mm³: 7-14 days If CD4 count < 200 cells/ mm³: 2-6 wk _For gastroenteritis with bacteremia:_ If CD4 count ≥ 200/mm³: 14 days; longer duration if bacteremia persists or if the infection is complicated (e.g., if metastatic foci of infection are present) If CD4 count < 200 cells/ mm³: 2-6 wk Secondary prophylaxis should be considered for: Patients with recurrent _Salmonella_ gastroenteritis ± bacteremia, or Patients with CD4 <200 cells/mm³ with severe diarrhea	Levofloxacin 750 mg (PO or IV) q24h, or Moxifloxacin 400 mg (PO or IV) q24h, or TMP-SMX (160 mg/800 mg) (PO or IV) q12h, or Ceftriaxone 1 g IV q24h, or Cefotaxime 1 g IV q8h	Oral or IV rehydration if indicated. Antimotility agents should be avoided. The role of long-term secondary prophylaxis in patients with recurrent _Salmonella_ bacteremia is not well established. Must weigh benefit against risks of long-term antibiotic exposure. Effective ART may reduce the frequency, severity, and recurrence of _Salmonella_ infections.

TABLE 69-1 Treatment of AIDS-Associated Opportunistic Infections—cont'd

OPPORTUNISTIC INFECTION	PREFERRED THERAPY	ALTERNATIVE THERAPY	OTHER COMMENTS
Mucocutaneous candidiasis	For oropharyngeal candidiasis; initial episodes (for 7-14 days): *Oral therapy:* Fluconazole 100 mg PO daily, *or* *Topical therapy:* Clotrimazole troches, 10 mg PO five times daily, *or* Miconazole mucoadhesive buccal 50-mg tablet— apply to mucosal surface over the canine fossa once daily (do not swallow, chew, or crush)	For oropharyngeal candidiasis; initial episodes (for 7-14 days): *Oral therapy:* Itraconazole oral solution 200 mg PO daily, *or* Posaconazole oral solution 400 mg PO bid for 1 day, then 400 mg daily *Topical therapy:* Nystatin suspension 4-6 mL qid or one to two flavored pastilles four to five times daily	Chronic or prolonged use of azoles may promote development of resistance. Higher relapse rate for esophageal candidiasis seen with echinocandins than with fluconazole use. Suppressive therapy usually not recommended unless patients have frequent or severe recurrences. If decision is to use suppressive therapy: *Oropharyngeal candidiasis:* Fluconazole 100 mg PO daily or three times a week *Esophageal candidiasis:* Fluconazole 100-200 mg PO daily Posaconazole 400 mg PO bid *Vulvovaginal candidiasis:* Fluconazole 150 mg PO once weekly
	For esophageal candidiasis (for 14-21 days): Fluconazole 100 mg (up to 400 mg) PO or IV daily, *or* Itraconazole oral solution 200 mg PO daily	For esophageal candidiasis (for 14-21 days): Voriconazole 200 mg PO or IV bid, *or* Posaconazole 400 mg PO bid, *or* Anidulafungin 100 mg IV one time, then 50 mg IV daily *or* Caspofungin 50 mg IV daily, *or* Micafungin 150 mg IV daily, *or* Amphotericin B deoxycholate 0.6 mg/kg IV daily *or* Lipid formulation of amphotericin B 3-4 mg/kg IV daily	Itraconazole oral solution 200 mg PO daily
	For uncomplicated vulvovaginal candidiasis: Oral fluconazole 150 mg for one dose, *or* Topical azoles (clotrimazole, butoconazole, miconazole, tioconazole, or terconazole) for 3-7 days	For uncomplicated vulvovaginal candidiasis: Itraconazole oral solution 200 mg PO daily for 3-7 days	
	For severe or recurrent vulvovaginal candidiasis: Fluconazole 100-200 mg PO daily for ≥7 days, *or* Topical antifungal ≥7 days		

Continued

TABLE 69-1 Treatment of AIDS-Associated Opportunistic Infections—cont'd

OPPORTUNISTIC INFECTION	PREFERRED THERAPY	ALTERNATIVE THERAPY	OTHER COMMENTS
Cryptococcosis	Cryptococcal meningitis: Induction therapy (for at least 2 wk, followed by consolidation therapy): Liposomal amphotericin B 3-4 mg/kg IV daily + flucytosine 25 mg/kg PO qid (Note: flucytosine dose should be adjusted in patients with renal dysfunction.)	Cryptococcal meningitis: Induction therapy (for at least 2 wk, followed by consolidation therapy): Amphotericin B deoxycholate 0.7 mg/kg IV daily + flucytosine 25 mg/kg PO qid, or Amphotericin B lipid complex 5 mg/kg IV daily + flucytosine 25 mg/kg PO qid, or Liposomal amphotericin B 3-4 mg/kg IV daily + fluconazole 800 mg PO or IV daily, or Amphotericin B deoxycholate 0.7 mg/kg IV daily + fluconazole 800 mg PO or IV daily, or Fluconazole 400-800 mg PO or IV daily + flucytosine 25 mg/kg PO qid, or Fluconazole 1200 mg PO or IV daily	Addition of flucytosine to amphotericin B has been associated with more rapid sterilization of CSF and decreased risk for subsequent relapse. Patients receiving flucytosine should have either blood levels monitored (peak level 2 hr after dose should be 30-80 µg/mL) or close monitoring of blood cell counts for development of cytopenia. Dosage should be adjusted in patients with renal insufficiency. Opening pressure should always be measured when an LP is performed. Repeated LPs or CSF shunting are essential to effectively manage increased intracranial pressure. Corticosteroids and mannitol are ineffective in reducing ICP and are *not* recommended. Some specialists recommend a brief course of corticosteroid for management of severe IRIS symptoms.
	Consolidation therapy (for at least 8 wk followed by maintenance therapy): Fluconazole 400 mg PO (or IV) daily	Consolidation therapy (for at least 8 wk followed by maintenance therapy): Itraconazole 200 mg PO bid for 8 wk—less effective than fluconazole	
	Maintenance therapy: Fluconazole 200 mg PO daily for at least 12 mo	Maintenance therapy: No alternative therapy recommendation	
	For non-CNS, extrapulmonary cryptococcosis and diffuse pulmonary disease: Treatment same as for cryptococcal meningitis Non-CNS cryptococcosis with mild-to-moderate symptoms and focal pulmonary infiltrates: Fluconazole, 400 mg PO daily for 12 mo		

TABLE 69-1 Treatment of AIDS-Associated Opportunistic Infections—cont'd

OPPORTUNISTIC INFECTION	PREFERRED THERAPY	ALTERNATIVE THERAPY	OTHER COMMENTS
Histoplasmosis	Moderately severe to severe disseminated disease: *Induction therapy (for at least 2 wk or until clinically improved):* Liposomal amphotericin B 3 mg/kg IV daily *Maintenance therapy:* Itraconazole 200 mg PO tid for 3 days, then 200 mg PO bid Less severe disseminated disease: *Induction and maintenance therapy:* Itraconazole 200 mg PO tid for 3 days, then 200 mg PO bid *Duration of therapy:* At least 12 mo Meningitis: *Induction therapy (4-6 wk):* Liposomal amphotericin B 5 mg/kg/day *Maintenance therapy:* Itraconazole 200 mg PO bid to tid for ≥1 year and until resolution of abnormal CSF findings Long-term suppression therapy: *For patients with severe disseminated or CNS infection after completion of at least 12 mo of therapy; and those who relapse despite appropriate therapy:* Itraconazole 200 mg PO daily	Moderately severe to severe disseminated disease: *Induction therapy (for at least 2 wk, or until clinically improved):* Amphotericin B lipid complex 3 mg/kg IV daily, or Amphotericin B cholesteryl sulfate complete 3 mg/kg IV daily Alternatives to itraconazole for maintenance therapy or treatment of less severe disease: Voriconazole 400 mg PO bid for 1 day, then 200 mg bid, or Posaconazole 400 mg PO bid, or Fluconazole 800 mg PO daily Meningitis: No alternative therapy recommendation Long-term suppression therapy: Fluconazole 400 mg PO daily	Itraconazole, posaconazole, and voriconazole may have significant interactions with certain ARV agents. These interactions are complex and can be bidirectional. Therapeutic drug monitoring and dosage adjustment may be necessary to ensure triazole antifungal and ARV efficacy and reduce concentration-related toxicities. Random serum concentration of itraconazole + hydroitraconazole should be >1 μg/mL. Clinical experience with voriconazole or posaconazole in the treatment of histoplasmosis is limited. Acute pulmonary histoplasmosis in HIV-infected patients with CD4 counts >300 cells/mm^3 should be managed as nonimmunocompromised host.

Continued

TABLE 69-1 Treatment of AIDS-Associated Opportunistic Infections—cont'd

OPPORTUNISTIC INFECTION	PREFERRED THERAPY	ALTERNATIVE THERAPY	OTHER COMMENTS
Coccidioidomycosis	Clinically mild infections (e.g., focal pneumonia): Fluconazole 400 mg PO daily, or Itraconazole 200 mg PO bid	Mild infections (focal pneumonia): *For patients who failed to respond to fluconazole or itraconazole:* Posaconazole 200 mg PO bid, or Voriconazole 200 mg PO bid)	Some patients with meningitis may develop hydrocephalus and require CSF shunting. Therapy should be continued indefinitely in patients with diffuse pulmonary or disseminated diseases because relapse can occur in 25%-33% of HIV-negative patients. It can also occur in HIV-infected patients with CD4 counts >250 cells/mm³. Therapy should be lifelong in patients with meningeal infections because relapse occurs in 80% of HIV-infected patients after discontinuation of triazole therapy. Itraconazole, posaconazole, and voriconazole may have significant interactions with certain ARV agents. These interactions are complex and can be bidirectional. Therapeutic drug monitoring and dosage adjustment may be necessary to ensure triazole antifungal and antiretroviral efficacy and reduce concentration-related toxicities. Intrathecal amphotericin B should only be given in consultation with a specialist and administered by an individual with experience with the technique.
	Severe, nonmeningeal infection (diffuse pulmonary infection or severely ill patients with extrathoracic, disseminated disease): Amphotericin B deoxycholate 0.7-1.0 mg/kg IV daily Lipid formulation amphotericin B 4-6 mg/kg IV daily *Duration of therapy:* Continue until clinical improvement, then switch to an azole.	Severe, nonmeningeal infection (diffuse pulmonary infection or severely ill patients with extrathoracic, disseminated disease): Some specialists will add a triazole (fluconazole or itraconazole, with itraconazole preferred for bone disease) 400 mg/day to amphotericin B therapy and continue triazole once amphotericin B is stopped.	
	Meningeal infections: Fluconazole 400-800 mg IV or PO daily	Meningeal infections: Itraconazole 200 mg PO tid for 3 days, then 200 mg PO bid, or Posaconazole 200 mg PO bid, or Voriconazole 200-400 mg PO bid, or Intrathecal amphotericin B deoxycholate, when triazole antifungal agents are ineffective	
	Chronic suppressive therapy: Fluconazole 400 mg PO daily, or Itraconazole 200 mg PO bid	Chronic suppressive therapy: Posaconazole 200 mg PO bid, or Voriconazole 200 mg PO bid	

TABLE 69-1   Treatment of AIDS-Associated Opportunistic Infections—cont'd

OPPORTUNISTIC INFECTION	PREFERRED THERAPY	ALTERNATIVE THERAPY	OTHER COMMENTS
Cytomegalovirus (CMV) disease	CMV retinitis: *Induction therapy for immediate sight-threatening lesions (adjacent to the optic nerve or fovea):* *Consult ophthalmologist because ganciclovir implant no longer available:* Ganciclovir 5 mg/kg IV q12h for 14-21 days followed by valganciclovir 900 mg PO bid *For small peripheral lesions:* Valganciclovir 900 mg PO bid for 14-21 days One dose of intravitreal ganciclovir can be administered immediately after diagnosis until steady-state plasma ganciclovir concentration is achieved with oral valganciclovir. Chronic maintenance (secondary prophylaxis): Valganciclovir 900 mg PO daily (for small peripheral lesion)	CMV retinitis: *Induction therapy:* Ganciclovir 5 mg/kg IV q12h for 14-21 days, *or* Foscarnet 90 mg/kg IV q12h or 60 mg q8h for 14-21 days, *or* Cidofovir 5 mg/kg/wk IV for 2 wk; saline hydration before and after therapy and probenecid, 2 g PO 3 hr before dose, followed by 1 g PO 2 hr and 8 hr after the dose (total of 4 g). (*Note:* This regimen should be avoided in patients with sulfa allergy because of cross-hypersensitivity with probenecid.) Chronic maintenance (secondary prophylaxis): Ganciclovir 5 mg/kg IV five to seven times weekly, *or* Foscarnet 90-120 mg/kg IV once daily, *or* Cidofovir 5 mg/kg IV every other week with saline hydration and probenecid as above	The choice of therapy for CMV retinitis should be individualized, based on location and severity of the lesions, level of immunosuppression, and other factors (e.g., concomitant medications and ability to adhere to treatment). The choice of chronic maintenance therapy (route of administration and drug choices) should be made in consultation with an ophthalmologist. Considerations should include the anatomic location of the retinal lesion, vision in the contralateral eye, the patients' immunologic and virologic status and response to ART. Patients with CMV retinitis who discontinue maintenance therapy should undergo regular eye examinations (optimally every 3 mo) for early detection of relapse IRU, and then annually after immune reconstitution. IRU may develop in the setting of immune reconstitution. Treatment of IRU: Periocular corticosteroid or short courses of systemic corticosteroid. Initial therapy in patients with CMV retinitis, esophagitis, colitis, and pneumonitis should include initiation or optimization of ART.
	CMV esophagitis or colitis: Ganciclovir 5 mg/kg IV q12h; may switch to valganciclovir 900 mg PO q12h once the patient can tolerate oral therapy *Duration:* 21-42 days or until symptoms have resolved Maintenance therapy is usually not necessary, but should be considered after relapses.	CMV esophagitis or colitis: Foscarnet 90 mg/kg IV q12h or 60 mg/kg q8h for patients with treatment-limiting toxicities to ganciclovir or with ganciclovir resistance, *or* Valganciclovir 900 mg PO q12h in milder disease and if able to tolerate PO therapy, *or* For mild cases, if ART can be initiated without delay, consider withholding CMV therapy. *Duration:* 21-42 days or until symptoms have resolved.	

Continued

TABLE 69-1   Treatment of AIDS-Associated Opportunistic Infections—cont'd

OPPORTUNISTIC INFECTION	PREFERRED THERAPY	ALTERNATIVE THERAPY	OTHER COMMENTS
	Well-documented, histologically confirmed CMV pneumonia: Experience for treating CMV pneumonitis in HIV patients is limited. Use of IV ganciclovir or IV foscarnet is reasonable (doses same as for CMV retinitis) The optimal duration of therapy and the role of oral valganciclovir have not been established.		
Herpes simplex virus (HSV) disease	Orolabial lesions (for 5-10 days): Valacyclovir 1 g PO bid, or Famciclovir 500 mg PO bid, or Acyclovir 400 mg PO tid Initial or recurrent genital HSV (for 5-14 days): Valacyclovir 1 g PO bid, or Famciclovir 500 mg PO bid, or Acyclovir 400 mg PO tid Severe mucocutaneous HSV: Initial therapy, acyclovir 5 mg/kg IV q8h After lesions begin to regress, change to PO therapy as above. Continue until lesions are completely healed. Chronic suppressive therapy: For patients with severe recurrences of genital herpes or patients who want to minimize frequency of recurrences: Valacyclovir 500 mg PO bid, or Famciclovir 500 mg PO bid, or Acyclovir 400 mg PO bid Continue indefinitely regardless of CD4 cell count.	For acyclovir-resistant HSV: Preferred therapy: Foscarnet 80-120 mg/kg/day IV in two to three divided doses until clinical response Alternative therapy: IV cidofovir (dosage as in CMV retinitis), or Topical trifluridine, or Topical cidofovir, or Topical imiquimod Duration of therapy: 21-28 days or longer	Patients with HSV infections can be treated with episodic therapy when symptomatic lesions occur or with daily suppressive therapy to prevent recurrences. Topical formulations of trifluridine and cidofovir are not commercially available. Extemporaneous compounding of topical products can be prepared using trifluridine ophthalmic solution and the IV formulation of cidofovir.

TABLE 69-1   Treatment of AIDS-Associated Opportunistic Infections—cont'd

OPPORTUNISTIC INFECTION	PREFERRED THERAPY	ALTERNATIVE THERAPY	OTHER COMMENTS
Varicella-zoster virus (VZV) disease	Primary varicella infection (chickenpox): *Uncomplicated cases (for 5-7 days):* Valacyclovir 1 g PO tid, *or* Famciclovir 500 mg PO tid *Severe or complicated cases:* Acyclovir 10-15 mg/kg IV q8h for 7-10 days May switch to oral valacyclovir, famciclovir, or acyclovir after defervescence if no evidence of visceral involvement	Primary varicella infection (chickenpox): *Uncomplicated cases (for 5-7 days):* Acyclovir 800 mg PO five times a day	In managing VZV retinitis consultation with an ophthalmologist experienced in management of VZV retinitis is strongly recommended. Duration of therapy for VZV retinitis is not well defined and should be determined based on clinical, virologic, and immunologic responses and ophthalmologic responses. Optimization of ART is recommended for serious and difficult-to-treat VZV infections (e.g., retinitis, encephalitis).
	Herpes zoster (shingles): *Acute localized dermatomal:* For 7-10 days consider longer duration if lesions are slow to resolve. Valacyclovir 1 g PO tid, *or* Famciclovir 500 mg tid	Herpes zoster (shingles): *Acute localized dermatomal:* For 7-10 days consider longer duration if lesions are slow to resolve. Acyclovir 800 mg PO five times a day	
	Extensive cutaneous lesion or visceral involvement: Acyclovir 10-15 mg/kg IV q8h until clinical improvement is evident May switch to PO therapy (valacyclovir, famciclovir, or acyclovir) after clinical improvement (i.e., when no new vesicle formation or improvement of signs and symptoms of visceral VZV), to complete a 10-14 day course.		
	Progressive outer retinal necrosis (PORN): (Ganciclovir 5 mg/kg + foscarnet 90 mg/kg) IV q12h + (ganciclovir 2 mg/0.05 mL ± foscarnet 1.2 mg/0.05 mL) intravitreal injection twice weekly, *or* Initiate or optimize ART.		
	Acute retinal necrosis (ARN): Acyclovir 10 mg/kg IV q8h for 10-14 days, followed by valacyclovir 1 g PO tid for 6 wk		

Continued

TABLE 69-1 Treatment of AIDS-Associated Opportunistic Infections—cont'd

OPPORTUNISTIC INFECTION	PREFERRED THERAPY	ALTERNATIVE THERAPY	OTHER COMMENTS
Progressive multifocal leukoencephalopathy (PML) (JC virus infections)	There is no specific antiviral therapy for JC virus infection. The main treatment approach is to reverse the immunosuppression caused by HIV. Initiate ART immediately in ART-naïve patients. Optimize ART in patients who develop PML in phase of HIV viremia on ART.	None	Corticosteroids may be used for PML-IRIS characterized by contrast enhancement, edema, or mass effect, and with clinical deterioration.

AIDS, acquired immunodeficiency syndrome; ART, antiretroviral therapy; ARV, antiretroviral; bid, twice daily; CD4, CD4+ lymphocyte cells; CFU, colony-forming unit; CNS, central nervous system; CSF, cerebrospinal fluid; CYP3A4, cytochrome P-450 3A4; DOT, directly observed therapy; DS, double strength; EMB, ethambutol; G6PD, glucose-6-phosphate dehydrogenase; HIV, human immunodeficiency virus; ICP, intracranial pressure; ICU, intensive care unit; IM, intramuscular; INH, isoniazid; IRIS, immune reconstitution inflammatory syndrome; IRU, immune recovery uveitis; IV, intravenous; LP, lumbar puncture; NSAIDs, nonsteroidal anti-inflammatory drugs; PI, protease inhibitor; PO, oral; PZA, pyrazinamide; q(n)h, every "n" hours; RFB, rifabutin; RIF, rifampin; SS, single strength; TB, tuberculosis; tid, thrice daily; TVR, telaprevir; TMP-SMX, trimethoprim-sulfamethoxazole; ZDV, zidovudine.
*Pyrimethamine and leucovorin doses are the same as for preferred therapy.
From Guidelines for Prevention and Treatment of Opportunistic Infections in HIV-Infected Adults and Adolescents: Recommendations from CDC, the National Institutes of Health, and the HIV Medicine Association of the Infectious Diseases Society of America. Available at http://aidsinfo.nih.gov/guidelines. Accessed May 5, 2014.

TABLE 69-2 Prophylaxis to Prevent First Episode of Opportunistic Disease

OPPORTUNISTIC INFECTIONS	INDICATION	PREFERRED	ALTERNATIVE
Pneumocystis pneumonia (PCP)	CD4 count <200 cells/mm³, or oropharyngeal candidiasis, or CD4 <14%, or history of AIDS-defining illness, or CD4 count >200 but <250 cells/mm³ if monitoring CD4 cell count every 3 mo is not possible Note: Patients who are receiving pyrimethamine-sulfadiazine for treatment or suppression of toxoplasmosis do not require additional PCP prophylaxis.	TMP-SMX 1 DS tablet PO daily, or TMP-SMX 1 SS tablet PO daily	TMP-SMX 1 DS tablet PO three times a week, or Dapsone 100 mg PO daily or 50 mg PO bid, or Dapsone 50 mg PO daily + pyrimethamine 50 mg + leucovorin 25 mg PO weekly, or Dapsone 200 mg + pyrimethamine 75 mg + leucovorin 25 mg PO weekly; or Aerosolized pentamidine 300 mg via Respirgard II nebulizer every month, or Atovaquone 1500 mg PO daily, or Atovaquone 1500 mg + pyrimethamine 25 mg + leucovorin 10 mg PO daily

TABLE 69-2 Prophylaxis to Prevent First Episode of Opportunistic Disease—cont'd

OPPORTUNISTIC INFECTIONS	INDICATION	PREFERRED	ALTERNATIVE
Toxoplasma gondii encephalitis	*Toxoplasma* IgG-positive patients with CD4 count <100 cells/mm³ Seronegative patients receiving PCP prophylaxis not active against toxoplasmosis should have *Toxoplasma* serology retested if CD4 count declines to <100 cells/mm³. Prophylaxis should be initiated if seroconversion occurred. *Note:* All regimens recommended for primary prophylaxis against toxoplasmosis are also effective as PCP prophylaxis.	TMP-SMX 1 DS tablet PO daily	TMP-SMX 1 DS tablet PO three times a week, *or* TMP-SMX 1 SS tablet PO daily, *or* Dapsone 50 mg PO daily + pyrimethamine 50 mg + leucovorin 25 mg PO weekly, *or* Dapsone 200 mg + pyrimethamine 75 mg + leucovorin 25 mg PO weekly; *or* Atovaquone 1500 mg PO daily; *or* Atovaquone 1500 mg + pyrimethamine 25 mg + leucovorin 10 mg PO daily
Mycobacterium tuberculosis infection (i.e., treatment of LTBI)	Positive screening test for LTBI, with no evidence of active TB, and no prior treatment for active TB or LTBI, *or* Close contact with a person with infectious TB, with no evidence of active TB, regardless of screening test results.	INH 300 mg + pyridoxine 25 mg PO daily × 9 mo, *or* INH 900 mg PO twice weekly (by DOT) + pyridoxine 25 mg PO daily × 9 mo.	Rifampin 600 mg PO daily × 4 mo, *or* Rifabutin (dose adjusted based on concomitant ART) × 4 mo. For persons exposed to drug-resistant TB, select anti-TB drugs after consultation with experts or public health authorities.
Disseminated *Mycobacterium avium* complex (MAC) disease	CD4 count <50 cells/mm³ after ruling out active disseminated MAC disease based on clinical assessment.	Azithromycin 1200 mg PO once weekly, *or* Clarithromycin 500 mg PO bid, *or* Azithromycin 600 mg PO twice weekly	Rifabutin (dose adjusted based on concomitant ART); rule out active TB before starting rifabutin.
Streptococcus pneumoniae infection	For individuals who have not received any pneumococcal vaccine, regardless of CD4 count, followed by: if CD4 count ≥ 200 cells/mm³ if CD4 count < 200 cells/mm³	PCV13 0.5 mL IM × 1. PPV23 0.5 mL IM at least 8 wk after the PCV13 vaccine. PPV23 can be offered at least 8 wk after receiving PCV13 or can wait until CD4 count increased to >200 cells/mm³.	PPV23 0.5 mL IM × 1
	For individuals who have previously received PPV23	One dose of PCV13 should be given at least 1 yr after the last receipt of PPV23.	
	Revaccination: If age 19-64 yr and ≥5 yr since the first PPV23 dose If age ≥ 65 yr, and if ≥5 yr since the previous PPV23 dose	PPV23 0.5 mL IM × 1 PPV23 0.5 mL IM × 1	

Continued

TABLE 69-2 Prophylaxis to Prevent First Episode of Opportunistic Disease—cont'd

OPPORTUNISTIC INFECTIONS	INDICATION	PREFERRED	ALTERNATIVE
Influenza A and B virus infection	All HIV-infected patients	Inactivated influenza vaccine annually (per recommendation for the season). Live-attenuated influenza vaccine is *contraindicated* in HIV-infected patients.	
Syphilis	For individuals exposed to a sex partner with a diagnosis of primary, secondary, or early latent syphilis within past 90 days, *or* For individuals exposed to a sex partner >90 days before syphilis diagnosis in the partner, if serologic test results are not available immediately after and the opportunity for follow-up is uncertain **(AIII)**	Benzathine penicillin G 2.4 million units IM for 1 dose	*For pencillin-allergic patients:* Doxycycline 100 mg PO bid for 14 days, *or* Ceftriaxone 1 g IM or IV daily for 8-10 days, or Azithromycin 2 g PO for 1 dose: **not recommended** for MSM or pregnant women
Histoplasma capsulatum infection	CD4 count ≤150 cells/mm^3 and at high risk because of occupational exposure or live in a community with a hyperendemic rate of histoplasmosis (>10 cases/100 patient-years)	Itraconazole 200 mg PO daily	
Coccidioidomycosis	A new positive IgM or IgG serologic test in patients who live in a disease-endemic area and with CD4 count <250 cells/mm^3	Fluconazole 400 mg PO daily	
Varicella-zoster virus	Preexposure prevention: Patients with CD4 counts ≥200 cells/mm^3 who have not been vaccinated, have no history of varicella or herpes zoster, or who are seronegative for VZV *Note:* Routine VZV serologic testing in HIV-infected adults and adolescents is not recommended.	Preexposure prevention: Primary varicella vaccination (Varivax), two doses (0.5 mL SQ each) administered 3 mo apart. If vaccination results in disease because of vaccine virus, treatment with acyclovir is recommended.	Preexposure prevention: VZV-susceptible household contacts of susceptible HIV-infected persons should be vaccinated to prevent potential transmission of VZV to their HIV-infected contacts.

TABLE 69-2   Prophylaxis to Prevent First Episode of Opportunistic Disease—cont'd

OPPORTUNISTIC INFECTIONS	INDICATION	PREFERRED	ALTERNATIVE
	Postexposure prevention: Close contact with a person with chickenpox or herpes zoster and is susceptible (i.e., no history of vaccination or of either condition, or known to be VZV seronegative)	Postexposure prevention: Varicella-zoster immune globulin (VariZIG) 125 IU/10 kg (maximum 625 IU) IM, administered as soon as possible and within 10 days after exposure. Note: VariZIG is available through Cangene, Canada. Individuals receiving monthly high-dose IVIG (>400 mg/kg) are likely to be protected if the last dose of IVIG was administered <3 wk before exposure.	Alternative postexposure prevention: Acyclovir 800 mg PO five times a day for 5-7 days, or Valacyclovir 1 g PO tid for 5-7 days These alternatives have not been studied in the HIV population. If antiviral therapy is used, varicella vaccines should not be given until at least 72 hr after the last dose of the antiviral drug.
Hepatitis A virus (HAV) infection	HAV-susceptible patients with chronic liver disease or who are injection drug users or MSM.	Hepatitis A vaccine 1 mL IM × two doses at 0 and 6-12 mo. IgG antibody response should be assessed 1 mo after vaccination; nonresponders should be revaccinated when CD4 count > 200 cells/mm³.	For patients susceptible to both HAV and hepatitis B virus (HBV) infection (see below): Combined HAV and HBV vaccine (Twinrix), 1 mL IM as a three-dose (0, 1, and 6 mo) or four-dose series (days 0, 7, 21 to 30 and at 12 mo)
Hepatitis B virus (HBV) infection	Vaccine nonresponders: Anti-HBs <10 IU/mL 1 mo after vaccination series. For patients with low CD4 counts at time of first vaccine series, some specialists might delay revaccination until after sustained increase in CD4 count with ART.	Revaccinate with a second vaccine series.	Some experts recommend revaccinating with 40-µg doses of either HBV vaccine.

ART, antiretroviral therapy; CD4, CD4⁺ lymphocyte count; DOT, directly observed treatment; DS, double strength; HBs, hepatitis B surface antibody; HIV, human immunodeficiency virus; IM, intramuscular; INH, isoniazid; IVIG, intravenous immune globulin; LTBI, latent tuberculosis infection; MSM, men who have sex with men; PCV13, 13-valent pneumococcal conjugate vaccine; PO, oral; PPV23, 23-valent pneumococcal polysaccharide vaccine; SQ, subcutaneous; SS, single strength; TB, tuberculosis; TMP-SMX, trimethoprim-sulfamethoxazole; VZV, varicella-zoster virus.

From Guidelines for Prevention and Treatment of Opportunistic Infections in HIV-Infected Adults and Adolescents: Recommendations from CDC, the National Institutes of Health, and the HIV Medicine Association of the Infectious Diseases Society of America. Available at http://aidsinfo.nih.gov/guidelines. Accessed May 5, 2014.

70 Chronic Fatigue Syndrome
N. Cary Engleberg

DEFINITION
- As defined in a 1994 Centers for Disease Control and Prevention/National Institutes of Health consensus conference, chronic fatigue syndrome (CFS) is a disorder involving 6 or more months of unexplained, profound fatigue with *at least four* of eight associated symptoms (see Table 70-1).
- A new name, "systemic exertion intolerance disease" was proposed by the Institute of Medicine in 2015, along with somewhat modified diagnostic criteria (see Table 70-2).
- Other names used for this disorder include "postinfectious fatigue," "chronic mononucleosis," "myalgic encephalomyelitis" (United Kingdom/Canada), and "chronic fatigue and immune dysfunction syndrome" (United States).

EPIDEMIOLOGY
- Prevalence is estimated at 0.2% to 1% of the population, depending on the definitions used.
- CFS occurs in women three to seven times more frequently than in men.
- It occurs in all socioeconomic strata and among all races.

ETIOLOGY
- CFS may be a sequel of various infectious diseases (e.g., herpesvirus infections, influenza, Q fever, brucellosis, Lyme disease, giardiasis) but is not known to be directly related to any ongoing chronic infection (see Table 70-3).
- Subtle disturbances of immune function are not consistent and not known to be causative of symptoms.
- Hypothalamus-pituitary-adrenal axis or autonomic disturbances may occur, but correcting these subtle anomalies does not improve symptoms of CFS.
- Prior or concurrent history of psychiatric disorders is common.

DIAGNOSIS
- Diagnosis is clinical and usually based on the 1994 consensus definition (see Table 70-1).
- Modified diagnostic criteria have also been proposed by the Institute of Medicine in 2015 (see Table 70-2).
- There is no valid laboratory test to rule in or to rule out CFS.

THERAPY
- Pharmacologic therapies are directed at relieving symptoms of pain, sleep disruption, and depression.
- No antimicrobial and immune therapies have been proven to be helpful.
- Nonpharmacologic therapies (cognitive-behavioral therapy and graded exercise therapy) have been repeatedly shown to be helpful in most patients.

PREVENTION
- There are no known preventive measures.

TABLE 70-1 CDC/NIH Consensus Conference Definition of Chronic Fatigue Syndrome

Clinically evaluated, unexplained chronic fatigue for >6 mo duration, which is not lifelong or the result of ongoing exertion and is not alleviated substantially by rest. Fatigue is associated with a significant reduction in occupational, educational, social, or personal activities *plus* ≥4 of the following concurrent symptoms:
Impaired memory or concentration
Sore throat
Tender cervical or axillary lymph nodes
Muscle pain
Multijoint pain
New headaches
Unrefreshing sleep
Postexertion malaise

CDC, Centers for Disease Control and Prevention; NIH, National Institutes of Health.
Modified from Fukuda K, Straus SE, Hickie I, et al. The chronic fatigue syndrome: a comprehensive approach to its definition and study. International Chronic Fatigue Syndrome Study Group. *Ann Intern Med.* 1994;121: 953-959.

TABLE 70-2 IOM Diagnostic Criteria for Systemic Exertion Intolerance Disease

Diagnosis requires that the patient have the following three symptoms:
1. A substantial reduction or impairment in the ability to engage in pre-illness levels of occupational, educational, social, or personal activities, that persists for more than 6 months and is accompanied by fatigue, which is often profound, is of new or definite onset (not lifelong), is not the result of ongoing excessive exertion, and is not substantially alleviated by rest, and
2. Postexertional malaise,* and
3. Unrefreshing sleep*
At least one of the following manifestations is also required:
1. Cognitive impairment* or
2. Orthostatic intolerance

*Frequency and severity of symptoms should be assessed. The diagnosis of systemic intolerance disease (myalgic encephalomyelitis/chronic fatigue syndrome) should be questioned if patients do not have these symptoms at least half of the time with moderate, substantial, or severe intensity.

TABLE 70-3 Proposed Infectious Causes of Chronic Fatigue Syndrome

	REFERENCES	
Proposed Etiologic Agent	**Suggestive Studies**	**Negative Studies**
Epstein-Barr virus	**6, 7**, 173	13, **14**, **15**, 16, 174-176
Cytomegalovirus	177, 178	13, **14**, 174-176
Human herpesvirus 6	45, 46, 179, 180	13, **14**, 175, 176, 181, 182
Human herpesvirus 7	183	46, 175, 179, 182
Human herpesvirus 8	—	46, 175, 184
Enteroviruses	185-187	13, **14**, 188-191
Parvovirus	39, 192	175, 193, 194
GB virus-C		195
Human spumavirus	196	—
Bornavirus	197, 198	199
Human retrovirus	200	201-203
Xenotropic murine retrovirus (XMRV)	49, 50	**54**, 56-58 59 (retraction of 49) 60 (retraction of 50)
Borrelia burgdorferi	204	205, 206
Brucella spp.	207	3
Mycoplasma spp.	208, 209	210
Candida albicans	211, 212	213

Infectious Diseases and their Etiologic Agents

71 Orthopoxviruses: Vaccinia (Smallpox Vaccine), Variola (Smallpox), Monkeypox, and Cowpox

Brett W. Petersen and Inger K. Damon*

DEFINITION

- Orthopoxvirus infections can cause a spectrum of febrile rash illnesses in humans, from fairly benign, localized skin infections to severe systemic infections.
- Vaccinia (smallpox vaccine), variola (smallpox), monkeypox, and cowpox are the four orthopoxvirus species known to cause human disease.

EPIDEMIOLOGY

- Most orthopoxvirus infections are zoonotic, with humans serving as accidental hosts.
- Vaccinia virus continues to be used as a vaccine, as well as a subject and tool for biomedical research, and it causes sporadic disease in vaccinees, contacts of vaccinees, and laboratory workers.
- Variola, the causative agent of smallpox, caused significant morbidity and mortality worldwide before its eradication in 1980.
- Monkeypox virus causes intermittent human infections, primarily in Central and West Africa, although isolated outbreaks have been identified in the United States and Sudan.
- Human cowpox virus infection is classically associated with occupational exposure to cattle; however, other animals, including rats, pet cats, and zoo and circus elephants, have been implicated.

MICROBIOLOGY

- Orthopoxviruses are a group of large, complex, double-stranded DNA viruses that replicate in the cytoplasm of the host cell.

DIAGNOSIS

- Diagnostic laboratory testing for orthopoxvirus infections can include polymerase chain reaction, viral culture, and electron microscopy of rash lesion material, as well as serologic testing of serum.

THERAPY

- Vaccinia Immune Globulin Intravenous (VIGIV) is licensed for the treatment of certain complications of vaccinia vaccine administration and is available through the Centers for Disease Control and Prevention.
- No antiviral drugs are currently licensed for use in the treatment of orthopoxvirus or other poxviral illnesses.
- The development and evaluation for therapeutics for orthopoxvirus infections is an active area of research.

---

*All material in this chapter is in the public domain, with the exception of any borrowed figures or tables.

PREVENTION

- Orthopoxviruses induce cross-reactive antibodies that protect against infection from other orthopoxvirus species.
- Vaccination with smallpox vaccine (i.e., vaccinia virus) can be used to protect individuals at high risk of orthopoxvirus disease.
- Other control measures focus on educational outreach to decrease the risk of exposure to likely zoonotic vectors.

72 Other Poxviruses That Infect Humans: Parapoxviruses (Including Orf Virus), Molluscum Contagiosum, and Yatapoxviruses

Brett W. Petersen and Inger K. Damon*

DEFINITION

- Parapoxviruses, molluscum contagiosum, and yatapoxviruses are among the nonorthopoxvirus infections of humans.

EPIDEMIOLOGY

- Parapoxvirus infections most commonly occur in individuals with occupational exposures to infected sheep, cattle, or goats.
- Molluscum contagiosum infection occurs worldwide and is spread through mild skin trauma, fomites, and sexual transmission.
- Yatapoxvirus infections are rarely reported; infections are acquired through exposure to infected animals and potentially arthropod vectors and are usually geographically restricted to Central and East Africa.

MICROBIOLOGY

- Poxviruses are a diverse group of large, complex double-stranded DNA viruses that replicate in the cytoplasm of the host cell.

DIAGNOSIS

- Parapoxvirus, molluscum contagiosum, and yatapoxvirus infections are often diagnosed clinically based on their characteristic clinical features in combination with appropriate exposure and travel histories.
- Diagnostic laboratory testing for poxviruses may include polymerase chain reaction assay, electron microscopy, viral culture, and serology.

THERAPY

- Parapoxvirus infections are usually self-limited; treatment with topical and intralesional cidofovir, as well as imiquimod, has been anecdotally reported.
- Multiple modalities for treatment of molluscum contagiosum have been described, including cryotherapy, mechanical curettage, and chemical treatments with podophyllin/podofilox, cantharidin, iodine, and tretinoin.

PREVENTION

- Transmission of parapoxviruses, molluscum contagiosum, and yatapoxviruses can be prevented by avoiding exposures to animal vectors, properly covering lesions, and observing good hand hygiene practices.

---

*All material in this chapter is in the public domain, with the exception of any borrowed figures or tables.

73 | Herpes Simplex Virus

Joshua T. Schiffer and Lawrence Corey

DEFINITION

- Herpes simplex virus (HSV) is a human α-herpesvirus of two types, HSV-1 and HSV-2.
- Both types cause common infections with varied clinical manifestations in otherwise healthy children and adults that are generally more severe in patients with immunosuppression.

EPIDEMIOLOGY

- HSV-1 and HSV-2 have a worldwide distribution and have no known animal reservoirs.
- HSV-1 is acquired more frequently and earlier than HSV-2. More than 90% of adults have antibodies to HSV-1 by the fifth decade of life.
- HSV-2 seroprevalence correlates with onset of sexual activity and is consistently higher in women than men.
- Global incidence of HSV-2 has been estimated at 23 million new cases per year.

MICROBIOLOGY

- HSV is a nonenveloped virus that is 160 nm in diameter and has a linear, double-stranded DNA genome.
- HSV-1 and HSV-2 have approximately 50% homology, and homologous sequences are distributed throughout the genome map.
- HSV infection occurs through attachment to cells via ubiquitous receptors, reflecting a wide tissue range of infections in the host, including sensory neurons, which can result in latency.
- Viral replication occurs through nuclear and cytoplasmic phases.
- Latency is associated with transcription of only a limited number of virus-encoded ribonucleic acids.

CLINICAL MANIFESTATIONS

- HSV has been isolated from nearly all visceral and mucosal sites. Clinical manifestations depend on the anatomic site, age, and immune status of the host and antigenic type (1 or 2) of the virus.
- Initial (primary) infections are more severe than recurrent ones, but reactivation of latent infection can result in frequent clinical manifestations.
- Orofacial infection (gingivostomatitis and pharyngitis) is the most frequent initial clinical manifestation of HSV-1 infection. Recurrent lesions on the vermilion border of the lip (herpes labialis) are the most frequent manifestation of latent infection.
- Clinical aspects of primary genital infections are clinically similar with HSV-1 or HSV-2, but recurrences are more frequent with HSV-2. Complications include aseptic meningitis, transverse myelitis, and sacral radiculopathy. Extragenital lesions may occur during the course of primary genital infection.
- HSV can cause various eye infections such as keratitis, blepharitis, conjunctivitis, and retinitis.

- Herpes simplex encephalitis is the most commonly identified cause of acute, sporadic viral encephalitis in the United States. Magnetic resonance imaging is the neuroimaging technique of choice to identify abnormalities.
- Esophagitis and pulmonary infections may be caused by HSV, most commonly in immunocompromised patients.
- Neonatal infections may occur through contact with HSV secretions. Infants younger than 6 weeks have the highest frequency of visual and central nervous system involvement.

DIAGNOSIS

- Clinical criteria are utilized for consideration of the diagnosis of HSV infection, but laboratory tests are needed to confirm the diagnosis.
- Diagnosis can be made by detection of HSV DNA by polymerase chain reaction assay in lesion scrapings, fluids, or tissue. Viral isolation can also be made in tissue culture, but this is three to four times less sensitive than by DNA molecular techniques.

TREATMENT

- Acyclovir, valacyclovir, or famciclovir is used to treat mucocutaneous and visceral infections (see Table 73-1).
- Genital infections may be treated as a primary infection when recognized or as a discrete recurrence. Individuals with frequent recurrences may be treated with suppressive therapy.
- Herpes simplex encephalitis is treated with high-dose acyclovir (10 mg/kg IV every 8 hours for 14 to 21 days).
- Acyclovir-resistant HSV strains can be treated with foscarnet or cidofovir.

TABLE 73-1 Antiviral Chemotherapy for Herpes Simplex Virus Infection

	DOSAGE/REGIMEN	COMMENT
Mucocutaneous HSV Infections		
Infections in Immunosuppressed Patients		
Acute symptomatic first or recurrent episodes	IV acyclovir, 5 mg/kg q8h, and oral acyclovir, 400 mg qid, famciclovir, 500 mg PO tid, or valacyclovir, 1 mg PO bid, for 7-10 days are effective	Treatment duration may vary from 7-14 days
Suppression of reactivation disease	IV acyclovir, 5 mg/kg q8h, valacyclovir, 500 mg PO bid, or oral acyclovir, 400-800 mg two to three times per day, prevents recurrences during the immediate 30-day post-transplantation period	Longer-term suppression is often used for persons with continued immunosuppression. In bone marrow and renal transplant recipients, valacyclovir, 2 g four times daily, is also effective in preventing CMV infection. Valacyclovir, 4 g four times daily, has been associated with TTP after extended use in HIV-positive persons. In HIV-infected persons, oral famciclovir, 500 mg bid, is effective in reducing clinical and subclinical reactivations of HSV-1 and HSV-2. If using acyclovir in HIV-infected patients, we generally start with the lower dose of 400 mg twice daily and increase to 800 mg twice daily if breakthrough recurrences occur. *Note:* Once-daily dosing of valacyclovir, 500 mg to 1 g, should be avoided in HIV-infected patients owing to concerns regarding lower efficacy.
Symptomatic recurrent genital herpes in HIV-1–infected patients	Oral acyclovir, 400 mg tid × 5-10 days Valacyclovir, 1000 mg bid × 5-10 days Famciclovir, 500 mg PO bid × 5-10 days	

TABLE 73-1 Antiviral Chemotherapy for Herpes Simplex Virus Infection—cont'd

	DOSAGE/REGIMEN	COMMENT
Infections in Immunocompetent Patients		
Genital Herpes		
First episodes	Oral acyclovir, 400 mg tid (V) or 200 mg five times per day (I) × 7-10 days Oral valacyclovir, 1000 mg bid × 7-10 days (I) Famciclovir, 250 mg tid × 5-10 days (I) IV acyclovir, 5 mg/kg q8h for 5 days, is given for severe disease or neurologic complications such as aseptic meningitis	
Symptomatic recurrent genital herpes	**Oral acyclovir,** 400 mg tid × 5 days (V), **800 mg PO tid × 2 days** or bid × 5 days (II) **Valacyclovir, 500 mg bid × 3 days (I)** or 1 g daily × 5 days (I) **Famciclovir,** 125 mg bid for 5 days (I), **1 g bid for 1 day (I), or 500 mg once then 250 mg PO bid × 3 doses (I)**	All these therapies are effective in shortening lesion duration. Short-course options (1, 2, or 3 days of therapy) should be considered based on increased convenience, likelihood of adherence and reduced cost and are **listed in bold.** Given the brief period of viral replication and rapid evolution of lesions, patients should be given drugs for self-administration when prodromal symptoms occur.
Suppression of recurrent genital herpes	**Oral acyclovir, 400 mg bid (I)** **Valacyclovir,** 500 mg daily (I) or 1000 mg daily (I) or 250-500 mg bid (I) prevents symptomatic reactivation. Persons with frequent reactivation (<9 episodes/yr) can take valacyclovir 500 mg daily; those with >9 episodes/yr should take valacyclovir 1000 mg/daily or 500 mg bid. **Famciclovir,** 250 mg bid (I)	Consider for patients with frequent (>6 episodes) or severe recurrences, in immunocompromised patients, or as an adjunct to prevent transmission
Orolabial HSV Infections		
First episode	Oral acyclovir, 15 mg/kg (up to 200 mg) five times per day (II) or 400 mg tid (V) × 7 days Famciclovir, 500 mg bid (V) Valacyclovir, 1000 mg bid (V) × 7 days	
Recurrent episodes	Oral acyclovir, 400 mg five times per day × 5 days (II) **Valacyclovir, 2000 mg bid × 1 day (I)** **Famciclovir, 1500 mg once (I)**	Self-initiated therapy with topical 1% penciclovir cream q2h during waking hours (I); topical acyclovir cream, 5% five times per day × 4 days (I). Short-course options should be considered based on increased convenience and likelihood of adherence and are **listed in bold.** Given the brief period of viral replication and rapid evolution of lesions, patients should be given drugs for self-administration when prodromal symptoms occur.
Suppression of reactivation of orolabial HSV	Oral acyclovir, 400 mg bid (II), or valacyclovir, 500 mg or 1000 mg daily (II), or famciclovir, 500 mg bid (V)	Consider for patients with frequent (>6 episodes) or severe recurrences, in immunocompromised patients, or as an adjunct to prevent transmission
Herpetic Whitlow		
	Oral acyclovir, 200 mg five times daily for 7-10 days	
HSV Proctitis		
	Oral acyclovir, 400 mg five times per day is useful in shortening the course of infection	In immunosuppressed patients or in patients with severe infection, IV acyclovir, 5 mg/kg q8h, may be useful

Continued

TABLE 73-1 Antiviral Chemotherapy for Herpes Simplex Virus Infection—cont'd

	DOSAGE/REGIMEN	COMMENT
Herpetic Eye Infections		
		In acute keratitis, topical trifluorothymidine, vidarabine, idoxuridine, acyclovir, penciclovir, and interferon are all beneficial. Débridement may be required; topical corticosteroids may worsen disease.
CNS HSV Infections		
HSV encephalitis	IV acyclovir, 10 mg/kg q8h (30 mg/kg/day) for 14-21 days	
HSV aseptic meningitis	IV acyclovir, 30 mg/kg/day for 7-10 days	No studies of systemic antiviral chemotherapy exist
Autonomic radiculopathy		No studies are available
Neonatal HSV Infections		
	Acyclovir, 60 mg/kg/day (divided into three doses) × 21 days	Monitoring for relapse should be undertaken; most authorities recommend continued suppression with oral acyclovir suspension for 3-4 mo
Visceral HSV Infections		
HSV esophagitis	IV acyclovir, 15 mg/kg per day	In some patients with milder forms of immunosuppression, oral therapy with valacyclovir or famciclovir is effective
HSV pneumonitis		No controlled studies exist. IV acyclovir, 15 mg/kg/day, should be considered.
Disseminated HSV Infections		
		No controlled studies exist. IV acyclovir, 10 mg/kg q8h, nevertheless should be given. No definite evidence indicates that therapy decreases the risk of death.
Erythema Multiforme–Associated HSV		
		Anecdotal observations suggest that oral acyclovir, 400 mg bid or tid, or valacyclovir, 500 mg bid, suppresses erythema multiforme
Surgical Prophylaxis		
		Several surgical procedures such as laser skin resurfacing, trigeminal nerve root decompression, and lumbar disk surgery have been associated with HSV reactivation. IV acyclovir, 3 mg/kg, and oral acyclovir, 800 bid, valacyclovir, 500 bid, or famciclovir, 250 bid, is effective in reducing reactivation. Therapy should be initiated 48 hr before surgery and continued for 3-7 days.
Infections with Acyclovir-Resistant HSV		
	Foscarnet, 40 mg/kg IV q8h, should be given until lesions heal. IV cidofovir, 5 mg/kg once weekly, might also be effective.	Imiquimod is a topical alternative, as is topical cidofovir gel 1%, which is not commercially available and must be compounded at a pharmacy. These topical preparations should be applied to the lesions once daily for 5 consecutive days.

CMV, cytomegalovirus; CNS, central nervous system; HIV, human immunodeficiency virus; HSV, herpes simplex virus; TTP, thrombotic thrombocytopenic purpura.

Note: I, II, III, IV, and V represent level of evidence.

Modified from Cernik C, Gallina K, Brodell RT. The treatment of herpes simplex infections: an evidence-based review. *Arch Intern Med.* 2008;168:1137-1144; and Spruance S, Aoki FY, Tyring S, et al. Short-course therapy for recurrent genital herpes and herpes labialis: entering an era of greater convenience, better treatment adherence, and reduced cost. *J Fam Pract.* 2007;56:30-36.

74 Chickenpox and Herpes Zoster (Varicella-Zoster Virus)

Richard J. Whitley

DEFINITION

- Varicella-zoster virus (VZV) is an alpha herpesvirus that causes chickenpox and herpes zoster.

EPIDEMIOLOGY

- Chickenpox is the primary infection occurring primarily in childhood.
- Chickenpox is usually a benign infection but can cause life-threatening disease in the immunocompromised host.
- Disease is more likely to occur in late winter and early spring.
- Herpes zoster is the consequence of reactivation of latent virus, occurring mainly in the elderly.
- Herpes zoster causes significant pain in many individuals.
- There is no seasonal predilection for occurrence of herpes zoster.

MICROBIOLOGY

- Varicella-zoster virus is a double-stranded DNA virus. Following primary infection, latency is established in sensory ganglia.

DIAGNOSIS

- The diagnosis of chickenpox and herpes zoster is usually clinical.
- Chickenpox is characterized by a maculopapular, vesicular, and papular rash in all stages of evolution.
- Herpes zoster is usually a unilateral vesicular rash. Dissemination can occur in immunocompromised patients.
- Tzanck smears of lesion scrapings may demonstrate intranuclear inclusions; however, the sensitivity is low.
- Polymerase chain reaction (PCR) can be applied to lesion scraping in order to detect VZV DNA and is the diagnostic procedure of choice.
- Viral culture can be used to make a diagnosis, but it is less sensitive than PCR.

THERAPY

- Three drugs are licensed for the treatment of VZV infections.
- Chickenpox in children 2 to 16 years of age can be treated with acyclovir at a dosage of 20 mg/kg 4 times per day for 5 days. For older patients, the dosage of acyclovir is 800 mg 5 times a day.
- By class effect, the prodrugs valacyclovir and famciclovir are used by some experts to treat chickenpox.
- Herpes zoster can be treated with acyclovir at 800 mg five times daily for 7 to 10 days.
- Herpes zoster can be treated with valacyclovir at 1 g three times daily for 7 to 10 days.
- Herpes zoster can be treated with famciclovir at 500 mg three times daily for 7 to 10 days.

- Herpes zoster will likely require control of pain with analgesics and medications such as pregabalin.

PREVENTION

- High-titered varicella-zoster immune globulin (VariZIG) can be administered to high-risk patients to attempt to prevent infection.
- A VZV vaccine is available to prevent chickenpox. It is a two-dose series with the first administered at 12 to 15 months of age and the second between 4 and 6 years. This two-dose series has dramatically decreased the incidence of chickenpox and its associated complications.
- A high-titered VZV vaccine is available for adults older than 50 years of age that will reduce the incidence of herpes zoster, the burden of illness, and postherpetic neuralgia.

75 Cytomegalovirus (CMV)

Clyde S. Crumpacker II

DEFINITION

- Human cytomegalovirus (HCMV) is a double-stranded DNA virus, a member of the Herpesviridae family, and infects a high percentage of humans worldwide. Recent evidence points to great genomic variability during replication in a single patient. HCMV infection is usually asymptomatic, but may cause severe congenital infection and severe disease in immunocompromised transplant and acquired immunodeficiency syndrome (AIDS) patients.

EPIDEMIOLOGY

- Infants infected in utero as a result of primary cytomegalovirus (CMV) infection in a pregnant woman are at risk for severe congenital abnormalities and sensorineural hearing loss. Healthy young adults can develop CMV mononucleosis. In immunocompromised AIDS patients, CMV retinitis leads to vision loss. In solid-organ and hematopoietic stem cell transplant patients, life-threatening CMV pneumonia and hepatitis, meningoencephalitis, colitis, and esophageal ulcers can occur. The potential role of HCMV in cardiovascular disease is being increasingly investigated.

MICROBIOLOGY

- HCMV grows only in human epithelial, endothelial, smooth muscle, neurologic, and fibroblast cells. Genomic analysis using high-throughput deep sequencing in congenitally infected infants reveals extensive genomic variability and diversity.

DIAGNOSIS

- The World Health Organization has standardized a CMV DNA polymerase chain reaction assay (COBAS Amplicor/COBAS Tagman CMV test) to detect CMV in blood and infected tissue. This assay uses international units and permits comparison among clinical trials. Detection of CMV pp65 antigen in infected neutrophils remains a valuable diagnostic tool.

THERAPY

- Ganciclovir (GCV) and valganciclovir (VGC) are the mainstays of treatment. Foscarnet is mainly useful for GCV-resistant CMV infection and disease. Cidofovir may be used for treatment of failures with other anti-CMV drugs. A lipid-coated version of cidofovir (CMX001), maribavir, and letermovir are experimental drugs for CMV undergoing clinical development.

PREVENTION

- GCV and VGC are used as prophylaxis in the transplantation setting. GCV and VGC are also used as preemptive therapy. An effective CMV vaccine has not yet been developed.

76 Epstein-Barr Virus (Infectious Mononucleosis, Epstein-Barr Virus–Associated Malignant Diseases, and Other Diseases)

Eric C. Johannsen and Kenneth M. Kaye

DEFINITION

- Infectious mononucleosis is a clinical syndrome characterized by pharyngitis, fever, lymphadenopathy, and the presence of atypical lymphocytes on a peripheral blood smear. Primary Epstein-Barr virus (EBV) infection is the most common cause of this syndrome.

VIROLOGY AND EPIDEMIOLOGY

- EBV is a herpesvirus that establishes lifelong latent infection in B lymphocytes.
- Replication occurs in oral epithelium, and infectious EBV is frequently present in the saliva of asymptomatic seropositive individuals.
- EBV is transmitted predominantly through exposure to infected saliva, frequently as a result of kissing.
- Seroprevalence approaches 95% in adults, and EBV is distributed throughout the world.
- In childhood, primary EBV infection is usually asymptomatic or a nonspecific illness.
- Frequency of presentation as infectious mononucleosis increases with age to about 50% of primary infections by adolescence.
- EBV is tightly linked with several malignancies, including endemic Burkitt's lymphoma, nasopharyngeal carcinoma, and lymphoproliferative disease.

MICROBIOLOGY

- EBV is a gamma-1 herpesvirus, genus *Lymphocryptovirus*.
- EBV is a double-stranded DNA virus that is enveloped.
- EBV is also known as human herpesvirus 4.

CLINICAL MANIFESTATIONS

- Infectious mononucleosis is generally a self-limited, spontaneously remitting syndrome.
- Complications may occur, including splenic rupture, neurologic manifestations such as encephalitis, autoimmune hemolytic anemia, and mild hepatocellular enzyme elevations.

DIAGNOSIS

- The appearance of nonspecific, heterophile antibodies (IgM reacting with sheep or horse red blood cells) can distinguish primary EBV infection from other causes of infectious mononucleosis.
- The presence of IgM viral capsid antigen (VCA) antibodies is closely correlated with acute EBV infection. Heterophile antibodies in a person with clinical infectious mononucleosis is sufficient to establish the diagnosis.
- EBV serology may be helpful in atypical cases and in children (who are frequently heterophile negative).
- Primary human immunodeficiency virus infection is the most important differential diagnostic consideration.
- Serial measurement of EBV viral loads may be useful in the detection of EBV-associated malignancies in immunosuppressed individuals, especially for lymphoproliferative disease.

THERAPY

- Treatment of mononucleosis is primarily supportive.
- Corticosteroids may be helpful in managing mononucleosis complications such as airway impingement from tonsillar enlargement.
- Antiviral therapy is of no proven benefit in infectious mononucleosis.

PREVENTION

- There is currently no EBV vaccine.

77 Human Herpesvirus Types 6 and 7 (Exanthem Subitum)

*Jeffrey I. Cohen**

DEFINITION

- Human herpesviruses 6 and 7 (HHV-6 and HHV-7) cause exanthem subitum or febrile seizures in young children and reactivate frequently in highly immunocompromised hosts. They can also cause encephalitis in immunocompromised hosts.

EPIDEMIOLOGY

- Most adults are seropositive for HHV-6 and HHV-7.
- The average age for infection with HHV-6 is about 1 year old and for HHV-7 is 2 years old.
- About 50% of hematopoietic transplant recipients and 20% to 33% of organ transplant recipients have HHV-6 and HHV-7 DNA in the blood.
- HHV-6 DNA is integrated in the chromosomes of 1% to 2% of persons and is transmitted in the germline DNA.

MICROBIOLOGY

- HHV-6 and HHV-7, like cytomegalovirus, are betaherpesviruses.

DIAGNOSIS

- Exanthem subitum is usually diagnosed clinically, but seroconversion to HHV-6 or HHV-7 antibody positivity can be used.
- Diagnosis of HHV-6 or HHV-7 disease in immunocompromised persons is difficult due to the high frequency of asymptomatic reactivation and the finding that up to 2% of persons have HHV-6 DNA integrated in their chromosomes.
- HHV-6 limbic encephalitis is diagnosed based on clinical signs and symptoms and HHV-6 DNA in the cerebrospinal fluid.
- Detection of HHV-6 protein or RNA in tissues is more specific than HHV-6 DNA for diagnosing virus-associated disease in immunocompromised persons.

THERAPY

- No therapy has been shown to be effective for treatment of HHV-6 or HHV-7, but both viruses are sensitive to ganciclovir, foscarnet, and cidofovir in vitro.
- Ganciclovir or foscarnet, or both, have been used to treat immunocompromised persons with HHV-6 or HHV-7 disease, especially with limbic encephalitis.

---

*All material in this chapter is in the public domain, with the exception of any borrowed figures or tables.

78 Kaposi's Sarcoma–Associated Herpesvirus (Human Herpesvirus 8)

Kenneth M. Kaye

DEFINITION

- Kaposi's sarcoma–associated herpesvirus (KSHV), or human herpesvirus 8 (HHV-8), is the etiologic agent of Kaposi's sarcoma, primary effusion lymphoma, and is also tightly linked with multicentric Castleman's disease.

VIROLOGY AND EPIDEMIOLOGY

- KSHV is a herpesvirus that establishes lifelong infection, primarily persisting in latently infected B lymphocytes.
- Replication occurs in oral epithelium, and infectious KSHV is present in the saliva of asymptomatic seropositive individuals.
- Transmission is predominantly the result of exposure to infected saliva.
- Primary infection is usually asymptomatic and rarely recognized.
- In contrast to other herpesviruses, seroprevalence varies significantly throughout the world and is highest in sub-Saharan Africa, the Mediterranean region, and in men who have sex with men in the United States.
- KSHV malignancy usually occurs in the setting of immune suppression.

MICROBIOLOGY

- KSHV is a gamma-2 herpesvirus, genus *Rhadinovirus*.
- KSHV is an enveloped, double-stranded DNA virus.
- KSHV is also known as HHV-8.

DIAGNOSIS

- KS can be diagnosed by its clinical appearance and confirmed by biopsy.
- Primary effusion lymphoma and multicentric Castleman's disease are diagnosed by biopsy.
- KSHV can be detected serologically, although assays are not standardized.

THERAPY

- Antiviral therapy is of no proven benefit in the treatment of KSHV malignancies, and therapy generally relies on cytotoxic approaches.

PREVENTION

- There is currently no KSHV vaccine.

79 Herpes B Virus

Jeffrey I. Cohen*

DEFINITION

- Herpes B virus is a macaque virus that can cause fatal encephalitis in humans.

EPIDEMIOLOGY

- Herpes B virus naturally infects Old World macaques, including rhesus and pig-tailed macaques and cynomolgus monkeys.
- Humans are infected with herpes B virus after bites, scratches, needlesticks, or mucosal splashes with fluids from Old World macaques.

MICROBIOLOGY

- Herpes B virus is an alphaherpesvirus and is the homolog of herpes simplex virus in macaques.

DIAGNOSIS

- A positive polymerase chain reaction (PCR) or culture for herpes B virus in skin lesions, conjunctival swabs, or cerebrospinal fluid in the presence of symptoms is diagnostic for herpes B virus infection.
- A positive PCR or culture for herpes B virus of wounds or mucosa shortly after injury indicates exposure to the virus but not necessarily infection.
- Human specimens for PCR, culture, or antibody testing should be sent to the National B Virus Resource Center in Atlanta, Georgia (www2.gsu.edu/~wwwvir/index.html).

THERAPY

- Persons with signs or symptoms of B virus, or positive cultures or PCR (other than wound or postcleansing PCR or culture) and exposure to Old World macaques should be treated.
- Intravenous acyclovir (12.5 to 15 mg/kg q8h) or ganciclovir (5 mg/kg q12h) is recommended for persons without central nervous system (CNS) disease.
- Intravenous ganciclovir (5 mg/kg q12h) is recommended for persons with CNS disease.
- Treatment is continued until symptoms resolve and two cultures over a 2-week period are negative; oral valacyclovir or acyclovir are often given after intravenous therapy is discontinued to prevent reactivation of latent virus.

PREVENTION

- First aid, with thorough cleansing of wounds or exposed mucosa, is important after injuries or mucosal splashes with macaque fluids.
- Persons who have high risk of exposure to B virus (see Table 79-1) should receive postexposure prophylaxis within 5 days of exposure with valacyclovir, 1 g tid, or acyclovir, 800 mg 5 times daily for 14 days.

---

*All material in this chapter is in the public domain, with the exception of any borrowed figures or tables.

TABLE 79-1 Recommendations for Postexposure Prophylaxis for Persons Exposed to Herpes B Virus

Prophylaxis Recommended

Skin exposure* (with loss of skin integrity) or mucosal exposure (with or without injury) to a high-risk source (e.g., a macaque that is ill, immunocompromised, or known to be shedding virus or that has lesions compatible with herpes B virus disease)

Inadequately cleaned skin exposure (with loss of skin integrity) or mucosal exposure (with or without injury)

Laceration of the head, neck, or torso

Deep puncture bite

Needlestick associated with tissue or fluid from the nervous system, lesions suspicious for herpes B virus, eyelids, or mucosa

Puncture or laceration after exposure to objects (a) contaminated either with fluid from monkey oral or genital lesions or with nervous system tissues, or (b) known to contain herpes B virus

A postcleansing culture is positive for herpes B virus

Prophylaxis Considered

Mucosal splash that has been adequately cleaned

Laceration (with loss of skin integrity) that has been adequately cleaned

Needlestick involving blood from an ill or immunocompromised macaque

Puncture or laceration occurring after exposure to (a) objects contaminated with body fluid (other than that from a lesion), or (b) potentially infected cell culture

Regimen for Prophylaxis

Valacyclovir, 1 g PO tid, or acyclovir, 800 mg PO 5 times daily × 14 days

Prophylaxis Not Recommended

Skin exposure in which the skin remains intact

Exposure associated with nonmacaque species of nonhuman primates

*Exposures include macaque bites or scratches, or contact with ocular, oral, or genital secretions, nervous system tissues, or materials contaminated by macaques (e.g., cages or equipment).
From Cohen JI, Davenport DS, Stewart JA, et al. Recommendations for prevention and therapy of persons exposed to B virus (Cercopithecine herpesvirus 1). *Clin Infect Dis.* 2002;35:1191-1203.

80 Adenoviruses

Elizabeth G. Rhee and Dan H. Barouch

DEFINITION

- Human adenoviruses (HAdVs) are DNA viruses that can cause a broad range of clinical syndromes, including respiratory tract infections, ocular disease, gastroenteritis, diarrhea, and cystitis.

EPIDEMIOLOGY

- HAdVs are ubiquitous; most humans have serologic evidence of prior infection by age 10 years.
- Transmission is via respiratory droplets or fecal-oral transmission. Virus secretion may persist for prolonged periods after acute infection resolves.
- Typically, the disease is subclinical or mildly symptomatic and self-limited.
- HAdVs are a common cause of febrile illness, respiratory tract infections (types 1 to 7), and gastroenteritis (types 2 to 5) in young children; sporadic pediatric outbreaks associated with daycare centers and summer camps.
- Acute respiratory disease, including pneumonia, is uncommon; sporadic outbreaks associated with military recruits (types 4 and 7); recent outbreak occurred in healthy adults (type 14).
- Epidemic keratoconjunctivitis (types 8, 19, and 37) has been linked to nosocomial transmission by infected instruments.
- HAdV is an emerging opportunistic pathogen in immunocompromised hosts, primarily hematopoietic stem cell transplant (HSCT) and solid organ transplant (SOT) recipients; it can result in disseminated disease or target grafted organ.
- There is interest in using HAdV as vectors for gene therapy, as vaccines being studied for infectious diseases (human immunodeficiency virus [HIV], malaria); and as immunomodulatory treatments for solid tumors.

MICROBIOLOGY

- HAdVs are nonenveloped, lytic DNA viruses, characterized by serologic responses to major capsid proteins and whole-genome analysis.
- HAdVs are classified into 7 groups (A to F); 60 types isolated from clinical specimens so far.
- HAdVs were originally isolated from adenoid tissues, leading to the virus name.

DIAGNOSIS

- Diagnosis is not routinely pursued because most infections are mild and self-limited.
- HAdVs are detected by routine viral tissue culture (except types 40 and 41) and can be recovered from swabs, samples, and tissues; immunofluorescence assay (IFA), enzyme-linked immunosorbent assay, acute/convalescent serum titers can establish diagnosis.
- Polymerase chain reaction is highly sensitive and specific (96% to 100%) in immunocompetent adults.

THERAPY

- There are no approved therapies available.
- Case series report partial clinical response but substantial toxicities to cidofovir in HSCT/SOT. Clinical trial of brincidofovir in transplant patients is underway.

PREVENTION

- Live oral vaccines (type 4 and 7) are administered to military personnel and are highly effective in preventing adenovirus-associated febrile respiratory diseases.

81 Papillomaviruses

William Bonnez

DEFINITION

- Human papillomavirus (HPV) infects the squamous stratified epithelia of the body and causes tumors that can be benign (warts, condylomas, papillomas) or malignant (squamous cell carcinomas, uterine cervical adenocarcinoma).
- They cause two main groups of diseases: (1) cutaneous (hand, foot, flat) warts and (2) lesions of the mucosal or genital surfaces, such as genital warts, laryngeal papillomas, as well as cancers of the cervix, vagina, vulva, anus, penis, and oropharynx, and their respective precursor lesions, called intraepithelial neoplasias (dysplasias).

EPIDEMIOLOGY

- Cutaneous warts are predominantly a disease of school-aged children. They are acquired from close contacts, predominantly in the family environment.
- Genital (or mucosal) HPV infections are mostly sexually transmitted, and their incidence peaks in late adolescence and early adulthood.
- Most of the sexually active population will have been exposed to genital HPV in a lifetime.
- Genital HPV infections in males and females are easily acquired, but most also disappear quickly. Persistence is a risk factor for the development of cancer.

MICROBIOLOGY

- HPVs are small, nonenveloped DNA viruses, classified according to the nucleotide sequence of the gene coding for the major capsid protein. These viruses are not routinely cultivatable.
- At least 184 types have been identified, but only a small number carry the bulk of the health burden.
- HPV types 1, 2, and 4 are the most common types found in cutaneous warts.
- HPV types 6 and 11 account for most genital warts.
- HPV types 16 and 18 cause the great majority of cancers of the anogenital tract and oropharynx and are defined as high-risk oncogenic.
- The more severe the grade of intraepithelial neoplasia, the more prevalent are high-risk oncogenic HPVs in the lesion.

DIAGNOSIS

- The diagnosis of cutaneous warts and of genital warts is typically clinical. A biopsy is indicated when the diagnosis is in doubt or a malignancy or its precursor is a consideration.
- For the screening of cervical cancer, cytology (Pap smear) is the primary diagnostic approach.
- HPV DNA testing supplements screening cytology.

THERAPY

- Many therapeutic modalities exist for the treatment of HPV-induced lesions, none of them fully satisfactory. They can be divided into medical and physical approaches.

- The chemical methods include salicylic acid solutions for cutaneous warts or podofilox or imiquimod for genital warts.
- The physical methods include cryotherapy, cold-blade excision, electrosurgery, and laser therapy, and they can be applied to most lesions.

PREVENTION

- Male condoms have some effectiveness in protecting against genital infections.
- Pap smears are essential for the prevention of cervical cancer.
- Vaccination is very effective and safe in preventing genital warts as well as intraepithelial neoplasias of the cervix, vagina, vulva, and the anus in males and females.
- Two highly effective vaccines are available. Gardasil is quadrivalent and protects against HPV-6, HPV-11, HPV-16, and HPV-18; Cervarix is bivalent, and it only covers HPV-16 and HPV-18. The vaccines are given intramuscularly in three doses.
- A 9-valent vaccine (Gardasil 9) has been approved by the U.S. Food and Drug Administration in December 2014. It covers HPV-31, HPV-33, HPV-45, HPV-52, and HPV-58, in addition to the four listed earlier.

JC, BK, and Other Polyomaviruses: Progressive Multifocal Leukoencephalopathy (PML)

C. Sabrina Tan and Igor J. Koralnik

JC VIRUS

Definition

- JC virus (JCV) is a ubiquitous human polyomavirus that causes central nervous system diseases in immunocompromised patients, including progressive multifocal leukoencephalopathy (PML), JCV granule cell neuronopathy, and JCV encephalopathy.

Epidemiology

- JCV infects 40% to 86% of the general population worldwide.
- JCV can be detected in the urine of one third of healthy and immunosuppressed individuals.
- PML can occur in up to 5% of untreated patients with acquired immunodeficiency syndrome.
- Up to 82% of PML patients are infected with human immunodeficiency virus.

Microbiology

- JCV is a member of the Polyomaviridae.
- It is a double-stranded DNA virus without an envelope.
- After primary infection, JCV remains latent in the kidney epithelial cells.
- Reactivation of JCV causes a lytic infection of oligodendrocytes in the brain, leading to PML.

Diagnosis

- *Definitive diagnosis of PML:* JCV is detected in cerebrospinal fluid by polymerase chain reaction (PCR) assay or JCV proteins are detected in brain tissues.
- *Possible diagnosis of PML:* Magnetic resonance imaging findings and clinical presentation are consistent with PML in the absence of JCV detection in cerebrospinal fluid.

Therapy

- There are no effective antiviral medications.
- Immune reconstitution can boost host cellular immune response to better control JC viral replication.

Prevention

- Measures should be taken to prevent immunosuppression.

BK VIRUS

Definition

- BK virus (BKV) is a ubiquitous human polyomavirus that causes hemorrhagic cystitis in hematopoietic stem cell transplantation patients and nephropathy in kidney transplantation recipients.

Epidemiology

- BKV infects 82% to 90% of the general population worldwide.
- BKV can be detected in the urine of asymptomatic healthy individuals.
- BKV nephropathy occurs in up to 10% of kidney transplant patients.
- BKV-associated disease can occur in up to 15.9% of allogeneic stem cell transplant recipients.

Microbiology

- BKV is a member of the Polyomaviridae.
- It is a double-stranded DNA virus without an envelope
- After primary infection, BKV remains latent in the kidney epithelial cells.
- Reactivation of BKV causes hemorrhagic cystitis and nephropathy.

Diagnosis

- BKV is detected by PCR assay in blood and sustained viruria in urine.
- Cytopathologic changes may be detected on a kidney biopsy specimen.

Therapy

- There is no effective antiviral medication.
- Reduction in immunosuppression can boost host cellular immune response to better control BKV replication.

Prevention

- Early detection of viral reactivation in urine and blood by PCR assay can be an indicator for a preemptive reduction in immunosuppression to help reduce occurrence of renal disease.

83 Hepatitis B Virus and Hepatitis Delta Virus

Chloe Lynne Thio and Claudia Hawkins

DEFINITION

- Hepatitis B virus (HBV) causes chronic hepatitis B, which can lead to progressive liver disease, including cirrhosis and hepatocellular carcinoma.
- Hepatitis delta virus (HDV) occurs as a coinfection or superinfection with HBV establishing a chronic infection in hepatocytes.

EPIDEMIOLOGY

- Five percent of the world's population has chronic hepatitis B, but prevalence varies widely (see Table 83-1).
- The highest HBV prevalence is in Asia, Africa, and parts of the Middle East.
- Chronic hepatitis B is the leading cause of end-stage liver disease worldwide.
- Transmission of HBV is through percutaneous or sexual routes. Perinatal transmission is also common.
- About 5% of people with chronic hepatitis B have evidence of exposure to HDV.
- HDV has a worldwide prevalence that generally mirrors HBV prevalence, although there are exceptions.
- HDV is primarily transmitted via the parenteral route, but there is some sexual transmission. Perinatal transmission is uncommon.

MICROBIOLOGY

- HBV is a partially double-stranded DNA virus in the *Hepadnavirus* family that primarily infects hepatocytes.
- HBV replication is through an RNA intermediate, so it has a reverse transcriptase.
- HDV is a small, defective RNA virus that relies on host cell machinery for replication.
- HDV requires the envelope of HBV for viral assembly and transmission.

CLINICAL PRESENTATION AND DIAGNOSIS

- Clinical presentation of HBV varies from asymptomatic to fulminant hepatitis with liver failure.
- The risk of developing chronic hepatitis B is inversely proportional to age of acquisition of infection. Chronic hepatitis B is also more likely in high-risk patient groups such as injection drug users, men who have sex with men, and human immunodeficiency virus–infected individuals.
- Laboratory diagnosis of HBV is by enzyme immunoassays, which detect various HBV antigens and antibodies, and by real-time polymerase chain reaction (PCR) to detect HBV DNA (see Table 83-2).
- Clinical presentation of HDV is also variable but can present as acute severe hepatitis.
- Laboratory diagnosis of HDV is with enzyme immunoassay for HDV antibodies and HDV RNA by real-time PCR.

TABLE 83-1 Global Seroprevalence Rates and Modes of Transmission of Hepatitis B

CHARACTERISTIC	HIGH	INTERMEDIATE	LOW
Carrier rate (%)	>8	2-7	<2
Distribution	Southeast Asia, China, Alaskan Eskimos, sub-Saharan Africa, Middle East except Israel, Haiti, Dominican Republic	Eastern and southern Europe, Mediterranean, central Asia, Latin and South America, Israel	United States, Canada, western Europe, Australia, New Zealand
Age at infection	Perinatal and early childhood	Childhood	Adult
Mode of transmission	Maternal and perinatal	Percutaneous	Sexual, percutaneous

TABLE 83-2 Interpretation of Serologic Tests in Hepatitis B

TEST	ACUTE HEPATITIS B	IMMUNITY THROUGH INFECTION*	IMMUNITY THROUGH VACCINATION	ACTIVE CHRONIC HEPATITIS B†	INACTIVE CHRONIC HEPATITIS B
HBsAg	+	–	–	+	+
Anti-HBs	–	+	+	–	–
HBeAg	+	–	–	±	–
Anti-HBe	–	±	–	±	+
Anti-HBc	+	+	–	+	+
IgM anti-HBc	+	–	–	–	–
HBV DNA	+	–	–	+	± (low)
ALT	Elevated	Normal	Normal	Elevated	Normal

ALT, alanine aminotransferase; anti-HBc, antibody to hepatitis B core antigen; anti-HBe, antibody to hepatitis B e antigen; anti-HBs, antibody to hepatitis B surface antigen; DNA, deoxyribonucleic acid; HBeAg, hepatitis B e antigen; HBsAg, hepatitis B surface antigen; HBV, hepatitis B virus; IgM, immunoglobulin M.
*Occasionally individuals with past infection have isolated anti-HBc only. The presence of an isolated immunoglobulin G anti-HBc may indicate a window period during acute infection or remote prior infection with loss of HBsAg or anti-HBs. In such cases, an HBV DNA test may prove useful.
†Chronic hepatitis B with a pre-core mutant is HBeAg– and anti-HBe+.

THERAPY

- Anti-HBV agents significantly reduce complications of chronic hepatitis B, including liver cirrhosis and hepatocellular carcinoma. These therapies are also effective in reducing the recurrence of HBV infection in transplant recipients and other immunocompromised hosts.
- HBV is treated with 180 μg of pegylated interferon-α (PEG IFN-α) weekly for 48 weeks or with nucleos(t)ide analogues often indefinitely (see Table 83-3).
- The first-line nucleos(t)ide agents are entecavir 0.5 mg daily or tenofovir 300 mg daily.
- HDV is treated with 180 μg PEG IFN-α weekly for a minumum of 48 weeks.

PREVENTION

- Vaccination with the hepatitis B vaccine is recommended in all infants and children and for nonimmune adults at high risk for infection (see Table 83-4).
- Infants born to mothers with chronic hepatitis B should receive the hepatitis B vaccine and hepatitis B immune globulin (HBIG) at birth.
- Nonimmune individuals who have percutaneous, sexual, ocular, or mucous membrane exposure to HBV-infected fluids should receive postexposure prophylaxis with HBIG and hepatitis B vaccine.

TABLE 83-3   Approved Agents for Treatment of Chronic Hepatitis B*

	PEG IFN-α	LAMIVUDINE	ADEFOVIR	ENTECAVIR	TELBIVUDINE	TENOFOVIR
Route	Subcutaneous	Oral	Oral	Oral	Oral	Oral
Dose	180 μg/wk	100 mg/day[†]	10 mg/day[†]	0.5 mg/day[†] (1 if lamivudine resistant)	600 mg/day[†]	300 mg/day[†]
Duration (wk)	48	≥48	≥48	≥48	≥48	≥48
Tolerability	Fair-poor: flulike symptoms	Good	Good: follow renal function	Good	Good	Good: follow renal function
HBeAg seroconversion	27%	16%-21%	12%	21%	22%	21%
Undetectable HBV DNA[‡]	25%-63%	40%-73%	21%-51%	67%-90%	60%-88%	76%-93%
ALT normalization	38%	41%-75%	53%	72%	65%	74%
HBsAg loss	3%	<1%	0%	2%	<1%	3%
Viral resistance	None	15%-30%	Minimal	None[§]	6%	0%

ALT, alanine aminotransferase; anti-HBe, antibody to hepatitis B e antigen; HBV, hepatitis B virus; HBsAg, hepatitis B surface antigen; PEG IFN-α, pegylated interferon-α.
*All data are for 1 year unless otherwise noted.
[†]Dose adjustment for creatinine clearance.
[‡]Higher end of range for HBeAg-negative disease.
[§]None; otherwise, 7% if preexisting lamivudine resistance.
Modified from Lok AS, McMahon BJ. Chronic hepatitis B. *Hepatology.* 2009;50:661-662.

TABLE 83-4 Doses and Schedules of Licensed Hepatitis B Vaccines*

HEPATITIS B VACCINES	AGE	DOSE	VOLUME	SCHEDULE
Engerix-B	<20 yr	10 μg	10 μg/ 0.5 mL	Infants[†]: birth, 1-4, 6-18 mo
				Older children: 0, 1-2, 4 mo
	>20 yr	20 μg	20 μg/1 mL	0, 1, 6 mo
	Diabetes 19-59 yr[¶]	20 μg	20 μg/1 mL	0, 1, 6 mo
	Dialysis and other immunocompromised	40 μg	2-20 μg/ 1 mL doses	0, 1, 2, 6 mo
Recombivax HB	<20 yr	5 μg	5 μg/0.5 mL	Infants[†]: birth, 1-4, 6-18 mo
				Older children: 0, 1-2, 4 mo
	11-15 yr	10 μg	10 μg/1 mL	0, 4-6 mo
	>20 yr	10 μg	10 μg/1 mL	0, 1, 6 mo
	Diabetes 19-59 yr[¶]	10 μg	10 μg/1 mL	0, 1, 6 mo
	Dialysis and other immunocompromised	40 μg[‡]	40 μg/1 mL	0, 1, 6 mo
COMBINATION VACCINES	**AGE[§]**	**ANTIGEN**	**VOLUME**	**SCHEDULE**
Comvax	6 wk-4 yr	PedvaxHIB[‖] and Recombivax	0.5 mL	2, 4, 12-15 mo
Pediarix	6 wk-6 yr	Engerix-B, Infanrix (DTaP), and IPV	0.5 mL	2, 4, 6 mo
Twinrix	>18 yr	Havrix (HAV) and Engerix-B (20 μg)	1 mL	0, 1, 6 mo

*All vaccines should be administered intramuscularly in the deltoid.
[†]Infants born to hepatitis B surface antigen (HBsAg)-positive mothers should have hepatitis B immune globulin (HBIG) within 12 hr of delivery, along with vaccine at a separate site. If mother's HBsAg status is unknown, administer vaccine within 12 hr and test mother. If mother is HBsAg positive, administer HBIG within 1 week.
[‡]Special formulation.
[§]Birth dose should be monovalent vaccine only; subsequent doses can be combination.
[‖]PedvaxHIB, licensed *Haemophilus influenzae* type b vaccine; Infarix, licensed diphtheria, tetanus, and acellular pertussis vaccine (DTaP); Havrix, licensed hepatitis A virus (HAV) vaccine.
[¶]Hepatitis B vaccination may be administered at the discretion of the treating clinician to unvaccinated adults with diabetes mellitus who are aged ≥60 years (see http://www.cdc.gov/mmwr/preview/mmwrhtml/mm6050a4.htm).

84 Human Parvoviruses, Including Parvovirus B19V and Human Bocaparvoviruses

Kevin E. Brown

DEFINITION

- At least four different types of parvovirus infect humans.
- Parvovirus B19 (B19V) can cause erythema infectiosum (slapped cheek disease), transient aplastic crisis, and pure red cell aplasia or fetal hydrops.
- Human bocaparvoviruses (HBoVs) can cause respiratory infections and may be associated with some cases of gastroenteritis.
- Human dependoparvovirus infections (adeno-associated viruses [AAVs]) are asymptomatic, and modified dependoparvoviruses are used as vectors for gene therapy.
- Disease associations with Parv4 infection are not clear.

EPIDEMIOLOGY

- Parvovirus B19 infection is a common infection in children and young adults. By age 15, 50% of children in America and Europe will have been infected and have IgG.
- B19V is mainly spread through the respiratory route, although it may also be transmitted through blood and blood products.
- B19V infections in temperate climates are more common in late winter, spring, and early summer, with increased rates of infection every 3 to 5 years.
- HBoV infections are ubiquitous in young children, with most if not all children being infected with HBoV1 by the age of 6.

DIAGNOSIS

- Although the slapped cheek rash of parvovirus B19 infection is classic, it is difficult to accurately diagnose outside of the context of an outbreak.
- Diagnosis of B19V rash is by detection of B19V IgM in serum.
- Hematologic disease due to B19 can be diagnosed by detection of high-titer B19V DNA ($>10^6$ IU/mL) in blood samples.
- Following infection, low levels of B19V DNA may be detected lifelong. Detection of low-level B19V DNA in samples therefore does not indicate recent or current infection.
- Similarly, long-term persistence of bocavirus DNA in respiratory and fecal samples indicates that detection of viral DNA alone does not correlate with infection. Respiratory HBoV1 infection should be diagnosed by detection of viral DNA in serum or serology, or both.

THERAPY

- Treatment for all parvovirus infections is mainly symptomatic.
- Intravenous immunoglobulin can be used for treatment of chronic anemia or pure red aplasia due to high-titer parvovirus B19 infection.

PREVENTION

- A vaccine for parvovirus B19 is in development.

85 Orthoreoviruses and Orbiviruses

Roberta L. DeBiasi and Kenneth L. Tyler

DEFINITION

- Reoviruses are linear double-stranded RNA viruses with broad host ranges.
- The term *reovirus* is an acronym for respiratory enteric orphan virus, which emphasizes the anatomic site from which these viruses were initially isolated.

EPIDEMIOLOGY

- Infection of humans is common but is rarely associated with significant disease.
- Asymptomatic infection is common; symptomatic infection usually consists of mild, self-limited upper respiratory tract and gastrointestinal illness.
- Reoviruses have been identified as the causative agent in rare human cases of meningitis, encephalitis, pneumonia, and myocarditis and are potentially associated with biliary atresia and choledochal cysts.

MICROBIOLOGY

- Five genera of the Reoviridae have been etiologically linked with diseases of humans: *Orthoreovirus, Orbivirus, Rotavirus, Coltivirus,* and *Seadornavirus.*
- Double-stranded RNA is organized into 10 to 12 segments, which are capable of reassortment and resultant generation of novel viruses.

DIAGNOSIS

- Laboratory diagnosis can be made serologically by a fourfold rise in acute and convalescent serum antibody response or by virus isolation from serum, stool, respiratory secretions, or cerebrospinal fluid.

THERAPY

- No specific therapy is available.

PREVENTION

- No specific preventative measures are recommended—reoviruses are ubiquitous.

86 Coltiviruses and Seadornaviruses

Roberta L. DeBiasi and Kenneth L. Tyler

DEFINITION

- *Coltivirus* and *Seadornavirus* are two of five genera of the Reoviridae virus family that have been documented to cause human disease.

EPIDEMIOLOGY

- Coltiviruses associated with human disease include the type-specific Colorado tick fever virus (CTFV; North America), Eyach virus (EYAV; France, Germany, Czech Republic), and Salmon River virus (SRV; North America).
- The only *Seadornavirus* implicated in human disease to date is Banna virus (BAV; Indonesia and China).
- Ticks are the principal vectors of coltiviruses but have also been isolated from mosquitoes, rodents, and humans.
- The distribution of CTFV coincides with the range of the principal tick vector. The virus has been isolated in 11 states, primarily within the Rocky Mountain region, as well as southwestern Canada.
- CTFV has been isolated from patients with acute febrile syndromes, meningitis, and encephalitis in North America.

MICROBIOLOGY

- Coltiviruses and seadornaviruses are nonenveloped double-stranded RNA viruses with a segmented genome. Coltiviruses have 12 gene segments enclosed within two capsids.

DIAGNOSIS

- CTFV should be considered in anyone presenting with a febrile illness following tick exposure in an endemic area.
- Patients may have cerebrospinal fluid pleocytosis. Leukopenia is common.
- Serologic methods, including enzyme-linked immunosorbent assay, as well as serum and cerebrospinal fluid reverse transcriptase–polymerase chain reaction have been used for diagnosis.
- Virus can also be isolated in cell culture.

THERAPY

- No specific therapy is available.

PREVENTION

- Preventative measures include tick and mosquito repellents such as diethyltoluamide, physical barriers, and reduction of standing water.
- CTFV patients should not be allowed to serve as blood product or hematopoietic stem cell donors until infection has fully resolved.

87 Rotaviruses

Philip R. Dormitzer

DEFINITION

- Rotavirus is a nonenveloped, double-stranded RNA virus that is the most important universal cause of dehydrating infant and childhood gastroenteritis.

VIRAL STRUCTURE AND REPLICATION

- The viral particle is a triple-layered icosahedron.
- Genome consists of 11 segments of double-stranded RNA.
- The outer layer glycoprotein VP7 and the spike protein VP4 mediate entry into cells and are the neutralization determinants.
- The virus binds cell surface carbohydrates.
- Cells are entered by viral penetration of the cellular membrane.
- After the outer layer is removed, a subviral particle transcribes and extrudes mRNA.
- New subviral particles assemble in viroplasms in the cytoplasm, and virions are completed by addition of the outer-layer proteins in the endoplasmic reticulum.

CLINICAL MANIFESTATIONS

- Gastroenteritis due to rotavirus is not readily distinguished from gastroenteritis caused by other agents on clinical grounds alone.
- Main symptoms are diarrhea and vomiting. Severe dehydration and death can result.

PATHOGENESIS

- The virus primarily infects epithelial cells at the tips of the intestinal villi.
- Multifactorial pathogenesis of rotavirus diarrhea includes malabsorption due to loss of intestinal epithelial cells, an enterotoxin, and enteric nervous system signaling to create a secretory state.

SEROLOGIC CLASSIFICATION

- Group A rotaviruses cause most human disease.
- There is an extensive diversity of antigenic types.
- Within group A, rotavirus has a dual serologic classification system with G type based on VP7 and P type based on VP4.
- Genetic classification is starting to replace serologic classification.

EPIDEMIOLOGY

- Infection is universal in the first years of life.
- Infection may be symptomatic or asymptomatic.
- Severe illness is most common between 6 months and 2 years of age.
- Reinfection occurs throughout life.
- There is a large burden of illness in all socioeconomic settings, but mortality is concentrated in developing countries.

- Annually, rotaviruses cause approximately 450,000 deaths of children younger than the age of 5 years.
- Exchange of strains and genome segments between human rotaviruses and animal rotaviruses maintains the diversity of circulating strains.

IMMUNITY

- Partial protection from reinfection is provided by previous infection, with generally decreasing severity of subsequent infections.
- Serotype influences but does not determine protection from reinfection.
- VP4 and VP7 each contain serotype-specific and heterotypic neutralizing epitopes.
- Neutralizing antibodies block the functions of the outer capsid proteins in cell entry.
- Non-neutralizing IgA against the middle layer protein, VP6, can interfere with intracellular virus replication, as the antibody is transcytosed across intestinal epithelial cells.
- Humoral immunity appears to be the most important determinant of protection from reinfection.
- Cellular immunity contributes to clearance of infection.
- Rotavirus interferes with the innate immune response by several mechanisms.

DIAGNOSIS

- Specific virologic diagnosis is not necessary for routine clinical care but is useful for epidemiologic study, in complicated or prolonged cases, and to reduce unnecessary antibiotic use.
- Antigen can be readily detected in the stool, most commonly by enzyme-linked immunosorbent assay.
- There is increasing use of nucleic acid–based testing for epidemiologic investigations.

THERAPY

- Therapy is primarily supportive and aimed at maintaining hydration until the infection resolves.
- No specific antiviral therapy is available.
- Mild and moderate dehydration can be treated effectively with oral rehydration solutions.
- Severe dehydration and treatment for patients with depressed consciousness or ileus require the use of intravenous fluids.
- In the context of malnutrition, zinc supplementation may be a useful adjunct to oral rehydration therapy.

IMMUNIZATION

- Two live-attenuated, oral rotavirus vaccines have been licensed and are currently in use—a monovalent vaccine (Rotarix) and a pentavalent vaccine (RotaTeq).
- A rare complication of immunization, intestinal intussusception, led to the withdrawal of a previous rotavirus vaccine, but there is consensus that the benefits of immunization with the current rotavirus vaccines far outweigh the risk for intussusception.
- Where the vaccines have been introduced, they have dramatically decreased severe rotavirus gastroenteritis and substantially decreased severe, dehydrating pediatric gastroenteritis overall.
- The next major challenge is distributing rotavirus vaccines to the developing countries where mortality is concentrated.
- Despite lower efficacy in impoverished settings than in affluent settings, rotavirus vaccines could have a large impact on infant mortality worldwide.
- Local production of new rotavirus vaccine candidates in developing countries could contribute to increased access.

88 Alphaviruses

Lewis Markoff

DEFINITION
- Alphaviruses, which constitute a genus of more than 30 viruses in the Togaviridae family, are lipid-enveloped, positive-sense RNA viruses.
- All human pathogenic alphaviruses are mosquito borne.

EPIDEMIOLOGY
- The presence of infected mosquitoes is required for disease outbreak. Human-to-human transmission does not occur.
- New World alphaviruses include Eastern, Western, and Venezuelan equine encephalitis viruses (EEEV, WEEV, and VEEV, respectively), which are found in North and South America.
- Old World alphaviruses, especially chikungunya (CHIK), Sindbis, Ross River, and O'nyong-nyong viruses, found in Europe, Africa, and Asia, cause a fever, arthralgia, and rash syndrome.
- In most cases, except for CHIK virus, the life cycle of the viruses requires mosquitoes and an animal host in nature, other than humans.

PATHOGENESIS
- Alphaviruses enter cells by receptor-mediated endocytosis and exit by budding from the plasma membrane.
- Alphaviruses enter the body via mosquito bites and replicate in various tissues, including Langerhans cells, which then migrate to lymph nodes, causing viremia. Viremia results in invasion of the central nervous system (CNS) by alphaviruses that cause encephalitis or of the joints and internal organs by viruses that cause fever, arthralgia, and rash.
- All alphaviruses suppress the innate immune response by inhibiting JAK/STAT signaling, a major early determinant of disease severity.
- At later times, recovery is mediated by virus-neutralizing antibodies and cytotoxic T cells.
- In the CNS, virus replication in neurons is suppressed indefinitely by antibody-secreting B cells.

DIAGNOSIS
- Knowledge of the patient's travel history is of major importance in diagnosis.
- The fever/arthralgia/rash syndrome caused by Old World alphaviruses can be confused with many other viral exanthems.
- Alphavirus encephalitis is similar in presentation to that caused by the flaviviruses, West Nile and St. Louis encephalitis viruses.
- Culture of virus from blood or detection by reverse-transcriptase polymerase chain reaction is not recommended for diagnosis of encephalitis but may occasionally yield positive results in the acute phase of fever/arthralgia/rash syndrome.
- Detection of virus-neutralizing antibodies in combination with recent travel history to an endemic area may be meaningful.

- Virus-specific IgM or IgG class antibodies, or both, can be detected by enzyme-linked immunosorbent assay; a greater than fourfold rise in titer between acute and convalescent sera or virus-specific IgM in cerebrospinal fluid, or both, are diagnostic.

THERAPY

- At present, there are no products licensed for treatment.
- Experimental therapies that seem promising include the use of human monoclonal antibodies, especially in treatment of alphavirus encephalitis.
- For encephalitis, supportive measures and intensive nursing care are currently indicated.
- For fever/arthralgia/rash syndrome, analgesics and nonsteroidal anti-inflammatory drugs are the main treatment options.

PREVENTION

- Veterinary vaccines are available for horses, and their immunization against WEE, EEE, and VEE is required in the United States.
- There are no licensed vaccines for prevention of alphavirus diseases in humans, but unlicensed vaccines against VEE, EEE, WEE, and CHIK are available for at-risk laboratory workers.
- Vaccines are under development, particularly against CHIK. One promising approach is the use of CHIK virus–like particles for immunization.
- The primary methods for disease prevention in humans are mosquito eradication programs, avoidance of mosquito-infested areas, and use of protection from mosquito bites, where exposure to possibly infected mosquitoes is unavoidable.

89 Rubella Virus (German Measles)

Anne A. Gershon

DEFINITION
- Rubella is an infectious illness characterized by fever and maculopapular rash, which may be accompanied by arthritis.
- Many postnatal infections are asymptomatic.
- Postnatal rubella is a rather benign illness, but congenital rubella can result in a variety of serious medical problems.
- Manifestations of congenital rubella include deafness, cataract or glaucoma, congenital heart disease, and mental retardation.
- Rubella vaccine was developed primarily to prevent congenital rubella from occurring.

EPIDEMIOLOGY
- In temperate climates, disease occurs mainly in the spring (if vaccine is not being used).
- Rubella is somewhat less contagious than measles.
- Widespread vaccination in the Americas led to the elimination of rubella as of 2009.
- Globally, rubella and congenital rubella remain serious medical problems, especially in Africa, some areas of Europe, Southeast Asia, and the Western Pacific.

MICROBIOLOGY
- Rubella is an RNA virus, a member of the Togaviridae family and the genus *Rubivirus*.

DIAGNOSIS
- Diagnosis can be made serologically (enzyme-linked immunosorbent assay) with acute and convalescent serum samples, or by demonstration of rubella IgM antibody on a single serum sample.
- A positive test for viral RNA using reverse-transcriptase polymerase chain reaction on throat swabs, cerebrospinal fluid, and/or amniotic fluid is especially useful for diagnosis of congenital rubella.

THERAPY
- None is available.

PREVENTION
- Live-attenuated rubella vaccine is effective and safe, usually administered along with measles and mumps vaccines (MMR).

90 Flaviviruses (Dengue, Yellow Fever, Japanese Encephalitis, West Nile Encephalitis, St. Louis Encephalitis, Tick-Borne Encephalitis, Kyasanur Forest Disease, Alkhurma Hemorrhagic Fever, Zika)

Stephen J. Thomas, Timothy P. Endy, Alan L. Rothman, and Alan D. Barrett*

DEFINITION

- The Flaviviridae incorporates the *Flavivirus, Pestivirus,* and *Hepacivirus* genera, which cause systemic febrile, central nervous system, and/or hemorrhagic fever syndromes.

EPIDEMIOLOGY

- Transmission and disease may occur with endemic, hyperendemic, and/or epidemic patterns.
- Yellow fever (YF) is found in tropical South America and sub-Saharan Africa. Disease is severe with high morbidity and mortality.
- Dengue is widely distributed throughout the tropics and subtropics. Severe disease is infrequent (~2% to 4% of apparent cases) but potentially fatal. Nonsevere disease (outpatient) accounts for much of dengue's global socioeconomic impact.
- Japanese encephalitis (JE) virus is a significant cause of encephalitis in Southeast and South Asia. Chronic morbidity and mortality are high in symptomatic cases.
- West Nile virus (WNV), St. Louis encephalitis (SLE) virus, JE virus, and tick-borne encephalitis (TBE) virus are the major neurotropic members of the genus *Flavivirus.* Infection with WNV is found worldwide, SLE is found in the Americas, whereas TBE occurs from Western Europe to Russia, Japan, and China. Most infections are subclinical. Clinically apparent cases with neurologic manifestations have a predilection for older individuals.
- Alkhurma hemorrhagic fever virus (AHFV), Kyasanur Forest disease virus (KFDV), and Zika virus (ZIKV) infections are emerging or reemerging in the Middle East, India, and Africa/Asia, respectively. All infections initially have nonspecific clinical findings; persons infected with AHFV and KFDV may develop hemorrhagic manifestations.

MICROBIOLOGY

- Flaviviruses are icosahedral, approximately (50 nm in diameter, approximately 11-kb single-stranded, positive-sense RNA viruses consisting of a lipid envelope covered densely with surface projections consisting of M (membrane) and E (envelope) glycoproteins. Nonstructural proteins make up the remainder of the genome.
- Mutations and replication errors are high.

DIAGNOSIS

- Diagnostic approaches are dictated by the disease course.
- During the viremic period, viral isolation and nucleic acid or antigen detection from blood are possible.
- During the subacute period, early-phase IgM antibodies may be detected in sera or cerebrospinal fluid using various assay platforms (e.g., enzyme-linked immunosorbent assay, hemagglutination inhibition).

---

*Disclaimer: The opinions or assertions contained herein are the private views of the author (SJT) and are not to be construed as reflecting the official views of the U.S. Army or the U.S. Department of Defense.

- During the convalescent period, a rise in IgG between acute and convalescent specimens is measured to identify a seroresponse (plaque reduction neutralization test).

THERAPY

- No licensed or specific antiviral therapies are available.
- Treatment is supportive, and outcomes are variable.

PREVENTION

- U.S.-licensed vaccines exist for YF and JE. Vaccines exist for TBE and KFDV.
- Two recently completed phase III studies in Asia and Latin America of a live-attenuated dengue tetravalent vaccine (CYD-TDV) demonstrated moderate efficacy against any dengue of any severity caused by any serotype and high efficacy against hospitalized and severe dengue.
- Numerous vaccine development efforts are underway for additional flaviviruses.

91 | Hepatitis C

Stuart C. Ray and David L. Thomas

DEFINITION

- Hepatitis C virus (HCV) is an enveloped, positive-strand RNA virus that is a member of the Flaviviridae family, *Hepacivirus* genus.
- It is a major worldwide cause of chronic liver disease, including cirrhosis and increased risk of hepatocellular carcinoma (HCC).

MICROBIOLOGY

- HCV is roughly spheroid and is 55 nm in diameter.
- The RNA genome is 9.6 kb in length and contains a single large open reading frame, which is processed into at least 10 proteins, including 3 structural proteins and 5 proteins of the viral RNA replicase complex (NS3, NS4A, NS4B, NS5A, and NS5B) (see Fig. 91-1).
- HCV has six major genotypes and provisionally a seventh.
- Extensive quasispecies variation is present in each infected individual.

EPIDEMIOLOGY

- More than 185 million persons are HCV antibody positive worldwide.
- Transmission occurs most commonly by percutaneous exposure to blood.
- In developed countries, most HCV infections are associated with IV drug abuse.
- In the developing world, transmission occurs from unsafe medical practices.
- HCV may be transmitted sexually, but this appears to be infrequent except in high-risk sexual activities.

CLINICAL MANIFESTATIONS

- Acute illness caused by HCV infection is unusual, but it is typical of acute hepatitis and consists of malaise, nausea, and right upper quadrant pain, followed by dark urine and jaundice.
- Fulminant hepatitis due to HCV infection is uncommon in Western countries.
- Chronic infection with HCV occurs in approximately 75% of patients after acute infection with HCV.
- Once established, chronic infection persists for decades and can be associated with cirrhosis, metabolic disorders such as insulin resistance and steatosis, and HCC.

DIAGNOSIS

- Diagnosis of HCV infection is usually made by assays of serum antibody to HCV followed by testing for HCV RNA.
- RNA tests are also used to assess the effects of treatment.
- Liver biopsies and noninvasive liver tests are used to assess the stage of liver diseases.

TREATMENT (SEE TABLE 91-1)

- The primary aim of treatment is to eradicate HCV in blood and liver and thus prevent complications of HCV infection.

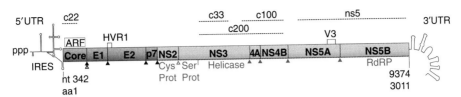

FIGURE 91-1 Organization of the hepatitis C virus (HCV) genome and viral polyprotein. The 5′ and 3′ untranslated region (UTR) RNA structures (curves) flank the major open reading frame (ORF). Unlike eukaryotic mRNA, the viral RNA genome has 5′ triphosphate ("ppp") and no 3′ polyadenylation. The 5′ UTR contains an internal ribosomal entry site (IRES). *Triangles* indicate sites of cleavage by host cellular signal peptidase (*black, open* indicating additional processing by signal peptide peptidase) and viral (*blue, open* indicating cleavage by the NS2/NS3 cysteine protease) proteases are shown as *triangles*. Putative structural (*gray*) and nonstructural (*blue*) mature proteins (*boxes*) generated by these cleavage events are labeled, below which in *blue* are viral enzymatic functions NS2/NS3 cysteine protease (Cys Prot), NS3 serine protease (Ser Prot), NS3 helicase, and the NS5B RNA-dependent RNA polymerase (RdRP). Positions of the first and last nucleotides (nt) and amino acids (aa) of the polyprotein ORF are shown, based on reference genome H77 (GenBank accession number AF009606). Above the ORF are positions of the alternate reading frame protein (ARFP), variable regions HVR1 and V3, and (indicated by *horizontal lines*) the antigens included in the enzyme immunoassay serologic assay.

TABLE 91-1 AASLD and IDSA Recommendations for HCV Treatment-Naïve Patients: January 2015

GENOTYPE	RECOMMENDATION*
1a	Daily fixed-dose combination of ledipasvir (90 mg)/sofosbuvir (400 mg) for 12 wk
	Daily fixed-dose combination of paritaprevir (150 mg)/ritonavir (100 mg)/ombitasvir (25 mg) plus twice-daily–dosed dasabuvir (250 mg) and weight-based RBV for 12 wk (no cirrhosis) or 24 wk (cirrhosis)
	Daily sofosbuvir (400 mg) plus simeprevir (150 mg) with or without weight-based RBV for 12 wk (no cirrhosis) or 24 wk (cirrhosis)
1b	Daily fixed-dose combination of ledipasvir (90 mg)/sofosbuvir (400 mg) for 12 wk
	Daily fixed-dose combination of paritaprevir (150 mg)/ritonavir (100 mg)/ombitasvir (25 mg) plus twice-daily–dosed dasabuvir (250 mg) for 12 wk. Weight-based RBV recommended for patients with cirrhosis
	Daily sofosbuvir (400 mg) plus simeprevir (150 mg) for 12 wk (no cirrhosis) or 24 wk (cirrhosis)
2	Daily sofosbuvir (400 mg) and weight-based RBV for 12 wk (no cirrhosis) or 16 wk (cirrhosis)
3	Daily sofosbuvir (400 mg) and weight-based RBV for 24 wk
4	Daily fixed-dose combination of ledipasvir (90 mg)/sofosbuvir (400 mg) for 12 wk
	Daily fixed-dose combination of paritaprevir (150 mg)/ritonavir (100 mg)/ombitasvir (25 mg) and weight-based RBV for 12 wk
	Daily sofosbuvir (400 mg) and weight-based RBV for 24 wk
5	Daily sofosbuvir (400 mg) and weight-based RBV plus weekly PEG IFN for 12 wk
6	Daily ledipasvir (90 mg)/sofosbuvir (400 mg) for 12 wk

AASLD, American Association for the Study of Liver Diseases; HCV, hepatitis C virus; IDSA, Infectious Diseases Society of America; PEG IFN, pegylated interferon; RBV, ribavirin.
*Listed alphabetically: see www.hcvguidelines.org for alternative treatments, treatments in experienced patients, and special populations.

- American Association for the Study of Liver Diseases (AASLD) and Infectious Diseases Society of America (IDSA) treatment recommendations for hepatitis C, January 2015:
  - See Table 91-1
  - Genotype 1a
    - Ledipasvir/sofosbuvir for 12 weeks
    - Paritaprevir/ritonavir/ombitasvir plus dasabuvir and weight-based ribavirin (RBV) for 12 weeks (no cirrhosis) or 24 weeks (cirrhosis)
    - Sofosbuvir plus simeprevir with or without RBV for 12 weeks (no cirrhosis) or 24 weeks (cirrhosis)
  - Genotype 1b
    - Ledipasvir/sofosbuvir for 12 weeks
    - Paritaprevir/ritonavir/ombitasvir plus dasabuvir for 12 weeks, plus RBV for patients with cirrhosis
    - Sofosbuvir plus simeprevir for 12 weeks (no cirrhosis) or 24 weeks (cirrhosis)
  - Genotype 2
    - Sofosbuvir and RBV for 12 weeks (no cirrhosis) or 16 weeks (cirrhosis)
  - Genotype 3
    - Sofosbuvir and RBV for 24 weeks
  - Genotype 4
    - Ledipasvir/sofosbuvir for 12 weeks
    - Paritaprevir/ritonavir/ombitasvir and RBV for 12 weeks
    - Sofosbuvir and RBV for 24 weeks
  - Genotype 5
    - Sofosbuvir and RBV and polyethylene glycol (PEG) for 12 weeks
  - Genotype 6
    - Ledipasvir/sofosbuvir for 12 weeks

Clinicians are urged to consult online guidelines for the latest recommendations on HCV treatment (www.hcvguidelines.org).

PREVENTION

- Strategies are primarily designed to reduce exposure to contaminated blood, through screening of blood products, application of precautions in health care settings, and reduction of IV drug abuse risks.
- Development of vaccines against HCV is challenging because of extensive viral diversity.

92 Coronaviruses, Including Severe Acute Respiratory Syndrome (SARS) and Middle East Respiratory Syndrome (MERS)

Kenneth McIntosh and Stanley Perlman

DEFINITION

- The coronaviruses (CoVs) commonly cause mild but occasionally more severe community-acquired acute respiratory infections in humans. CoVs also infect a wide variety of animals, and several CoVs (e.g., severe acute respiratory syndrome [SARS], Middle East respiratory syndrome [MERS]) have crossed the species barrier, producing outbreaks of severe respiratory disease. As of January 23, 2015, 956 cases of laboratory-confirmed MERS were reported to the World Health Organization, with 351 deaths.

EPIDEMIOLOGY

- Community-acquired CoV infections cause about 15% of common colds. They are typically epidemic in the winter months. MERS has occurred in patients in the Arabian Peninsula and those who recently traveled from this locale.

MICROBIOLOGY

- CoVs are members of the Nidovirales order, single-stranded, positive-sense RNA viruses with a large genome. They mutate and also recombine frequently.

DIAGNOSIS

- Laboratory diagnosis is best accomplished by finding viral RNA through polymerase chain reaction.

THERAPY

- There are no accepted effective antiviral drugs for CoVs.

PREVENTION

- Prevention is through epidemiologic methods. The SARS epidemic was halted through careful case finding, quarantine, and use of barrier precautions.

93 Parainfluenza Viruses

Michael G. Ison

DEFINITION
- Parainfluenza virus (PIV) causes acute respiratory illness, including colds, croup, bronchiolitis, and pneumonia.

EPIDEMIOLOGY
- PIV-1 and PIV-2 cause seasonal outbreaks in the fall, with PIV-1 causing epidemics in odd-numbered years. Clinically, PIV-1 is strongly associated with croup in children.
- PIV-3 causes annual epidemics in the spring; in years where PIV-1 does not circulate, the season is typically more active and prolonged. PIV-3 is associated with more severe infections, particularly among immunocompromised adults and children.
- PIV-4 is associated with milder disease, typically limited to the upper airway.
- Although antibodies are produced in response to clinical disease, reinfection is common throughout life.
- Disease, particularly associated with PIV-3, frequently progresses to the lower airway in immunocompromised adults and children and is associated with significant morbidity and mortality.

MICROBIOLOGY
- Parainfluenza is a single-stranded, enveloped RNA virus belonging to the Paramyxoviridae family. It includes PIV-1, PIV-2, PIV-3, and PIV-4.

DIAGNOSIS
- National parainfluenza virus trends are available at www.cdc.gov/surveillance/nrevss/human-paraflu/natl-trend.htm.
- Laboratory diagnosis can be made by culture or polymerase chain reaction (PCR) assay, with improved sensitivity with molecular diagnostic methods.

THERAPY
- Croup is generally treated with glucocorticoids and nebulized epinephrine in young children.
- Although ribavirin and intravenous immunoglobulin have been used in the treatment of immunocompromised adults and children, their efficacy is uncertain.
- A number of novel antivirals are currently under development.

PREVENTION
- Standard and contact precautions are recommended to avoid nosocomial spread of PIV in the health care setting.
- A number of live-attenuated vaccine candidates are undergoing development.

94 Mumps Virus

Nathan Litman and Stephen G. Baum

DEFINITION

- Mumps is an acute viral infection most commonly manifest as nonsuppurative swelling and tenderness of the parotid or other salivary glands caused by the mumps virus.
- Less common manifestations of mumps include meningitis, encephalitis, epididymo-orchitis, oophoritis, and pancreatitis.

EPIDEMIOLOGY

- Mumps is endemic throughout the world, and humans are the only natural hosts for the virus.
- Incubation period is usually 16 to 18 days with a range of 2 to 4 weeks.
- Before the introduction of the mumps vaccine in the United States in 1967, epidemics occurred every 2 to 5 years with peak incidence between January and May.
- Since 1967, there has been more than a 99% decline in the annual U.S. incidence of mumps.
- Outbreaks of mumps have been reported throughout the world, including the United States, even in populations who have received the recommended two-dose measles-mumps-rubella (MMR) series.

MICROBIOLOGY

- Mumps is an enveloped, single-stranded RNA virus.
- Only one serotype of mumps virus exists, but there are 13 genotypes.

DIAGNOSIS

- The clinical diagnosis is made on the basis of a history of exposure and of parotid swelling and tenderness.
- The diagnosis is confirmed by isolation of mumps virus or detection of mumps nucleic acid by polymerase chain reaction from clinical specimens or the presence of mumps-specific IgM antibodies or a fourfold rise in mumps IgG antibodies in serum.

THERAPY

- Therapy for mumps is symptomatic and supportive.

PREVENTION

- Immunization with live, attenuated mumps virus vaccine as part of the standard MMR vaccine at 12 months and 4 to 6 years of age is recommended for all children; a two-dose series of MMR is recommended for individuals beyond childhood who have not received the childhood series.

95 Respiratory Syncytial Virus (RSV)

Edward E. Walsh and Caroline Breese Hall*

DEFINITION

- Respiratory syncytial virus (RSV) causes acute upper and lower tract respiratory illnesses.

EPIDEMIOLOGY

- RSV circulates annually during the winter months in temperate climates.
- RSV is the leading cause of bronchiolitis in infants.
- Reinfection is common throughout life and can be severe in elderly and immunocompromised persons.
- RSV is primarily transmitted by direct contact with infected persons or their secretions.

MICROBIOLOGY

- RSV is an enveloped nonsegmented RNA virus in the Paramyxoviridae family.
- RSV isolates can be classified into antigenically distinct groups, A and B.

DIAGNOSIS

- Clinical diagnosis in infants is relatively accurate during the winter months; however, in older children and adults, laboratory confirmation by culture, antigen detection, or reverse-transcriptase polymerase chain reaction is necessary.

THERAPY

- Treatment for most infants and adults is supportive only.
- Aerosolized ribavirin, a nucleoside analogue, can be considered for administration to high-risk infants. It is also used to treat RSV in highly immunocompromised persons, with or without anti-RSV immunoglobulin, but its efficacy is not established.

PREVENTION

- Attention to infection control measures, such as hand hygiene and contact precautions, can reduce the spread of RSV.
- Palivizumab, a humanized neutralizing monoclonal antibody to RSV, is beneficial for specific high-risk infants, including those with underlying cardiac and pulmonary disease and low gestational age.

---

*Caren Hall passed away in 2012. She was the author for this and other chapters for previous editions of this book. This chapter is dedicated to her memory.

96 Human Metapneumovirus

Ann R. Falsey

DEFINITION

- Human metapneumovirus (hMPV) is a paramyxovirus that causes acute respiratory tract infections.

EPIDEMIOLOGY

- Distribution is worldwide.
- Infection is most common in winter and spring in temperate climates.
- hMPV cocirculates with other seasonal viruses, including influenza and respiratory syncytial virus (RSV).
- Infection is universal by age 5 years.
- Reinfections occur throughout life.

MICROBIOLOGY

- Virus is in family Paramyxoviridae, subfamily Pneumovirinae, genus *Metapneumovirus;* has nonsegmented single-stranded RNA (ssRNA).
- Diverged from avian metapneumoviruses 200 to 300 years ago.
- Two major genotypes (A and B) and four subgroups (A1, A2, B1, and B2).

DIAGNOSIS

- Clinical syndrome is not distinct and ranges from common cold to acute respiratory distress syndrome.
- Bronchiolitis, asthma exacerbations, and pneumonia occur in children.
- Diagnosis is best accomplished by reverse-transcriptase polymerase chain reaction (RT-PCR) of respiratory secretions.
- Immunofluorescence assay of respiratory secretions is less sensitive than RT-PCR but is an acceptable method of diagnosis.

THERAPY

- Therapy is supportive.
- Intravenous gamma globulin and ribavirin have been used in severely ill immunocompromised patients, but efficacy, if any, is unclear.

PREVENTION

- No vaccine is available.
- Infection control measures include hand hygiene and use of masks, gowns, and gloves in outbreak situations.

97 Measles Virus (Rubeola)

Anne A. Gershon

DEFINITION

- Measles is a highly contagious viral infection, usually of childhood.
- The disease presents with a nonpruritic rash that begins on the head and face and spreads down the body, with fever and malaise.
- Initially, before the rash appears, measles can resemble influenza.
- There is usually accompanying conjunctivitis, cough, and coryza.
- Complications include infections of the respiratory tract and central nervous system involvement.

EPIDEMIOLOGY

- Measles is very contagious before the rash appears, which enhances the chance of spread before the disease is identified.
- Measles is also contagious for a few days after rash onset.
- The virus spreads by droplets and also by the airborne route.
- Widespread vaccination with two vaccine doses in the Americas has reduced the incidence of measles so that the virus is no longer endemic in these regions.
- However, measles outbreaks continue to occur in the United States (34 outbreaks in 2013 to 2014, and a large outbreak in 2015 related to exposure at Disneyland in California).
- When vaccination rates fall below 95%, measles outbreaks can occur if the virus is reintroduced into a population.
- Immunosuppressed patients are at high risk to develop severe measles without necessarily manifesting a rash.
- Measles vaccination has been shown to be unrelated to development of autism.

MICROBIOLOGY

- Measles is caused by an RNA virus classified as a *Morbillivirus* of the Paramyxoviridae family.

DIAGNOSIS

- Clinically, measles may be confused with Kawasaki disease.
- Measles virus is difficult to culture.
- Diagnosis is usually made clinically, particularly if Koplik spots on the oral mucosa are observed.
- Laboratory diagnosis can be made by reverse-transcriptase polymerase chain reaction (RT-PCR) on just about any body fluid or tissue.

THERAPY

- No specific therapy has been proven to be useful.
- Administration of vitamin A once daily by mouth for 2 days should be considered for patients with measles.
- The mechanism of action of vitamin A is thought to be by immunomodulation.

PREVENTION

- Live-attenuated measles vaccine is administered to healthy children at 12 to 15 months of age and again at age 4 to 6 years.
- Passive immunization with immunoglobulin G should be given to high-risk children and adults exposed to measles but having no history of measles.

98 Zoonotic Paramyxoviruses: Nipah, Hendra, and Menangle

Anna R. Thorner and Raphael Dolin

DEFINITION

- Hendra and Nipah viruses are highly pathogenic zoonotic paramyxoviruses that emerged during the 1990s in Australia and Southeast Asia, respectively.

EPIDEMIOLOGY

- In 1994, in Queensland, Australia, Hendra virus caused two outbreaks of fatal illness in horses and their human caretakers. Additional outbreaks involving humans occurred in 2004, 2008, and 2009.
- Nipah virus was first recognized when it caused an outbreak of severe encephalitis in pig farmers in Malaysia and abattoir workers in Singapore in 1998 and 1999. Multiple outbreaks have been detected subsequently in Bangladesh and India, including cases that have involved human-to-human transmission.
- Menangle virus, another paramyxovirus, caused decreased farrowing rates and stillbirths in pigs, as well as illness in two humans in Australia in 1997.
- The *Pteropus* species of fruit bat, also known as the flying fox, is the reservoir of all three viruses.

CLASSIFICATION

- Nipah and Hendra viruses are members of the *Henipavirus* genus within the Paramyxovirinae subfamily of the Paramyxoviridae family.

CLINICAL MANIFESTATIONS

- Nipah virus causes a severe and often fatal meningoencephalitis. Clinical manifestations of Hendra virus infection range from a self-limited influenza-like syndrome to a fatal respiratory illness or encephalitis. Menangle virus has caused an influenza-like illness in two people.

DIAGNOSIS

- Diagnostic tests that can be used to detect Nipah and Hendra viruses include culture, electron microscopy, immunohistochemistry, serology, and real-time reverse-transcriptase polymerase chain reaction.

THERAPY

- Because no specific antiviral therapies have been evaluated for the treatment of Nipah virus or Hendra virus infection, treatment involves only supportive care, such as intravenous hydration and mechanical ventilation, when indicated.
- A recombinant human monoclonal antibody, m102.4, directed against the henipavirus glycoprotein protects animals from disease after inoculation with Hendra virus or Nipah virus.

PREVENTION

- Several vaccines have been developed against Nipah virus and Hendra virus, but none is currently available for use in humans.
- A Hendra virus subunit vaccine was shown to be highly effective at preventing Hendra virus infection in horses following a lethal challenge; it became available for use in horses in Australia in 2012.

99 Vesicular Stomatitis Virus and Related Vesiculoviruses

Steven M. Fine

DEFINITION

- Vesicular stomatitis virus (VSV) is a vesiculovirus that causes outbreaks of stomatitis, mainly in livestock but sometimes also in humans.

EPIDEMIOLOGY

- A large percentage of people who live in endemic areas are infected and usually have had mild or subclinical disease.
- Seasonal outbreaks among horses, cattle, and other livestock have the potential to cause large economic losses, particularly in the southwestern United States.
- Endemic disease occurs in areas of Central and South America.
- The mode of transmission is not known, although the virus is believed to be introduced to a herd by an insect vector, and it can then spread from animal to animal by direct contact.

MICROBIOLOGY

- VSV is a single-stranded, negative-strand RNA virus that is a member of the Rhabdoviridae family, genus *Vesiculovirus*.

DIAGNOSIS

- Samples from lesions can be tested by enzyme-linked immunosorbent assay, complement fixation, or isolation of virus in tissue culture, as well as by polymerase chain reaction assays.
- The main purpose of diagnosis is to quickly distinguish the disease from the more dangerous foot-and-mouth disease in livestock.

THERAPY

- Therapy in humans is generally not required.
- There is no known antiviral treatment, so therapy consists of supportive measures.

PREVENTION

- Quarantine of animals from infected ranches is commonly instituted.
- Protective clothing and gloves should be worn when handling infected animals.
- An experimental vaccine is in trials. A killed vaccine for animals is approved, but its efficacy is unknown.

100 Rabies (Rhabdoviruses)

Kamaljit Singh, Charles E. Rupprecht, and Thomas P. Bleck

DEFINITION

- Rabies is a zoonotic encephalitis caused by different species of neurotropic viruses in the Rhabdoviridae family.

EPIDEMIOLOGY

- Rabies is one of the oldest human diseases, with the highest case fatality rate.
- Approximately 3.3 billion people live in regions where rabies is enzootic.
- An estimated 55,000 people die from rabies each year.
- Although all age groups are susceptible, rabies is most common in children younger than 15 years.
- Bites by rabid dogs cause 99% of human deaths globally.
- In the United States, bats account for most human rabies cases.
- Rabies virus transmission may also occur through tissue or organ transplantation.

MICROBIOLOGY

- Rhabdoviruses are bullet-shaped, single-stranded RNA viruses of the order Mononegavirales, family Rhabdoviridae, and genus *Lyssavirus*.
- Rabies virus is the type species of the *Lyssavirus* genus.

DIAGNOSIS

- Development of an acute neurologic syndrome after the bite of a rabid animal is classically recognized in developing countries.
- Encephalitic rabies occurs in the majority of patients with fever, hydrophobia, aerophobia, agitation, autonomic overactivity with hypersalivation, coma, and paralysis.
- Paralytic rabies is characterized by ascending flaccid quadriparesis and coma.
- Antemortem diagnosis can be made by direct immunofluorescent staining of skin biopsy specimens, reverse-transcriptase polymerase chain reaction of saliva or skin biopsy, or detection of antirabies virus antibodies in serum or cerebrospinal fluid.

THERAPY

- There is no proven antiviral therapy.
- Most patients with rabies virus infection die within a few days to 2 weeks after the onset of coma.

PREVENTION

- Annually, more than 10 million people receive rabies postexposure prophylaxis.
- After exposure to a rabid animal, prevention consists primarily of prompt wound cleansing.
- Postexposure prophylaxis consists of prompt administration of rabies immune globulin and rabies vaccine according to the Advisory Committee on Immunization Practices and World Health Organization guidelines.

- Bat rabies causes the majority of human cases in the United States, and postexposure prophylaxis depends on the type of exposure and availability of the animal for rabies diagnosis.
- Preexposure prophylaxis should be targeted to high-risk groups, including veterinarians, laboratory workers, and certain travelers.

101 Marburg and Ebola Hemorrhagic Fevers (Marburg and Ebola Viral Diseases) (Filoviruses)

Thomas W. Geisbert

DEFINITION

- Marburg viral disease and Ebola viral disease are severe and often fatal diseases characterized by fever, headache, malaise, myalgia, vomiting, diarrhea, coagulation disorders, and multi-organ failure.

EPIDEMIOLOGY

- Human outbreaks occur sporadically in regions of Central Africa.
  - In 2014, an extraordinarily large outbreak of Ebola viral disease developed in West Africa and still continues in early 2015.
- Recent evidence suggests that bats may play a role as a reservoir host.
- The manner in which filovirus outbreaks are initiated is unknown; however, it is thought that the initial cases occur as a result of contact with an infected animal.
- Nosocomial transmission has occurred frequently during outbreaks of filovirus disease in endemic areas.

DIAGNOSIS

- Clinical symptoms are nonspecific, but a constellation of symptoms, including fever, headache, malaise, myalgia, sore throat, vomiting, diarrhea, and the appearance of a maculopapular rash may indicate infection with a filovirus.
- Reverse-transcriptase polymerase chain reaction (RT-PCR) is the most frequently used assay to diagnose filovirus infection.

TREATMENT

- There are no approved postexposure treatments for filovirus infections.
- Treating patients infected with Marburg or Ebola viruses consists primarily of intensive supportive care that is directed toward maintaining effective blood volume and electrolyte balance.
- Several experimental treatments have shown promise in nonhuman primate models of filovirus infection, including vesicular stomatitis virus–based postexposure vaccines, small interfering RNAs, antisense oligonucleotides, and pools of monoclonal antibodies.

PREVENTION

- There are no approved vaccines against Marburg or Ebola viruses, but significant progress has been made in the development of ChAd3- and recombinant vesicular stomatitis virus (rVSV)-based vaccines.
- Appropriate personal protection equipment (PPE) is essential for health care workers.
- Isolation of infected patients and close contacts is essential.
- Avoid contact with bush meat and sick animals, particularly nonhuman primates, in endemic regions.

102 Influenza (Including Avian Influenza and Swine Influenza)
John J. Treanor

DEFINITION

- Influenza viruses are enveloped, negative-sense, single-stranded RNA viruses whose genome is segmented. They cause epidemic acute respiratory disease characterized by fever, cough, and systemic symptoms. Three types (A, B, and C) are recognized, as well as many subtypes within the type A viruses.

EPIDEMIOLOGY

- Influenza viruses are transmitted by the respiratory route and cause large epidemics, which generally occur during the winter in temperate climates. In addition to infecting humans, influenza A viruses infect a wide variety of animals, particularly migratory waterfowl. New influenza A virus subtypes sporadically emerge in humans to cause widespread disease, or pandemics.

MICROBIOLOGY

- Influenza viruses are readily isolated in eggs or mammalian cell culture at 33°C. They undergo constant antigenic evolution, referred to as antigenic drift or shift that allows them to reinfect individuals who have had previous infections.

DIAGNOSIS

- In the context of recognized epidemics, influenza is usually diagnosed clinically on the basis of characteristic symptoms of fever and cough. Rapid detection of virus in respiratory secretions also can be accomplished by antigen detection or molecular techniques such as polymerase chain reaction assay.

THERAPY

- Antiviral therapy with oseltamivir, zanamivir, or peramivir is available and may shorten the duration of illness and reduce the rate of complications. Therapy is most effective when used early in the course of illness (see Table 102-1).

PREVENTION

- Influenza vaccines are effective in the prevention of influenza illness, although improved vaccines are needed.
- Inactivated and live-attenuated vaccines are available in trivalent and quadrivalent formulations (see Table 102-2).
- The objectives of vaccination include protection of the individual, as well as protection of the population through herd immunity. Antiviral drugs can also be used prophylactically in selected circumstances.

TABLE 102-1 Antiviral Chemotherapy and Chemoprophylaxis for Influenza

INFECTION	DRUG	ROUTE	DOSAGE
Influenza A and B: treatment	Oseltamivir	Oral	Adults: 75 mg bid × 5 days Children aged 1-12 years: 30-75 mg bid, depending on weight†, × 5 days
	Zanamivir	Inhaled orally	Adults and children aged ≥7 yr: 10 mg bid × 5 days
Influenza A: treatment	Amantadine*	Oral	Adults: 100 mg qd or bid × 5-7 days Children aged 1-9 yr: 5 mg/kg/day (maximum, 150 mg/day) × 5-7 days
	Rimantadine*	Oral	100 mg qd or bid × 5-7 days in adults
Influenza A and B: prophylaxis	Oseltamivir	Oral	Adults: 75 mg/day Children aged ≥1 yr: 30-75 mg/day, depending on weight†
	Zanamivir	Inhaled orally	Adults and children aged ≥5 yr: 10 mg/day
Influenza A: prophylaxis	Amantadine* or rimantadine*	Oral	Adults: 200 mg/day Children aged 1-9 yr: 5 mg/kg/day (maximum, 150 mg/day)

*Amantadine and rimantadine are not considered for use because of widespread resistance in influenza A/H3N2 and A/H1N1 viruses currently circulating (2012-2013). They may be considered if sensitivities become reestablished.

†For detailed dosage recommendations in children aged <1 yr, see www.cdc.gov/flu/professionals/antivirals/summary-clinicians.htm.

TABLE 102-2   Influenza Vaccines Available in the United States, 2013-2014 Influenza Season*

VACCINE	TRADE NAME	MANUFACTURER	AGE INDICATIONS	ROUTE
Inactivated influenza vaccine, trivalent (IIV3), standard dose	Afluria	CSL Limited	≥9 yr	IM[†]
	Fluarix	GlaxoSmithKline	≥3 yr	IM[†]
	Flucelvax	Novartis Vaccines	≥18 yr	IM[†]
	FluLaval	ID Biomedical Corporation of Quebec (distributed by GlaxoSmithKline)	≥3 yr	IM[†]
	Fluvirin	Novartis Vaccines	≥4 yr	IM[†]
	Fluzone	Sanofi Pasteur	≥6 mo	IM[†]
	Fluzone Intradermal	Sanofi Pasteur	18-64 yr	ID
Inactivated influenza vaccine, trivalent (IIV3), high dose	Fluzone High-Dose	Sanofi Pasteur	≥65 yr	IM[†]
Inactivated influenza vaccine, quadrivalent (IIV4), standard dose	Fluarix Quadrivalent	GlaxoSmithKline	≥3 yr	IM[†]
	FluLaval Quadrivalent	ID Biomedical Corporation of Quebec (distributed by GlaxoSmithKline)	≥3 yr	IM[†]
	Fluzone Quadrivalent	Sanofi Pasteur	≥6 mo	IM[†]
Recombinant influenza vaccine, trivalent (RIV3)	FluBlok	Protein Sciences	18-49 yr	IM[†]
Live-attenuated influenza vaccine, quadrivalent (LAIV4)	FluMist Quadrivalent	MedImmune	2-49 yr	IN

ID, intradermal; IIV, Inactivated influenza vaccine; IIV3, inactivated influenza vaccine, trivalent; IIV4, inactivated influenza vaccine, quadrivalent; IM, intramuscular; IN, intranasal; LAIV, live attenuated influenza vaccine; RIV, recombinant influenza vaccine.

*Immunization providers should check U.S. Food and Drug Administration-approved prescribing information for 2013-2014 influenza vaccines for the most complete and updated information, including (but not limited to) indications, contraindications, and precautions. Package inserts for U.S.-licensed vaccines are available at http://www.fda.gov/BiologicsBloodVaccines/Vaccines/ApprovedProducts/ucm093833.htm.

†For adults and older children, the recommended site of vaccination is the deltoid muscle. The preferred site for infants and young children is the anterolateral aspect of the thigh. Specific guidance regarding site and needle length for intramuscular administration may be found in the Advisory Committee on Immunization Practices General Recommendations on Immunization.

Modified from Centers for Disease Control and Prevention. Summary Recommendations: Prevention and Control of Influenza with Vaccines: Recommendations of the Advisory Committee on Immunization Practices—(ACIP)—United States, 2013-14. Available at http://www.cdc.gov/flu/professionals/acip/2013-summary-recommendations.htm#table1.

103 California Encephalitis, Hantavirus Pulmonary Syndrome, and Bunyavirus Hemorrhagic Fevers

Dennis A. Bente

DEFINITION

- This largest family of RNA viruses has more than 350 named isolates that can be found worldwide, and its members are able to infect invertebrates, vertebrates, and plants.

EPIDEMIOLOGY

- Multiple members are significant human pathogens with the ability to cause severe disease, ranging from febrile illness, encephalitis, and hepatitis to hemorrhagic fever.
- With exception of hantaviruses, bunyaviruses are transmitted by hematophagous arthropods, including ticks, mosquitoes, and phlebotomine flies.
- Hantaviruses are maintained in nature through persistent infection of rodents.

DIAGNOSIS

- Early diagnosis is based on reverse-transcriptase polymerase chain reaction assay of blood samples. In most cases, the diagnosis is based on serologic investigation of acute and early convalescent sera. Diagnostic tests are typically performed in reference laboratories.

THERAPY

- No specific therapy is available, and treatment is typically supportive. Ribavirin treatment has been studied only in some bunyavirus infections, and data from in vitro and in vivo models hold promise. Ribavirin has shown clinical benefit in hemorrhagic fever with renal syndrome (HFRS) and in Crimean-Congo hemorrhagic fever (CCHF). However, comprehensive clinical trials have not been conducted.

PREVENTION

- No specific preventive measures are available, yet experimental vaccines for some bunyaviruses have been developed. Individual protective measures such as arthropod repellents and insecticide-impregnated mosquito bed nets are recommended in endemic areas.

104 Lymphocytic Choriomeningitis, Lassa Fever, and the South American Hemorrhagic Fevers (Arenaviruses)

Alexey Seregin, Nadezhda Yun, and Slobodan Paessler

EPIDEMIOLOGY

- Lymphocytic choriomeningitis virus (LCMV) is worldwide in distribution; Lassa fever is found in Africa, and the New World complex viruses circulate in South and North America and can cause hemorrhagic fevers.
- Transmission is by rodents, with generally high species specificity of reservoir vectors.

MICROBIOLOGY

- These pleomorphic viruses are 50 to 300 nm in diameter with two single RNA segments with ambisense gene organization.

CLINICAL MANIFESTATIONS

- *LCMV:* Febrile illness is accompanied by headache and systemic symptoms; course may be biphasic with meningitis presenting during second phase in 5 to 10 days; full recovery is usual, but immunosuppression may result in disseminated and fatal disease.
- *Lassa fever:* The illness is usually mild, but in 5% to 10% it may result in severe multisystem disease, resulting in death in 15% to 25% of hospitalized patients; fever, pharyngitis, retrosternal pain, and proteinuria are the most common features; fatal cases usually occur in the second week of illness, with hypotension, vasoconstriction, mucosal hemorrhages, and capillary leak syndrome.
- *South American hemorrhagic fevers:* Argentinean, Bolivian, and Venezuelan hemorrhagic fevers have progressive fever, malaise, and myalgias, most frequently affecting the lower back; petechiae and small vesicles are frequent; vascular disease (capillary leak), vasoconstriction, and shock may occur; various blood and neurologic abnormalities can be seen; overall mortality is 15% to 30%; and convalescence may take weeks, but recovery is usually without sequelae.

DIAGNOSIS

- Detection of virus is evident in acute blood specimens by reverse-transcriptase polymerase chain reaction assay or virus culture, depending on the particular viral agent.
- IgM antibodies may be detected by serology, and increases in antibody titers (seroconversion) can be noted by comparing acute and convalescent serum specimens.

TREATMENT

- Supportive treatment may be lifesaving.
- Convalescent human plasma has been shown to be effective in Argentinean hemorrhagic fever but has not been as successful in Lassa fever.
- Ribavirin treatment of patients hospitalized with Lassa fever as well as in patients with Argentinean and Bolivian hemorrhagic fevers is beneficial.

PREVENTION

- Reduction of transmission from rodents to humans is needed.
- Person-to-person transmission in hospitals is a problem with Lassa fever, and use of gloves and gowns and careful disposal of patients' wastes and fomites should be implemented. If available, single rooms with negative pressure should be utilized.
- Steps should be taken to avoid infection in laboratory workers who examine samples that may contain arenaviruses.
- A live-attenuated vaccine is available against Argentinean hemorrhagic fever and is licensed in Argentina.

105 Human T-Lymphotropic Virus (HTLV)

Edward L. Murphy and Roberta L. Bruhn

DEFINITION

- Human T-lymphotropic virus (HTLV) is a human retrovirus of the subfamily Retroviridae and genus *Deltaretrovirus*.
- It causes chronic human infection by integration of proviral DNA into the somatic DNA of host T lymphocytes, with expansion of infectious burden by proliferation of infected lymphocytes more importantly than by production of free virus particles.
- To date, four types of the virus have been discovered: HTLV-1 and HTLV-2 infections are estimated in millions of humans, and HTLV-3 and HTLV-4 have occurred in only a few isolates since their discovery in the past decade.
- HTLV-1 causes adult T-cell leukemia, and both HTLV-1 and HTLV-2 cause HTLV-associated myelopathy (HAM).

EPIDEMIOLOGY

- HTLV-1 is endemic to central Africa, the Caribbean basin, parts of South America, and southwestern Japan as well as other discrete geographic areas. There is limited genetic variation and close homology to primate T-lymphotropic viruses, suggesting several instances of cross-species transmission.
- HTLV-2 is endemic to Amerindian tribes in North, Central, and South America as well as Central African pygmies. It is hyperendemic among injection drug users in North America and Europe.
- Both HTLV-1 and HTLV-2 are transmitted by mother-to-child transmission predominantly by breast-feeding, by sexual transmission, and by parenteral infection.
- In endemic populations, both retroviruses show an increased prevalence in older individuals, and prevalence is frequently higher in females than in males.

DIAGNOSIS AND PATHOGENESIS

- HTLV antibodies may be detected using screening enzyme immunoassays and supplemental Western blot/recombinant immunoblot, with differentiation of HTLV-1 from HTLV-2 using type-specific antigens in supplemental assays.
- Polymerase chain reaction (PCR) assay to detect HTLV-1 or HTLV-2 proviral DNA in peripheral blood mononuclear cells may be performed in cases where serology is inconclusive. PCR assay is also useful in detecting infection in infants carrying passive maternal antibodies.
- Most infected individuals are asymptomatic. Two to 4 percent of those infected with HTLV-1 will develop adult T-cell leukemia/lymphoma (ATL), characterized by monoclonal integration of HTLV-1 provirus into a T-lymphocytic malignancy.
- One to 4 percent of those infected with either HTLV-I or HTLV-2 will develop HAM, a spastic paraparesis affecting predominantly the lower limbs and hyperactive bladder in a person infected with HTLV.

THERAPY

- No treatment is currently recommended for persons with asymptomatic HTLV-1 or HTLV-2 infection. Periodic follow-up should include physical examination and complete blood cell count to detect ATL or HAM.
- The lymphoma type of ATL is often treated initially with vincristine, cyclophosphamide, prednisolone, and doxorubicin; survival is poor. Chronic, smoldering, and leukemia types of ATL often respond better to a combination of zidovudine and interferon-α.
- Therapy for HAM is currently unsatisfactory. Corticosteroids may produce improvement, but side effects limit the duration of therapy. Interferon-α and interferon-1β have been used with some success. The anabolic steroid danazol may relieve bladder symptoms.

PREVENTION

- To interrupt mother-to-child transmission, HTLV-infected pregnant women in middle- and high-income countries should not breastfeed their infants if this can be accomplished safely. Limiting the duration of breast-feeding to less than 6 months may be attempted in low-income countries.
- The use of condoms should be recommended to prevent sexual transmission.
- Injection drug users with HTLV infection should be instructed not to share needles.
- The U.S. Food and Drug Administration recommends HTLV testing of all donated blood and tissue. No vaccine is currently available.

106 Human Immunodeficiency Viruses

Marvin S. Reitz, Jr., and Robert C. Gallo

DEFINITION

- Human immunodeficiency virus (HIV) is a *Lentivirus*, family Retroviridae, that causes acquired immunodeficiency syndrome (AIDS). There are two types, HIV-1 and HIV-2, of which HIV-1 is the more widely distributed and more pathogenic.

EPIDEMIOLOGY

- HIV infection is worldwide in distribution and is transmitted by sexual activity and intravenous drug use.

MICROBIOLOGY

- HIV is a single-stranded positive-sense RNA virus that contains three structural genes *(gag, pol, env)* and six regulatory genes. HIV infects $CD4^+$ T cells and uses its reverse transcriptase to transcribe its RNA genome into double-stranded DNA, which is integrated into the host cell genome.

DIAGNOSIS

- Infection is established by detection of viral RNA (virus load) or of immunologic responses to viral proteins (Western blot).

THERAPY AND PREVENTION

- Antiretroviral therapy (ART) has been developed using nucleoside and non-nucleoside reverse-transcriptase inhibitors, protease inhibitors, integrase inhibitors, and entry inhibitors. ART can also decrease the rate of transmission of infection. Vaccine development seeks to stimulate immune responses to HIV antigens that will inhibit transmission and/or replication of virus.

107 Poliovirus

José R. Romero and John F. Modlin

DEFINITION

- Polioviruses are the cause of poliomyelitis, a systemic viral infection that predominantly affects the central nervous system, causing paralysis. Only three serotypes exist (1 to 3). The name of the disease (polios, "gray"; myelos, "marrow" or "spinal cord"), now commonly shortened to polio, is descriptive of the pathologic lesions that involve neurons in the gray matter, especially in the anterior horns of the spinal cord.

EPIDEMIOLOGY

- Wild-type poliovirus type 2 no longer circulates worldwide. Serotypes 1 and 3 have been eradicated from most of the world. They remain endemic in three countries (Afghanistan, Nigeria, and Pakistan) and have recently been reintroduced in several sub-Saharan African and Eastern Mediterranean countries. In 2012, the annual number of cases of poliomyelitis (223) was the lowest since the initiation of the global poliovirus eradication effort in 1988.

MICROBIOLOGY

- The polioviruses are members of the genus *Enterovirus*, family Picornaviridae. Morphologically, they are small (30 nm in diameter), nonenveloped, icosahedral-shaped viruses that possess a single-stranded, positive-sense RNA genome.

DIAGNOSIS

- Polioviruses can be isolated from throat secretions and from feces but rarely from the cerebrospinal fluid. Characterization is accomplished by sequencing of the major capsid protein VP1 and is available only in public health reference laboratories.

THERAPY

- No specific therapy is available. Supportive measures to ensure airway patency, adequate respiratory effort, and clearance of secretions are the mainstay of treatment for severe cases of paralysis.

PREVENTION

- Vaccination using inactivated or live-attenuated oral vaccines has been essential in the elimination of the polioviruses. Public health measures, such as provision of potable water and proper sewage disposal, play major roles in the community-wide control of the polioviruses.

108 Coxsackieviruses, Echoviruses, and Numbered Enteroviruses (EV-D68)

José R. Romero and John F. Modlin

DEFINITION

- The coxsackieviruses, echoviruses, and numbered enteroviruses are members of the genus *Enterovirus*.
- The four species (human enterovirus [EV] A to D) within the genus contain more than 100 serotypes.
- Enteroviruses are responsible for a wide array of clinical syndromes involving multiple organ systems, including acute meningitis, encephalitis, paralysis, exanthems, hand-foot-and-mouth disease, herpangina, myopericarditis, pleurodynia, and acute hemorrhagic conjunctivitis.

EPIDEMIOLOGY

- The enteroviruses are found worldwide.
- In regions with temperate climates, the majority of enteroviral infections occur during the summer and early autumn months. In tropical regions, infections occur year-round, with increased frequency during the rainy season.
- A large outbreak of EV-D68 occurred in the United States in 2014.

MICROBIOLOGY

- Morphologically, they are small (30 nm in diameter), nonenveloped, icosahedral-shaped viruses that possess a single-stranded, positive-sense RNA genome.

DIAGNOSIS

- Enteroviruses can be isolated or their genomic RNA detected from throat secretions, feces, cerebrospinal fluid, and blood, as well as various tissues (heart, brain) and fluids (urine, pericardial, vesicle).
- Nucleic acid amplification testing has been shown to be quicker and more sensitive than cell culture for enterovirus detection.
- Serotype identification is accomplished by sequencing of the major capsid protein VP1.

THERAPY

- Therapy is supportive.
- No specific antiviral therapy is currently available for the treatment of enterovirus infections.
- The investigational compound pleconaril, an inhibitor of viral binding and uncoating, has undergone clinical studies in enteroviral-associated disease but is no longer under development.

PREVENTION

- Contagion can be prevented by hand washing and, in the case of certain serotypes, avoidance of enterovirus-contaminated fomites.
- Investigational vaccines are under development for the prevention of human EV-A71 infection.

109 Human Parechoviruses

José R. Romero and John F. Modlin

DEFINITION

- The human parechoviruses (HPeVs) are members of a relatively newly created genus designated *Parechovirus* in the Picornaviridae family. At least 16 types have been identified.
- HPeVs are responsible for multiple clinical syndromes involving many organ systems, including undifferentiated febrile illness, meningitis, encephalitis, paralysis, and respiratory illnesses.

EPIDEMIOLOGY

- HPeVs are found worldwide.
- The majority of HPeV infections occur during the summer and autumn months.

MICROBIOLOGY

- Morphologically they are small (28 nm in diameter), nonenveloped, icosahedral-shaped viruses that possess a single-stranded, positive-sense RNA genome.

DIAGNOSIS

- HPeVs can be isolated, or their genomic RNA can be detected from oral secretions, feces, cerebrospinal fluid, and blood.
- Nucleic acid amplification has been quicker and more sensitive than cell culture for their detection.
- Type identification is accomplished by sequencing of the major capsid protein, VP1.

THERAPY

- Therapy is supportive. No specific antiviral therapy is available.

PREVENTION

- Contagion can be prevented by hand washing.

110 Hepatitis A Virus

Francisco Averhoff, Yury Khudyakov, and Beth P. Bell*

DEFINITION
- Hepatitis A is an acute inflammatory condition of the liver caused by hepatitis A virus and characterized by constitutional symptoms including anorexia, fatigue and weight loss, and jaundice.

MICROBIOLOGY
- Hepatitis A virus (HAV) is a nonenveloped RNA virus member of the picornavirus family. Three genotypes infect humans (I, II, and III).
- HAV is relatively resistant to heat but can be inactivated at higher temperatures.
- HAV is resistant to organic solvents and detergents and can survive in acidic environments to a pH of 3.
- HAV can be inactivated by hypochlorite (bleach) and quaternary ammonium formulations containing HCI (found in many toilet cleaners).

EPIDEMIOLOGY
- Transmission is fecal-oral with peak viral shedding before onset of symptoms.
- Humans are the only important reservoir for HAV.
- Spread is most commonly person to person (including sexual contact) but can occur as foodborne and waterborne transmission, among injection drug users and men who have sex with men, and rarely by infected blood products.
- Most common risk factors in the United States include international travel and close contact (sexual or household) with a hepatitis A–infected person.
- In the United States, the incidence of hepatitis A has plummeted over the past 15 years as a result of implementation of routine vaccination of children. Large community-wide epidemics previously common are now rare.
- Globally, hepatitis A is one of the leading causes of vaccine-preventable deaths. Disease incidence paradoxically may increase as improvement in living conditions delays infection to older ages, when symptoms are likely to be more severe.

DIAGNOSIS
- Hepatitis A is not clinically distinguishable from other forms of viral hepatitis.
- Laboratory diagnosis is made by detection of IgM antibodies to HAV in a single, acute-phase serum sample.

THERAPY
- Most illnesses are self-limited and can be managed with supportive and symptomatic measures.

---

*All material in this chapter is in the public domain, with the exception of any borrowed figures or tables.

- Fulminant cases are rare but need to be managed appropriately and may require transplantation in extremely ill patients.
- Chronic hepatitis A does not occur.

PREVENTION

- In the United States, vaccination with hepatitis A vaccine is recommended for all children at age 12 to 23 months. Vaccination of older children and adults may be warranted, including patients with chronic hepatitis B and C (see Table 110-1).
- Vaccination of international travelers and persons in selected high-risk groups is recommended (see Table 110-1).
- Administer postexposure prophylaxis with hepatitis A vaccine (preferred) or immune globulin if exposure occurred within the previous 2 weeks, if patient is immunosuppressed, or if patient is younger than 1 year of age (see Table 110-2).

TABLE 110-1 Recommendations for Routine Preexposure Use of Hepatitis A Virus Vaccine

GROUP	COMMENTS
Children	Vaccine should be given to all children at age 1 yr (12-23 mo).* Vaccination of children 2-18 yr may also be warranted.†
International travelers‡	IG may be given in addition to or instead of vaccine; children <12 mo should receive IG (see Table 176-2)
Close contacts of newly arriving international adoptees	All persons who anticipate close personal contact (e.g., household contact or regular babysitter) during the first 60 days after arrival
Men who have sex with men	Includes adolescents
Illicit drug users	Includes adolescents
Persons with chronic liver disease, such as those with hepatitis B or C	Increased risk of fulminant hepatitis A with HAV infection
Persons receiving clotting factor concentrates	
Persons who work with HAV in research laboratory settings	

HAV, hepatitis A vaccine; IG, immune globulin.

*Hepatitis A vaccine is not licensed for children <12 months.

†States and communities with existing vaccination programs for children age 2 to 18 years are encouraged to maintain these programs. Catch-up vaccination for this age group may be warranted elsewhere in the context of ongoing outbreaks among children.

‡Persons traveling to Canada, Western Europe, Japan, Australia, or New Zealand are at no greater risk than in the United States.

From Centers for Disease Control and Prevention. Prevention of hepatitis A through active or passive immunization. Recommendations of the Advisory Committee on Immunization Practices. *MMWR Morb Mortal Wkly Rep.* 2006;55(RR-7):1-23; and Centers for Disease Control and Prevention. Updated recommendations from the Advisory Committee on Immunization Practices (ACIP) for use of hepatitis A vaccine in close contacts of newly arriving international adoptees. *MMWR Morb Mortal Wkly Rep.* 2009;58:1006-1007.

TABLE 110-2   Recommendations for Hepatitis A Postexposure Prophylaxis

GROUP*	RECOMMENDED PROPHYLAXIS[†]
Persons 12 mo–40 yr	Single antigen hepatitis A vaccine at age-appropriate dose
Persons >40 yr	IG 0.02 mL/kg is preferred; vaccine can be used if IG cannot be obtained
Children <12 mo	IG 0.02 mL/kg[‡]
Immunocompromised persons, persons who have chronic liver disease, and persons for whom vaccine is contraindicated	IG 0.02 mL/kg[‡]

IG, immune globulin.

*Persons recently exposed to hepatitis A virus who have not previously received hepatitis A vaccine.

†Postexposure prophylaxis should be given as soon as possible after exposure. The efficacy of immune globulin or vaccine administered more than 2 weeks after exposure has not been established.

‡In the event of ongoing exposure, persons for whom immune globulin is recommended should receive immune globulin 0.06 mL/kg, repeated every 5 months during exposure.

111 Rhinovirus

Ronald B. Turner

VIROLOGY AND EPIDEMIOLOGY

- Rhinoviruses are unenveloped RNA viruses in the family Picornaviridae.
- One-hundred one serotypes have been detected, now divided into two phylogenetic species (human rhinovirus [RV]-A and RV-B); a third species, RV-C, also exists.
- Rhinoviruses are among the most common pathogens of man, with an incidence of 0.5 infections per year in adults and 2 infections per year in children.
- Infections occur year-round, with seasonal peaks in the spring and fall in temperate climates.

DIAGNOSIS

- The common cold is the characteristic clinical manifestation.
- Exacerbations of asthma in children are frequently associated with rhinovirus infection.
- Rhinoviruses may cause bronchiolitis in young children.
- Specific virologic diagnosis is best accomplished with polymerase chain reaction but is rarely useful for patient management.

THERAPY

- Despite multiple studies, no specific antiviral therapy has been established.

PREVENTION

- There is no proven intervention to prevent rhinovirus infection.

112 Noroviruses and Sapoviruses (Caliciviruses)

Raphael Dolin and John J. Treanor

DEFINITION

- The genera *Norovirus* and *Sapovirus,* of the family *Caliciviridae,* cause acute gastroenteritis.

EPIDEMIOLOGY

- Noroviruses are the major worldwide cause of viral gastroenteritis, cause both foodborne and person-to-person outbreaks, and can be spread via fomites.
- Noroviruses account for 21 million cases of gastroenteritis in the United States annually and for up to 200,000 deaths in the developing world among children younger than 5 years.
- Sapoviruses cause gastroenteritis less frequently than noroviruses.

MICROBIOLOGY

- Noroviruses and sapoviruses are single-stranded, positive-sense RNA viruses. Each is divided into five genogroups and has multiple genotypes.
- Neither noroviruses nor sapoviruses have been cultivated in vitro.

CLINICAL MANIFESTATIONS

- Illness caused by noroviruses and sapoviruses consists of combinations of vomiting and diarrhea, often accompanied by abdominal cramps, nausea, and low-grade fever.
- Illness usually lasts 12 to 60 hours and remits spontaneously.
- More severe disease and even fatalities can occur in young children and in the elderly. Immunocompromised patients may have prolonged shedding of virus, along with severe and persistent gastrointestinal illness.

DIAGNOSIS

- Noroviruses may be suspected as a cause of outbreaks of gastrointestinal illness if the above clinical features are present, particularly if a large number of individuals are involved. However, the illness is not sufficiently distinctive in individual cases to permit a clinical diagnosis to be made on clinical grounds alone.
- Specific diagnosis is made by detection of virus in stool specimens by reverse-transcriptase polymerase chain reaction assay. Enzyme immunoassays are also available, but they are generally of low sensitivity, although high specificity.

THERAPY

- Only supportive therapy is available, particularly maintaining hydration, which is all that is needed.

PREVENTION

- The main control measures are to prevent contamination of food supplies and water by good hygiene and by restriction of food handling by ill individuals until at least 2 to 3 days after gastrointestinal illness has resolved.

- Vigorous hand washing by ill individuals should be maintained.
- Decontamination of exposed surfaces should be carried out with Environmental Protection Agency–recommended disinfectants; for example, household bleach should be carried out at 1:10 to 1:50 dilutions.
- An initial clinical study of an investigational norovirus vaccine, consisting of virus-like particles, reduced experimentally induced gastroenteritis by 47%.

113 | Astroviruses and Picobirnaviruses

Raphael Dolin and John J. Treanor

DEFINITION

- Astrovirus causes acute gastroenteritis. Picobirnaviruses have been detected in stools but have not been established as causes of illness in humans.

EPIDEMIOLOGY

- Astroviruses are worldwide in distribution, cause disease most frequently in young children, but can also cause gastroenteritis in adults and in immunosuppressed patients. Transmission is likely by the fecal-oral route.

MICROBIOLOGY

- Astroviruses are single-stranded RNA viruses, comprising 8 serotypes, with a characteristic star-shaped morphology seen on electron micrographs. Picobirnaviruses are double-stranded RNA viruses with a bisegmented genome.

CLINICAL MANIFESTATIONS

- Illness induced by astroviruses consists of diarrhea, headache, malaise, nausea, low-grade fever, and, less commonly, vomiting. Illness may be somewhat less severe than that seen with rotaviruses.

DIAGNOSIS

- Astroviruses in stools can be detected by electron microscopy, enzyme immunoassay, and by reverse-transcriptase polymerase chain reaction assay, which is the most sensitive technique.

THERAPY

- Treatment is supportive. Intravenous immune globulin has been used in immunosuppressed patients, but its efficacy is not established.

PREVENTION

- Although virus-like particles from astroviruses have been produced, vaccines have not been developed.

114 Hepatitis E Virus

Stephen R. Walsh

DEFINITION

- Hepatitis E virus (HEV) is a member of the Hepeviridae family, genus *Hepevirus,* which causes acute hepatitis in the normal host and chronic hepatitis in immunosuppressed patients.

EPIDEMIOLOGY

- HEV may be the most common form of acute viral hepatitis and occurs in both sporadic and epidemic forms.
- HEV is transmitted by waterborne spread of fecally contaminated water or by fecally transmitted zoonotic infection. Person-to-person transmission is uncommon.
- HEV is unique among the hepatitis viruses because of its disproportionately high mortality rate in pregnant women (25% in the third trimester).
- HEV infection is uncommon, but likely underdiagnosed in developed countries, and zoonotic infections may be responsible for many of the cases that are locally acquired in developed countries.
- Chronic hepatitis E infection has recently been described in immunosuppressed patients.

MICROBIOLOGY

- HEV virions are nonenveloped, icosahedral particles of approximately 32-nm diameter.
- HEV has a single-stranded positive-sense RNA genome that contains three open reading frames (ORFs).
- Four genotypes and 24 subgenotypes have been described.

DIAGNOSIS

- Diagnosis of HEV had previously been made serologically, but molecular diagnosis via polymerase chain reaction has better sensitivity and specificity and is the diagnostic technique of choice, if available.

THERAPY

- Acute HEV infection is generally self-limited and requires only supportive care. Severe acute cases have been treated successfully with ribavirin.
- Ribavirin monotherapy appears to be highly effective in treatment of chronic hepatitis E in solid-organ transplant recipients.

PREVENTION

- Protecting water supplies from contamination with human feces is the most important means to prevent HEV infection.
- A vaccine using the ORF2 capsid protein that assembles into virus-like particles (Hecolin) has been shown to be safe and effective and is licensed in China.

115 Prions and Prion Diseases of the Central Nervous System (Transmissible Neurodegenerative Diseases)

Patrick J. Bosque and Kenneth L. Tyler

DEFINITION

- Prion diseases are transmissible neurodegenerative conditions of mammals characterized by a rapidly progressive decline of cognitive, motor, and other brain functions.
- Prion diseases are biochemically defined by the accumulation of an abnormal form of a normally expressed brain protein, the prion protein (PrP).

EPIDEMIOLOGY

- Human prion disease is rare; its incidence is 1×10^{-6} worldwide.
- About 90% of cases are sporadic.
- About 10% of cases are genetic.
- Infectious transmission accounts for less than 1% of human cases.

MICROBIOLOGY

- The causative agent is composed of an aggregate of misfolded forms of PrP.
- The aggregate serves as a catalytic template for the further aggregation of PrP and thus replicates.
- The prion contains no information-bearing nucleic acid.

DIAGNOSIS

- Treatable mimics of prion disease should be excluded before making the diagnosis.
- Certain diagnosis can only be made by detecting abnormal PrP aggregates in tissue, typically brain.
- Diagnosis is usually made by history and clinical signs and supported by ancillary tests, including magnetic resonance imaging, electroencephalography, and cerebrospinal fluid analysis.

THERAPY

- No effective therapy exists for prion infection.

PREVENTION

- Only standard precautions are needed for most procedures, to prevent iatrogenic transmission of prion disease.
- Additional precautions are needed for neurosurgical cases.
- Transfusion of red blood cells and plasma protein products can transmit one form of prion disease, variant Creutzfeldt-Jakob disease.
- Tissue from persons with prion disease must not be transplanted.
- Dietary exposure to ruminant animal prions should be avoided.

116 *Chlamydia trachomatis* (Trachoma, Genital Infections, Perinatal Infections, and Lymphogranuloma Venereum)

Byron E. Batteiger and Ming Tan

DEFINITION

- *Chlamydia trachomatis* is an obligate intracellular bacterium that mainly infects ocular and genitourinary epithelium.
- The ocular disease trachoma is the leading infectious cause of blindness worldwide.
- Chlamydial genital infections are the most common bacterial sexually transmitted infections in the world.
- Lymphogranuloma venereum (LGV), caused by distinct serovars of *C. trachomatis,* is a less common disease characterized by enlarged inguinal lymph nodes or severe proctocolitis.

EPIDEMIOLOGY

- Trachoma is common in poor, rural areas of developing countries, with an estimated 40 million active cases worldwide.
- Active infection in trachoma largely affects young children, often those younger than 1 year of age, whereas the scarring sequelae that produce blindness occur later in life.
- The sexually transmitted urogenital infections are common worldwide with an estimated 105.7 million new cases in 2008.
- Chlamydial genital infections are most prevalent among adolescent women and men, where repeated infections are common.
- Chlamydial genital infections are often asymptomatic but can cause reproductive sequelae in women, including involuntary infertility and ectopic pregnancy.
- Transmission during vaginal delivery can lead to neonatal conjunctivitis and pneumonia.
- *C. trachomatis* infections are reportable to the Centers for Disease Control and Prevention and all state health departments in the United States.

PATHOPHYSIOLOGY

- Disease manifestations are largely mediated by the host response to the infection, which is initiated and sustained by actively infected nonimmune host epithelial cells.
- In a substantial minority of persons with trachoma and genital infections, the host inflammatory response leads to tissue scarring, resulting in end-organ dysfunction and sequelae.

MICROBIOLOGY

- *C. trachomatis* is a gram-negative bacterium, but Gram stain is not used for identification.
- The organism is cultivated in cell culture because it does not grow and divide axenically.
- The bacterium replicates within a cytoplasmic inclusion in the host cell.
- The two morphologic forms are the infectious but nondividing elementary body and the reticulate body, which is an intracellular, replicating form.

DIAGNOSIS

- Diagnosis of trachoma in endemic areas is typically by physical examination of the eye according to criteria established by the World Health Organization.

- Diagnosis of genital infections requires microbiologic testing, ideally by nucleic acid amplification tests of first-catch urine in men and vaginal swabs in women.

THERAPY (SEE TABLE 116-1)

- Therapy of trachoma is generally provided by repeated mass treatment of hyperendemic communities with single-dose azithromycin.
- Recommended treatment of uncomplicated urogenital infection is either azithromycin 1 g orally as a single dose or doxycycline 100 mg orally twice daily for 7 days. Treatment of sex partners is crucial to prevent repeated infection.
- Treatment of complicated infections requires longer durations of therapy: for salpingitis, 14 days; for epididymitis, 10 days; and for proctitis, 7 days.
- LGV is treated with doxycycline for 21 days.

PREVENTION

- Trachoma can be prevented by face washing, access to clean water, and improvements in sanitation.
- In the United States and other developed countries, prevention of sexually transmitted genital infections and complications is largely focused on screening and treating nonpregnant sexually active women aged 25 years or younger on an annual basis. Uptake of screening in the United States is relatively low.
- Screening of all pregnant women is recommended.
- Screening and treatment of women older than 25 years of age is recommended if risk factors are identified, such as new or multiple sexual partners.
- One-time screening and treatment in women decreases risk of symptomatic pelvic inflammatory disease in the following year. Data are currently lacking as to whether screening programs reduce population prevalence of chlamydial genital infection.
- Screening of young men in high-risk settings (sexually transmitted disease and adolescent clinics, correctional facilities) should be considered if resources allow.
- No vaccine is currently available for either trachoma or chlamydial genital infections. Induction of sterilizing immunity appears unlikely, and future vaccine efficacy evaluation may be based on demonstrating reduced risk of inflammatory sequelae in the eye and symptomatic pelvic inflammatory disease in women.

TABLE 116-1 Clinical Characteristics of Common *Chlamydia trachomatis* Infections

	INFECTION	SYMPTOMS AND SIGNS	PRESUMPTIVE DIAGNOSIS	DEFINITIVE DIAGNOSIS	TREATMENT
Men	Nongonococcal urethritis	Urethral discharge, dysuria	Urethral leukocytosis; no gonococci seen	Urine or urethral NAAT	Azithromycin, 1 g PO (single dose) *or* Doxycycline, 100 mg PO bid, for 7 days
	Epididymitis	Unilateral epididymal tenderness, swelling; pain; fever, presence of NGU	Urine or urethral NAAT	Urethral leukocytosis; pyuria on urinalysis	STI likely: Ceftriaxone 250 mg IM plus doxycycline, 100 mg PO bid, for 10 days *History of insertive anal intercourse:* Ceftriaxone, 250 mg IM, plus levofloxacin, 500 mg bid for 10 days
	Proctitis (non-LGV)	Rectal pain, discharge and bleeding; history of receptive anal intercourse	≥1 PMN/OIF on rectal Gram stain; no gonococci seen	Urine or urethral NAAT; rectal culture or NAAT	Doxycycline, 100 mg PO bid, for 7 days
	LGV	Painful, tender inguinal lymphadenopathy, fever	"Groove sign"	Urine, urethral, lymph node or rectal NAAT; rectal or lymph node culture; LGV-specific testing if available	Doxycycline, 100 mg PO bid, for 21 days
	LGV proctitis	Rectal pain, discharge, and bleeding in MSM; absence of inguinal lymphadenopathy	≥1 PMN/OIF on rectal Gram stain; no gonococci seen	Urine, urethral, or rectal NAAT; rectal culture; LGV-specific testing if available	Doxycycline, 100 mg PO bid, for 21 days
	Conjunctivitis	Ocular pain, redness, discharge; simultaneous genital infection	Gram stain of conjunctival swab negative for bacterial pathogens; PMNs on smear	Rectal culture or NAAT; NAAT of conjunctivae	Azithromycin, 1 g PO (single dose) *or* Doxycycline, 100 mg PO bid, for 7 days

Continued

TABLE 116-1 Clinical Characteristics of Common *Chlamydia trachomatis* Infections—cont'd

	INFECTION	SYMPTOMS AND SIGNS	PRESUMPTIVE DIAGNOSIS	DEFINITIVE DIAGNOSIS	TREATMENT
Women	Cervicitis	Mucopurulent cervical discharge; ectopy, easily induced bleeding	≥20 PMN/OIF on cervical Gram stain	Urine or cervical NAAT	Azithromycin, 1 g PO (single dose) *or* Doxycycline, 100 mg PO bid, for 7 days
	Urethritis	Dysuria, frequency; no hematuria	Pyuria on UA; negative urine Gram stain and culture	Urine, cervical, or urethral NAAT	Azithromycin, 1 g PO (single dose) *or* Doxycycline, 100 mg PO bid for 7 days
	PID	Lower abdominal pain, adnexal pain, cervical motion tenderness	Evidence of mucopurulent cervicitis	Urine or cervical NAAT	Outpatient: Ceftriaxone 250 mg IM as a single dose, plus doxycycline 100 mg PO bid for 14 days, with or without metronidazole, 500 mg PO bid for 14 days
Adults	Conjunctivitis	Ocular pain, redness, discharge; simultaneous genital infection	Gram stain of conjunctival swab negative for bacterial pathogens; PMNs on smear	DFA or NAAT on conjunctival swab	Azithromycin, 1 g PO (single dose) *or* Doxycycline, 100 mg PO bid for 7 days
Newborns	Conjunctivitis	Ocular pain, redness, discharge; simultaneous genital infection	Gram stain of conjunctival swab negative for bacterial pathogens; PMNs on smear	DFA or NAAT on conjunctival swab; vagina, rectum, pharynx also often positive	Erythromycin base 50 mg/kg/day, orally divided into four doses daily for 14 days; evaluate and treat parents as well
	Pneumonia	Staccato cough, tachypnea, hyperinflation	Diffuse interstitial infiltrate, eosinophilia	Nasopharyngeal NAATs or culture; MIF serology (IgM)	Erythromycin base 50 mg/kg/day, orally divided into four doses daily for 14 days; evaluate and treat parents as well

DFA, direct fluorescent antibody; IgM, immunoglobulin M; LGV, lymphogranuloma venereum; MIF, microimmunofluorescence; MSM, men who have sex with men; NAAT, nucleic acid amplification test; NGU, nongonococcal urethritis; OIF, oil immersion field; PMN, polymorphonuclear neutrophil; STI, sexually transmitted infection; UA, urinalysis.

117 Psittacosis (Due to *Chlamydia psittaci*)

David Schlossberg

DEFINITION
- A systemic infection that frequently causes pneumonia.

EPIDEMIOLOGY
- Acquired by inhalation, after exposure to infected birds, although not all infected birds appear ill, and occasional patients provide no history of bird exposure.

MICROBIOLOGY
- The etiologic agent is *Chlamydia psittaci* of the family Chlamydiaceae.

DIAGNOSIS
- Diagnosis is made serologically in most cases; when available, polymerase chain reaction may be positive. Because diagnostic methods are imperfect, treatment should not await definitive diagnosis.

THERAPY
- Doxycycline or tetracycline is treatment of choice. Macrolides and fluoroquinolones have good in vitro activity, but there is limited clinical experience.

PREVENTION
- Treat imported birds and birds that have suspected infection.

118 *Chlamydia pneumoniae*

Margaret R. Hammerschlag, Stephan A. Kohlhoff, and Charlotte A. Gaydos

MICROBIOLOGY AND EPIDEMIOLOGY

- Obligate intracellular bacterium, must be grown in tissue culture
- Capable of causing persistent infection, often subclinical
- Worldwide distribution, infects many animals as well as humans
- Primarily a respiratory pathogen in humans, causing community-acquired pneumonia
- Can cause epidemics in enclosed populations: military bases, schools, nursing homes

DIAGNOSIS

- *Chlamydia pneumoniae* causes pneumonia; clinically it cannot be differentiated from other causes of atypical pneumonia, especially *Mycoplasma pneumoniae.*
- The most accurate method of diagnosis is identification of the organism in respiratory samples by culture or nucleic acid amplification test (NAAT).
- Serology is of limited value, requires paired sera, and many patients who are positive by culture or NAAT will be seronegative.

THERAPY

- *C. pneumoniae* is susceptible to macrolides, quinolones, and tetracyclines. Data on efficacy are limited, including optimal dose and duration of therapy.
- Ten- to 14-day courses of erythromycin, clarithromycin, doxycycline, levofloxacin, or moxifloxacin or 5 days of azithromycin are clinically effective and result in approximately 80% microbiologic eradication.

119 *Mycoplasma pneumoniae* and Atypical Pneumonia

Robert S. Holzman and Michael S. Simberkoff

DEFINITION

- Atypical pneumonia caused by *Mycoplasma pneumoniae* is a syndrome that in contrast to lobar pneumonia is:
  - Slower in onset
  - Generally milder
  - Not associated with lobar consolidation
  - Not associated with resolution by crisis
- Many other viral and bacterial agents can produce an atypical pneumonia syndrome.

ETIOLOGIC AGENT

- *M. pneumoniae*
  - Bacterium lacking cell wall
  - Adhesins and adhesion organelle important in pathogenesis
  - Fastidious
  - May be cultivable from sputum after symptoms of illness resolve

EXTRAPULMONARY SITES AND MANIFESTATIONS OF INFECTION

- Skin (maculopapular or vesicular rashes, Stevens-Johnson syndrome)
- Cardiac (pericarditis, myocarditis)
- Central nervous system (encephalitis or meningitis, myelitis, radiculopathy)
- Musculoskeletal (myalgia/arthralgia, rhabdomyolysis, arthritis)
- Raynaud's phenomenon
- Renal (glomerulonephritis, nephrotic syndrome)
- Hematologic

DIAGNOSIS

- Clinical suspicion by syndrome
- Presence of cold agglutinins in the absence of another explanation
- Detection of rising titers of antibodies to *M. pneumoniae*
- Detection of *M. pneumoniae*–specific antigens
- Detection of *M. pneumoniae*–specific genetic components

TREATMENT

- Macrolides (e.g., azithromycin, 500 mg day 1, 250 mg day 2 to 5)
  - Macrolide resistance is increasing and may limit usefulness
- Tetracyclines (e.g., doxycycline, 100 mg twice daily for 14 days)
- Fluoroquinolones (e.g., moxifloxacin, 400 mg daily for 14 days)

120 Genital Mycoplasmas: *Mycoplasma genitalium*, *Mycoplasma hominis*, and *Ureaplasma* Species

David H. Martin

MICROBIOLOGY AND TAXONOMY

- The genital mycoplasmas include *Mycoplasma hominis*, *Mycoplasma genitalium*, *Ureaplasma urealyticum*, and *Ureaplasma parvum*. The latter two only recently were assigned to separate species.
- The genital mycoplasmas lack cell walls and have the smallest genomes of known free-living microorganisms.

EPIDEMIOLOGY

- All of these organisms are primarily sexually transmitted but also may be transmitted to infants at birth. There is evidence that they may persist in children into adulthood.
- The epidemiology of infection with *M. genitalium* closely parallels that of *Chlamydia trachomatis* and *Neisseria gonorrhoeae*.

CLINICAL MANIFESTATIONS

- *U. urealyticum* causes urethritis, whereas *U. parvum* appears to be a colonizer. Only relatively sexually inexperienced men are susceptible to *U. urealyticum* disease, which is likely due to the development of immunity after multiple exposures to this common urethral organism.
- Although the pathogenesis is unclear, the ureaplasmas are strongly associated with bronchopulmonary dysplasia in very-low-birth-weight infants.
- *M. hominis* plays a minor role in genital tract disease but is implicated in postpartum fever, bacteremia, and postoperative mediastinal and wound infections.
- *M. genitalium* is a cause of urethritis in men and endocervicitis in women. It is likely a cause of pelvic inflammatory disease but appears to cause milder disease than *N. gonorrhoeae* and *C. trachomatis*.

DIAGNOSIS

- Most clinical laboratories are not equipped to diagnose infections caused by these organisms. Only *M. hominis* is detectable using methods routinely employed in clinical laboratories, but sensitivity is poor. The ureaplasmas require special media for growth, and *M. genitalium* cannot be cultured at all outside research laboratories. Nucleic acid amplification assays for this organism have been developed but are not in general use.

THERAPY

- Tetracycline class drugs are active against most ureaplasmas and *M. hominis* but not against *M. genitalium*. Macrolides are effective for the ureaplasmas but not for *M. hominis* and are only partially effective for *M. genitalium*. Quinolones, especially moxifloxacin, are active against all of the genital mycoplasmas.

121 *Rickettsia rickettsii* and Other Spotted Fever Group Rickettsiae (Rocky Mountain Spotted Fever and Other Spotted Fevers)

David H. Walker and Lucas S. Blanton

ETIOLOGY

- Spotted fever group (SFG) rickettsiae are small, gram-negative, obligately intracellular bacteria that cause tick-, mite-, and flea-borne human infections.
- In humans, rickettsiae infect endothelial cells and exert their pathophysiologic effects through endothelial injury, with a resultant increase in vascular permeability.

EPIDEMIOLOGY

- *Rickettsia rickettsii* is the agent that causes Rocky Mountain spotted fever (RMSF). *Dermacentor variabilis*, *Dermacentor andersoni*, and *Rhipicephalus sanguineus* ticks transmit the infection in the eastern two thirds, western, and southwestern United States, respectively. RMSF also occurs in Central and South America.
- In the United States, RMSF is most prevalent in the South Atlantic and South Central regions. Infections usually occur during the late spring and summer, when ticks are most active. Other tick-borne SFG rickettsiae with a broad range of distribution include *R. conorii* (Europe, Africa, and South Asia), *R. sibirica* (eastern Russia and Asia), *R. africae* (sub-Saharan Africa and West Indies), *R. parkeri* (North and South America), and *R. slovaca* (Europe).
- *Rickettsia felis* causes flea-borne spotted fever and has a worldwide distribution.

CLINICAL MANIFESTATIONS

- RMSF typically manifests with fever early in the course. Other manifestations include headache, myalgias, nausea, vomiting, and abdominal pain.
- Rash is common but may not occur in the first few days of illness. Rash typically starts on the wrists and ankles before spreading proximally. Involvement of the palms and soles occurs in 36% to 82% but is often a late sign.
- Skin necrosis, gangrenous digits, neurologic complications, azotemia, pulmonary edema, and acute respiratory distress syndrome are manifestations of severe infection.
- The case fatality rate of RMSF is 23% without appropriate antimicrobial treatment and up to 4% despite appropriate antimicrobials.
- Other SFG rickettsioses manifest with a wide spectrum of disease severity but are generally less severe than RMSF and often have an associated eschar at the tick bite site.

DIAGNOSIS

- The indirect immunofluorescence assay is the serologic method of choice. A fourfold rise in immunoglobulin G titer from acute illness to convalescence retrospectively confirms the diagnosis.
- Immunohistochemical detection of SFG rickettsiae in skin biopsy can establish the diagnosis during acute illness.
- Polymerase chain reaction amplification of rickettsial nucleic acids in blood, skin or eschar biopsy, or eschar swab is a useful tool for diagnosis and species identification.
- Treatment should not be withheld while awaiting laboratory confirmation.

TREATMENT AND PREVENTION

- Doxycycline, 100 mg twice daily for 7 to 10 days is the treatment of choice for RMSF and other SFG rickettsioses.
- Chloramphenicol is an alternative, but its use is associated with a higher case fatality in those with RMSF.
- Azithromycin and clarithromycin are alternatives for less severe SFG rickettsioses.
- Prevention is aimed toward the avoidance of contact with vectors through repellents and protective clothing.

122 *Rickettsia akari* (Rickettsialpox)

Didier Raoult

DEFINITION
- Vesicular fever with eschar caused by mite bites; may be confused with anthrax.

EPIDEMIOLOGY
- Found worldwide but is particularly common in New York City.

MICROBIOLOGY
- Infection caused by intracellular *Rickettsia akari*.

DIAGNOSIS
- Based on serology and polymerase chain reaction assay of swab from a vesicle or eschar.

THERAPY
- Doxycycline, 100 mg twice daily for 7 days.

PREVENTION
- Mouse eradication from buildings will prevent transmission to humans.

123 Coxiella burnetii (Q Fever)

Thomas J. Marrie and Didier Raoult

DEFINITION

- Q fever can be manifest as a self-limited febrile illness, pneumonia, endocarditis, or hepatitis. There are many other less common manifestations, such as meningitis, encephalitis, and osteomyelitis. Infections are divided into acute and chronic forms.

EPIDEMIOLOGY

- Q fever is a zoonosis that is usually acquired by inhalation or, much less commonly, by ingesting unpasteurized milk.
- Cattle, sheep, and goats are the most common reservoirs. Infected parturient cats are important in the spread of *Coxiella* in some areas.
- There is an extensive wildlife reservoir.
- The environment is contaminated at the time of parturition by an infected animal.
- Windborne spread from the contaminated environment can occur over a distance of at least 10 km.
- The distribution is worldwide, with the exception of New Zealand, Antarctica, and the Arctic.

MICROBIOLOGY

- Pleomorphic gram-negative (structurally—does not stain with Gram stain) coccobacillus
- *Coxiella burnetii*—only species in the genus
- Intracellular pathogen
- Spore former
- Undergoes phase variation; acute infection leads to antibody predominantly against phase II antigens, whereas chronic infections, such as endocarditis, are characterized by immunoglobulin G (IgG) antibody predominantly against phase I antigens.

DIAGNOSIS

- In most instances, an indirect immunofluorescent serologic test is the best one.
- A fourfold rise in titer between acute and convalescent samples is diagnostic of acute disease.
- Chronic infection is diagnosed on the basis of clinical manifestations (e.g., endocarditis) in conjunction with an IgG phase I titer that is equal to or exceeds phase II and is at least 1:1600.
- Isolation of *C. burnetii* by using a shell vial technique can be done in Biosafety Level 3 laboratories.
- Polymerase chain reaction assay can be used to amplify *C. burnetii* DNA from a variety of clinical specimens, such as heart valves and joint fluid. Fluorescent in situ hybridization can identify organisms in tissue, although standard histopathologic stains are negative.

THERAPY

- Acute Q fever: 10 days of doxycycline, a fluoroquinolone or a macrolide
- Chronic Q fever: Doxycycline plus hydroxychloroquine until phase I IgG antibody titers have declined to 1:800 or less

PREVENTION

- Good animal husbandry practices
- Use of seronegative sheep or goats in research facilities

124 Rickettsia prowazekii (Epidemic or Louse-Borne Typhus)

Lucas S. Blanton and David H. Walker

MICROBIOLOGY

- *Rickettsia prowazekii* is a small obligately intracellular gram-negative coccobacillus.
- Its 1.1-Mb genome has undergone evolutionary reduction, resulting in the reliance on the host cell cytosol for many biosynthetic functions.
- An extracellular dormant form remains infectious in louse feces for months or longer.

EPIDEMIOLOGY

- The agent is transmitted between patients by the human body louse *(Pediculus humanus corporis)*.
- Lice become infected while feeding on rickettsemic patients. The organism is inoculated into a new host by scratching rickettsiae-laden louse feces into louse-bitten skin or by rubbing into mucous membranes.
- Recovered patients remain latently infected, are susceptible to reactivation with rickettsemia, and can serve as a source for an epidemic.
- Epidemics are associated with conditions that promote louse infestations through poor hygiene—poverty, cold climate, jails, and displacement of populations by wars and other calamities.
- In North America, an extrahuman reservoir of *R. prowazekii* exists in flying squirrels *(Glaucomys volans),* with infections transmitted to humans by mucous membrane or inhalational exposure to the squirrel's flea or louse feces.

CLINICAL MANIFESTATIONS

- Frequent symptoms include fever, headache, chills, myalgia, and rash (see Table 124-1).
- Untreated illness may progress to cause pulmonary edema, encephalitis, and death.
- Recrudescent typhus and flying squirrel–associated typhus manifest similarly but are less severe.

DIAGNOSIS

- The indirect immunofluorescence assay is the mainstay of serologic diagnosis. A fourfold rise in immunoglobulin G (IgG) titer from acute illness to convalescence confirms the diagnosis.
- Polymerase chain reaction assay and immunohistochemical detection of *R. prowazekii* in blood or tissue, respectively, can establish the diagnosis during acute illness.
- Treatment should not be withheld while awaiting laboratory confirmation.

TREATMENT AND PREVENTION

- Doxycycline, 100 mg twice daily for 7 to 10 days, is the treatment of choice. Chloramphenicol is an alternative treatment.
- Control of body lice by changing and washing garments in hot water is essential for prevention and outbreak control.

TABLE 124-1 Clinical Manifestations of Epidemic Typhus		
	PLACE	
Manifestation	**Burundi**	**Ethiopia**
Number of cases	102	60
Fever >39°C	100%	100%
Headaches	100%	100%
Any rash	25%	38%
Purpuric rash	11%	33%
Stupor	81%	35%
Coma	4%	—
Cough	70%	38%
Nausea, vomiting	57%	43%
Conjunctivitis	15%	53%
Diarrhea	13%	—
Splenomegaly	8%	13%
Photophobia	—	33%
Myalgias	100%	70%

Data for Burundi from Fournier PE, Ndihokubwayo JB, Guidran J, et al. Human pathogens in body and head lice. *Emerg Infect Dis.* 2002;8:1515-1518; data for Ethiopia from Perine PL, Chandler BP, Krause DK, et al. A clinico-epidemiological study of epidemic typhus in Africa. *Clin Infect Dis.* 1992;14:1149-1158.

Chapter 124 *Rickettsia prowazekii* (Epidemic or Louse-Borne Typhus)

125 *Rickettsia typhi* (Murine Typhus)

Lucas S. Blanton, J. Stephen Dumler, and David H. Walker

DEFINITION

- Murine typhus is caused by *Rickettsia typhi*.
- *R. typhi* is an obligately intracellular gram-negative bacterium.
- The organism infects endothelial cells in mammalian hosts and midgut epithelial cells in flea hosts.

EPIDEMIOLOGY

- Murine typhus is distributed worldwide and is prevalent in tropical and subtropical seaboard regions where rats (*Rattus* spp.) and their fleas *(Xenopsylla cheopis)* serve as reservoirs and vectors, respectively.
- In the United States, most cases are reported in south Texas and southern California where the cat flea *(Ctenocephalides felis)* is the predominant vector and where opossums are the suspected reservoir.
- The disease is transmitted by the inoculation of infected flea feces into a flea bite wound.
- Murine typhus is increasingly recognized as an illness in travelers returning from endemic regions throughout the world.

CLINICAL MANIFESTATIONS

- Common symptoms in early illness include fever, headache, nausea, and vomiting.
- Rash is common as illness progresses. It is usually described as macular or maculopapular, and it is most commonly observed on the trunk.
- The clinical course is usually uncomplicated, but, occasionally, central nervous system abnormalities, renal insufficiency, respiratory failure, and death occur.
- Elevations in serum hepatic aminotransferase levels are frequent laboratory findings. Vascular injury often leads to hypoproteinemia, hypoalbuminemia, and electrolyte abnormalities (e.g., hyponatremia and hypocalcemia).

DIAGNOSIS

- Early diagnosis of murine typhus is based on clinical suspicion and epidemiology.
- Immunofluorescence assay is the mainstay of serologic diagnosis, which is generally retrospective. A fourfold rise in IgG titer from acute illness to convalescence confirms the diagnosis.
- Immunohistochemical detection of *R. typhi* in a skin biopsy specimen or polymerase chain reaction assay amplification of rickettsial nucleic acids in blood or skin biopsy samples can establish the diagnosis during acute infection.
- To avoid severe or potentially fatal infection, treatment should not be withheld while awaiting laboratory confirmation.

TREATMENT AND PREVENTION

- Doxycycline, 100 mg twice daily for 7 to 10 days, is the treatment of choice. Chloramphenicol is an alternative treatment.
- Prevention is directed toward the control of flea vectors and potential flea hosts.

126 Orientia tsutsugamushi (Scrub Typhus)

Didier Raoult

DEFINITION

- Mite-borne rickettsiosis, presenting one or more papular lesions that form an eschar at bite sites, followed in several days by rapid onset of fever, headache, myalgia, and local and then generalized adenopathy, often followed by rash

EPIDEMIOLOGY

- Extremely common in rural Asia and western Australia

MICROBIOLOGY

- Caused by intracellular *Orientia tsutsugamushi*

DIAGNOSIS

- Indirect fluorescent antibody assay is standard serology. Polymerase chain reaction assay of swab or tissue of eschar pretreatment is very sensitive. The Weil-Felix test is unreliable but widely used.

THERAPY

- Based on doxycycline, 100 mg twice daily for 7 days

PREVENTION

- Avoiding mite bite in rural Asia with vector control

127 Ehrlichia chaffeensis (Human Monocytotropic Ehrlichiosis), Anaplasma phagocytophilum (Human Granulocytotropic Anaplasmosis), and Other Anaplasmataceae

J. Stephen Dumler and David H. Walker

DEFINITION
- Infection by intracellular bacteria in the Anaplasmataceae family

MICROBIOLOGY
- Organisms of the family Anaplasmataceae of the order Rickettsiales are obligately intracellular gram-negative bacteria.
- *Ehrlichia chaffeensis, Ehrlichia canis, Ehrlichia muris,* and *Neorickettsia helminthoeca* infect mostly monocytes and macrophages in blood and tissues of mammalian hosts.
- *Anaplasma phagocytophilum* and *Ehrlichia ewingii* infect mostly neutrophils and other granulocytes in the blood of mammalian hosts.
- The mammalian target cell of *Neoehrlichia mikurensis* is not known.

EPIDEMIOLOGY
- Human monocytotropic ehrlichiosis (HME) and human *E. ewingii* infection are distributed predominantly in south-central and eastern North America, where *Amblyomma americanum* ticks and white-tailed deer *(Odocoileus virginianus)* serve as vectors and reservoirs, respectively.
- Human granulocytic anaplasmosis (HGA) is distributed worldwide, especially in northern latitudes of North America, Europe, and Asia, where *Ixodes persulcatus* clade ticks or *Haemaphysalis longicornis* ticks (China) and multiple small mammals serve as vectors and reservoirs.
- Human *E. muris*–like agent infection is distributed in the upper Midwest of the United States (Wisconsin and Minnesota), where *Ixodes scapularis* ticks and white-footed mice and other small mammals serve as vectors and reservoirs.
- Human *N. mikurensis* infection occurs in Europe and northern China, where *I. persulcatus* clade ticks and small mammals serve as vectors and reservoirs.
- Sennetsu neorickettsiosis occurs in eastern and southeastern Asia, where digenean trematodes serve as vectors and aquatic animals, mostly fish, serve as reservoirs through which infection is acquired by oral transmission. All members of the Anaplasmataceae are obligately intracellular bacteria that survive within vacuoles of host cells generally derived from the bone marrow, but also occasionally endothelial cells.

CLINICAL MANIFESTATIONS
- Frequent early manifestations include fever, headache, myalgia, nausea, and vomiting.
- Rash is infrequent or rare.
- The clinical course is usually uncomplicated, but severe complications can include a septic shock–like syndrome, respiratory distress, meningoencephalitis, renal failure, and death, particularly for HME.
- Leukopenia, thrombocytopenia, and elevations in serum hepatic aminotransferase levels are frequent findings.

DIAGNOSIS

- Early diagnosis of HME, HGA, and other human infections caused by bacteria in the Anaplasmataceae family is based on clinical suspicion and epidemiologic clues.
- Rapid laboratory confirmation can sometimes be achieved by blood smear examination for morulae (inclusions) in circulating leukocytes or by detection of bacterial DNA in blood by polymerase chain reaction assay.
- Seroconversion or fourfold increase in antibody titer from acute to convalescent phase confirms the diagnosis retrospectively.
- Early therapy improves outcomes and prevents severe complications or sequelae.

THERAPY

- Doxycycline, 100 mg twice daily for 5 to 10 days until fever is resolved, is the treatment of choice.
- Chloramphenicol should not be used.
- Rifampin has been successfully used in children.

PREVENTION

- Prevention is directed toward avoidance of tick exposures and bites and early removal of attached ticks. Neorickettsiosis could be prevented by avoidance of uncooked or fermented fish food products in regions where the disease occurs.

128 Staphylococcus aureus (Including Staphylococcal Toxic Shock Syndrome)

Yok-Ai Que and Philippe Moreillon

DEFINITION

- Gram-positive pathogen responsible for superficial and deep-seated infections
- Frequent colonizer of asymptomatic carriers
- Responsible for both pyogenic and toxin-related diseases
- Primary cause of community- and hospital-acquired bloodstream infections
- First cause of invasive infections, including infective endocarditis and osteomyelitis
- Frequently resistant to methicillin (methicillin-resistant *S. aureus* [MRSA]) and all β-lactam drugs (in up to 50% of hospital isolates)
- Often co-resistant to many clinically available antibiotics

EPIDEMIOLOGY

- Colonizer of the anterior nostrils in 20% to 40% of the normal population
- Number one public health problem in drug-resistant nosocomial infections
- Clonal spread of MRSA from health care (HCA-MRSA) and other permissive environments (see Fig. 128-1)
- Polyclonal dispersion of susceptible strains in the community; but successful clones of community-acquired (CA)-MRSA may spread worldwide (e.g., USA300)
- Superantigen producer responsible for toxic shock syndrome and food poisoning

MICROBIOLOGY

- Most virulent species of the more than 40 *Staphylococcus* spp. taxa
- Conserved core genome of approximately 2.8 million bp
- Multiple mobile genetic elements (MGEs); pathogenic and genomic islands, transposons, and prophages encoding virulence and antibiotic-resistance genes (see Tables 128-1, 128-2, and 128-3)
- Evolution of successful clones via mutations and acquisition of MGEs
- Methicillin resistance conferred by a polymorph family of SCC*mec* cassettes

DIAGNOSIS

- Conventional cultures mandatory and critical to detect new resistance phenotypes
- Prolonged incubation needed for small-colony variants responsible for chronic infection
- Molecular tests useful for rapid identification of known drug-resistance genes
- Molecular typing critical to manage MRSA epidemics and infection control

THERAPY

- First choice for methicillin-susceptible *S. aureus:* penicillinase-resistant β-lactam or first-generation cephalosporin, for instance, cephalexin or dicloxacillin orally; nafcillin or oxacillin intravenously; or, outside the United States, flucloxacillin. Alternatives include clindamycin or trimethoprim-sulfamethoxazole orally or intravenously).
- First choice for MRSA would be vancomycin or daptomycin intravenously, or, if susceptible, trimethoprim-sulfamethoxazole or clindamycin orally or intravenously. Alternatives include

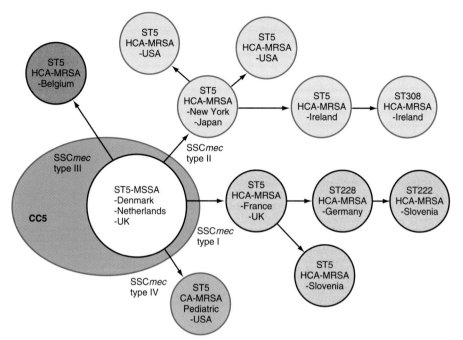

FIGURE 128-1 Evolution of methicillin-susceptible *Staphylococcus aureus* (MSSA) into methicillin-resistant *S. aureus* (MRSA) as exemplified by sequence type 5 (ST5). ST5 belongs to clonal cluster 5 (CC5), which gathers *S. aureus* isolates sharing homologies in five of the seven genes (*arcC, aroE, glpF, gmk, pta, tpi,* and *yqiL*) compared with method of multilocus sequence typing (MLST). Parental ST5 is an MSSA that has been isolated in several countries, including Denmark, the Netherlands, and the United Kingdom. It acquired various types of SCC*mec* at several independent occasions, probably from CoNS donor strains. After SCC*mec* acquisition, new MRSA clones followed their own geographic and genetic evolution, spreading either as HCA-MRSA (SCC*mec* I, II, or III) or CA-MRSA clones (SCC*mec* IV) and sometimes evolving into new ST types (e.g., ST222, ST228, and ST308). Three clonal clusters (CC5, CC8, and CC30) generated six of the seven major pandemic MRSA clones described over the past 3 decades. (Modified from Robinson DA, Enright MC. Evolutionary models of the emergence of methicillin-resistant *Staphylococcus aureus*. *Antimicrob Agents Chemother*. 2003;47:3926-3934.)

ceftaroline, linezolid, or telavancin; or, for acute bacterial skin and skin structure infections, dalbavancin, oritavancin, or tedizolid.

- Partner drug for combinations: rifampin.
- Benefit of aminoglycosides not well demonstrated.

PREVENTION

- Decolonization of staphylococcal carriers (see Table 128-4)
- Detection of HCA-MRSA and epidemic CA-MRSA
- Hospital hygiene measures
- Vaccines in development

Part II Infectious Diseases and their Etiologic Agents

TABLE 128-1 *Staphylococcus aureus* Extracellular Factors Involved in Pathogenesis and Response to Global Regulatory Elements during Bacterial Growth

Gene	Location	Product	Activity/Function	Timing*	ACTION OF REGULATORY GENES†			
					agr	saeRS	rot	sarA
Surface Proteins								
spa	Chromosome	Protein A	Anti-immune, anti-PMN	Exp	−	‡	+	
cna	Chromosome	Collagen BP	Collagen binding	Exp	−			
fnbA	Chromosome	Fibronectin BPA	Fibronectin binding	Exp	−			+
fnbB	Chromosome	Fibronectin BPB	Fibronectin binding	Exp	−			+
clfA	Chromosome	Clumping factor A	Fibrinogen binding	Exp	0			
clfB	Chromosome	Clumping factor B	Fibrinogen binding	Exp	0		+	0
lfb	Chromosome	Lactoferrin BP	Lactoferrin binding	Exp				
Capsular Polysaccharides								
cap5	Chromosome	Polysaccharide capsule type 5	Antiphagocytosis?	Pxp	+			+
cap8	Chromosome	Polysaccharide capsule type 8	Antiphagocytosis?	Pxp	+			
Cytotoxins								
hla	Chromosome	α-Hemolysin	Hemolysin, cytotoxin	Pxp	+	+	−	‡
hlb	Chromosome	β-Hemolysin	Hemolysin, cytotoxin	Pxp	+	+	−	‡
hld	Chromosome	δ-Hemolysin	Hemolysin, cytotoxin	Pxp	+	0		+
hlg	Chromosome	γ-Hemolysin	Hemolysin, cytotoxin	Pxp	+		−	‡
lukS/F	PVL phage	PVL	Leucolysin	Pxp	+		−	
Superantigens								
sea	Bacteriophage	Enterotoxin A	Food poisoning, TSS	Xp	0			
seb	SaPI3§	Enterotoxin B	Food poisoning, TSS	Pxp	+			‡
sec	SaPI4§	Enterotoxin C	Food poisoning, TSS	Pxp	+			
sed	Plasmid	Enterotoxin D	Food poisoning, TSS	Pxp	+			
eta	ETA phage	Exfoliatin A	Scalded skin syndrome	Pxp	+			
etb	Plasmid	Exfoliatin B	Scalded skin syndrome	Pxp	+			
tst	SaPI1,2, bov1§	Toxic shock toxin-1	Toxic shock syndrome	Pxp	+			‡
Enzymes								
SplA-F	Chromosome	Serine protease-like	Putative protease		+		−	
ssp	Chromosome	V8 protease	Spreading factor	Pxp	+	0		−
aur	Chromosome	Metalloprotease (aureolysin)	Processing enzyme?	Pxp	+			−
sspB	Chromosome	Cysteine protease	Processing enzyme?	?			−	
scp	Chromosome	Staphopain (protease II)	Spreading, nutrition	Pxp	+			−
geh	Chromosome	Glycerol ester hydrolase	Spreading, nutrition	Pxp	+	0	−	‡
lip	Chromosome	Lipase (butyryl esterase)	Spreading, nutrition	Pxp	+	0		‡
fme	Chromosome	FAME	Fatty acid esterification	Pxp	+			‡
plc	Chromosome	PI-phospholipase C		Pxp	+			
nuc	Chromosome	Nuclease	Nutrition	Pxp	+	+		

TABLE 128-1 *Staphylococcus aureus* **Extracellular Factors Involved in Pathogenesis and Response to Global Regulatory Elements during Bacterial Growth—cont'd**

Gene	Location	Product	Activity/Function	Timing*	ACTION OF REGULATORY GENES[†]			
					agr	*saeRS*	*rot*	*sarA*
has	Chromosome	Hyaluronidase	Spreading factor	Xp	[‡]			
coa	Chromosome	Coagulase	Clotting, clot digestion	Exp		+	+	+
sak	Bacteriophage	Staphylokinase	Plasminogen activator	Pxp	+	0		

BP, binding protein; FAME, fatty acid modifying enzyme; PMN, polymorphonuclear neutrophil.

*Timing: Xp, throughout exponential phase; Exp, early exponential phase only; Pxp, postexponential phase; 0, no effect of gene on. Expression: +, upregulated; –, downregulated.

[†]*agr*, accessory gene regulator; PVL, Panton-Valentine leukocidin; *saeRS*, *S. aureus* exoproteins; *rot*, repressor of toxins; *sarA*, *Staphylococcus* accessory regulator.

[‡]Controversial.

[§]*SaPI*, *S. aureus* pathogenic island.

Modified from Cheung AL, Projan SJ, Gresham H. The genomic aspect of virulence, sepsis, and resistance to killing mechanisms in *Staphylococcus aureus*. *Curr Infect Dis Rep*. 2002;4:400-410; and Novick RP, Geisinger E. Quorum sensing in staphylococci. *Ann Rev Genet*. 2008;42:541-564.

TABLE 128-2 *Staphylococcus aureus* **MSCRAMMs Belonging to Sortase-Mediated Cell Wall–Associated Proteins**

GENE	PROTEIN	AA	SORTASE	MOTIF	LIGAND SPECIFICITY	POTENTIAL IMPLICATION IN DISEASE
Spa	Protein A	508	SrtA	LPETG	Antibody Fc fragment (IgG, IgM) von Willebrand's factor, TNFR1, platelets	Experimental sepsis, experimental osteoarthritis
clfA	Clumping factor A	933	SrtA	LPDTG	Fibrinogen, platelets	Experimental endocarditis
clfB	Clumping factor B	913	SrtA	LPETG	Fibrinogen, cytokeratin 10, platelets	Colonization of nasal mucosa
cna	Collagen-binding protein	1183	SrtA	LPKTG	Collagen	Experimental osteomyelitis, septic arthritis
fnA	Fibronectin-binding protein A	1018	SrtA	LPETG	Fibronectin, fibrinogen, elastin	Experimental endocarditis
					Platelets	Cell invasion, experimental mastitis
fnB	Fibronectin-binding protein B	914	SrtA	LPETG	Fibronectin, fibrinogen, elastin, platelets	Experimental mastitis
sdrC	Serine-aspartate repeat protein	947	SrtA	LPETG	Undetermined	—
sdrD	Serine aspartate repeat protein	1315	SrtA	LPETG	Undetermined	—

Continued

TABLE 128-2 *Staphylococcus aureus* MSCRAMMs Belonging to Sortase-Mediated Cell Wall–Associated Proteins—cont'd

GENE	PROTEIN	AA	SORTASE	MOTIF	LIGAND SPECIFICITY	POTENTIAL IMPLICATION IN DISEASE
sdrE	Serine aspartate repeat protein	1166	SrtA	LPETG	Platelets	—
pls	Plasmin-sensitive protein	1637	SrtA	LPDTG	Cellular lipids, ganglioside M3; nasal epithelial cells	Colonization of nasal mucosa
sraP (sasA)	Serin-rich adhesin for platelets	2261	SrtA	LPDTG	Platelets	Experimental endocarditis
IsdA (sasE)	Iron-regulated surface determinant A	354	SrtA	LPKTG	Fibrinogen, fibronectin Hemoglobin/transferrin	Nasal colonization
IsdB (sasJ)	Iron-regulated surface determinant B	645	SrtA	LPQTG	Hemoglobin/hemin	—
isdC	Iron-regulated surface determinant C	227	SrtB	NPQTN	Hemin	—
isdH (harA) (sasI)	Iron-regulated surface determinant H	895	SrtA	LPKTG	Haptoglobin Haptoglobin/hemoglobin complex	Nasal colonization
sasB	S. aureus surface protein B	937	SrtA	LPDTG	Undetermined	—
sasC	S. aureus surface protein C	2186	SrtA	LPNTG	Undetermined	—
sasD	S. aureus surface protein D	241	SrtA	LPAAG	Undetermined	—
sasF	S. aureus surface protein F	637	SrtA	LPKAG	Undetermined	—
sasG	S. aureus surface protein G	1117	SrtA	LPKTG	Nasal epithelial cells	Associated to invasive disease
sash (adsA)	S. aureus surface protein H	308	SrtA	LPKTG	Cell-wall associated adenosine, synthase	Escape phagocyte-induced killing
sasK	S. aureus surface protein K	211	SrtA	LPKTG	Undetermined	—
fmtB	Formyl transferase B		SrtA	LPXTG	Cell wall synthesis, β-lactam resistance	Antibiotic resistance

AA, protein length in amino acids; Srt, sortase; IgM, immunoglobulin M; MSCRAMMs, microbial surface components recognizing adhesive matrix molecules; TNFR1, TNF-receptor 1.

Modified from Roche FM, Massey R, Peacock SJ, et al. Characterization of novel LPXTG-containing proteins of *Staphylococcus aureus* identified from genome sequences. *Microbiology*. 2003;149:643-654; Clarke S, Foster S. Surface adhesins of *Staphylococcus aureus*. *Adv Microb Physiol*. 2006;51:187-224; and Dedent A, Marraffini L, Schneewind O. Staphylococcal sortases and surface proteins. In: Fischetti V, Novick RP, Ferretti J, et al, eds. *Gram-Positive Pathogens*. 2nd ed. Washington, DC: ASM Press; 2006:486-495.

TABLE 128-3 Summary of Major Mobile Genetic Elements in Sequenced *Staphylococcus aureus* Strains

	S. AUREUS STRAIN										
	MRSA252	N315	Mu50	COL	8325	MW2	MSSA476	FPR3757	JH1/JH9	Newman	RF122
Clonal cluster	30	5	5	8	8	1	1	8	5	8	151
Bacteriophage											
ΦSa1			NI								*lukFM*
ΦSa2	NI				NI (Φ12)	PV-*luk*		PV-*luk*	NI		
ΦSa3	*chip scin sak sea*	*chip scin sak sep*	*chip sak sea*		*chip scin* Sak	*scin sak sea seg sek*	*scin sak sea seg sek*	*chip scin sak*	*chip scin sak*	*chip scin sak sea*	
ΦSa4							NI		NI		
ΦSa5					NI (Φ11)					NI	
ΦSa6				NI (L54a)					NI	NI	NI
ΦSA7										NI	
ΦSa8											NI
SAPIs											
SAPI1				*seb ear seq sek*				*ear seq sek*			
SAPI2		*sel sec tst*	*sel sec tst*								*Mdr*
SAPI3			*fhuD*			*ear sel sec*					
SAPI4	NI						NI				
SAPIbov											*tst sel*
Plasmids											
I	*ble kn**	*ble kn**	*ble kn**	*tet*					*tetK;* NI		
II	*cadAC arsBC**	*cadDX arsBC*				*blaZ cadD*	*blaZ cadD*		*blaZ arsR cadD aac/aph*		
III			*aac/aph qacA*						*erm ileS*		
Transposons											
Tn552	*blaZ*										
Tn554	*erm spc*	*erm spc*	*erm spc*								
Tn5801			*tetM*								
Tn976-like	NI			NI							

Continued

TABLE 128-3 Summary of Major Mobile Genetic Elements in Sequenced *Staphylococcus aureus* Strains—cont'd

	S. AUREUS STRAIN										
	MRSA252	N315	Mu50	COL	8325	MW2	MSSA476	FPR3757	JH1/JH9	Newman	RF122
SCC											
mec I				mecA							
mec II	mecA	mecA	mecA							mecA	
mec III											
mec IV						mecA		mecA arc opp			
non-mec							far1				

aac/aph, aminoglycoside resistance; *arc*, arginine catabolism; *arsBC*, arsenic resistance genes; *blaZ*, penicillin resistance; *bsa*, bacteriocin biosynthesis genes; *cadACDX*, cadmium resistance genes; *chip*, chemotaxis inhibitory protein; *ear*, putative β-lactamase type protein; *erm*, erythromycin resistance; *far1*, fusidic acid resistance; *fhuD*, siderophore transporter; *ileS*, mupiricin resistance; *lukFM*, leukocidin; *mdr*, multidrug resistance; *opp*, oligopeptide uptake; *mecA*, penicillin-binding protein 2a conferring resistance to methicillin; *qacA*, quaternary ammonium compound (antiseptic) resistance; *PV-luk*, Panton-Valentine leukocidin; *sak*, staphylokinase; *SaPI*, *S. aureus* pathogenicity island; *SCC*, staphylococcal cassette chromosome; *scin*, staphylococcal chemotaxis inhibitory protein; *sea* to *sep*, enterotoxin A to enterotoxin P; *spc*, spectinomycin resistance; *tst*, toxic shock syndrome toxin-1; *tet* and *tetM*, tetracycline resistance.

Note: Phage and SaPI families based on homology of integrase genes and insertion site. NI, Element present but no identified virulence or resistance gene. FPR3757 SCC*mec* is fused to ACME element; SaPIS belongs to SaPI1 family based on integrase and insertion site. RF122 has two phage fragments.

*Integrated plasmid.

Modified from Lindsay J. *S. aureus* evolution: lineages and mobile genetic elements (MGEs). In: Lindsay J, ed. *Staphylococcus aureus Molecular Genetics*. Norfolk, UK: Casiter Academic Press; 2008:45-69.

TABLE 128-4 Example of Decontaminating Scheme for Patients Colonized or Infected with Methicillin-Resistant *Staphylococcus aureus* (MRSA)

Protective Measures

Put patient in contact isolation (one or several contaminated patients in single room with restricted access)
Use protective gown and gloves
Use protective mask and glasses if risk for projection of contaminated liquids
Clean hands with alcoholic solution at glove removal and between caregiving procedures
Leave any disposable item in room and discard for sterilization in special containers

Decontamination Measures

Apply nasal mupirocin (2%) every 8 hours for 5-7 days
Apply chlorhexidine-based oral spray three to four times a day for 5-7 days
Take daily shower or clean body thoroughly with chlorhexidine-based soap for 5-7 days
In the case of dental prostheses, clean and soak the prosthesis daily in chlorhexidine-based solution for 5-7 days

Control Cultures and Decision

Take control swabs of any contaminated sites 48 and 96 hours after the end of treatment
Keep isolation measures in force until laboratory results are available
If no MRSA is present in control cultures, consider patient decontaminated. Relieve isolation and swab weekly for follow-up cultures.
If MRSA is present in control cultures, pursue isolation measures and repeat whole decontamination scheme

Modified from Current Recommendations at the University Hospital of Lausanne, Switzerland.

129 Staphylococcus epidermidis and Other Coagulase-Negative Staphylococci

Mark E. Rupp and Paul D. Fey

MICROBIOLOGY

- More than 40 species of coagulase-negative staphylococci are gram-positive cocci that are closely related to the intrinsically more virulent *Staphylococcus aureus* and differentiated from *S. aureus* by their inability to produce coagulase.
- *Staphylococcus epidermidis,* the most common clinically encountered species of coagulase-negative staphylococci, is a prominent part of the normal commensal flora of human skin. *S. epidermidis* owes its pathogenic success to three factors: (1) its normal niche on human skin, giving it access to any device inserted or passed through the skin; (2) its ability to adhere to biomaterials and elaborate biofilm; and (3) changes in the human host population resulting in greater numbers of immunosuppressed patients and greater use of bioprosthetic devices.
- Other noteworthy species of coagulase-negative staphylococci include *S. saprophyticus,* a common cause of uncomplicated urinary tract infection in sexually active women; *S. haemolyticus,* often resistant to glycopeptides; and *S. lugdunensis,* a more virulent coagulase-negative staphylococcus that mimics infections due to *S. aureus.*

EPIDEMIOLOGY

- *S. epidermidis* is a prominent cause of intravascular catheter-related infection and infection of a variety of medical devices, such as prosthetic joints, artificial heart valves, and cerebrospinal fluid shunts.
- Strains of *S. epidermidis* can establish predominance in hospital environments and spread from unit to unit, hospital to hospital, and country to country.

DIAGNOSIS

- Differentiating "true" infection-causing coagulase-negative staphylococci from contaminants can, at times, be a diagnostic challenge. Finding coagulase-negative staphylococci at high numbers or repetitively in situations clinically consistent with infection is indicative of a true infection. Unfortunately, in some situations, infections due to coagulase-negative staphylococci can be indolent and diagnosis is difficult.

THERAPY

- Most nosocomial *S. epidermidis* strains are multidrug resistant, and glycopeptide or alternative antistaphylococcal antibiotics directed at methicillin-resistant strains are employed in treatment. Isolates of *S. epidermidis* with an oxacillin minimal inhibitory concentration (MIC) of 0.25 µg/mL or less may be treated with oxacillin or nafcillin. Vancomycin is the drug with which there is the most clinical experience in coagulase-negative staphylococcal infections, although case reports support use of daptomycin and linezolid. Most species are susceptible in vitro to the newer agents: telavancin, dalbavancin, oritavancin, ceftaroline, and tedizolid, as well as to the older agents, quinupristin-dalfopristin, and tigecycline, but their clinical utility for coagulase-negative staphylococcal infections remains to be defined.

- In some situations, rifampin is added to the regimen for better activity against biofilm-associated organisms.
- Information is accruing with regard to treatment of biomaterial-based infections with the device in situ, but most of these data are anecdotal. In general, infected devices should be removed whenever possible. A number of biofilm-directed therapeutic modalities appear to hold promise.

PREVENTION

- Biomedical devices must be inserted or implanted with scrupulous attention to aseptic practices. There is great interest in developing biomedical devices that are less prone to bacterial adherence and infection.

130 *Streptococcus pyogenes*

Amy E. Bryant and Dennis L. Stevens

DEFINITION

- *Streptococcus pyogenes* is an important global human pathogen that causes a wide variety of acute infections, such as soft tissue infections and pharyngitis; severe life-threatening infections, such as streptococcal toxic shock syndrome; and devastating postinfectious sequelae, such as rheumatic fever and glomerulonephritis.

EPIDEMIOLOGY

- The most common infection is streptococcal pharyngitis.
- Superficial skin and soft tissue infections include impetigo, erysipelas, and cellulitis.
- Severe life-threatening infections include scarlet fever, bacteremia, pneumonia, necrotizing fasciitis, myonecrosis, and streptococcal toxic shock syndrome.
- Postinfectious sequelae include acute rheumatic fever and poststreptococcal glomerulonephritis.

MICROBIOLOGY

- *S. pyogenes* is a gram-positive, β-hemolytic streptococcus that is catalase negative. More than 150 different strains have been identified based on different M-protein types. It is a group A streptococcus based on its carbohydrate structure, according to Lancefield typing of β-hemolytic strains. Mucoid strains are rich in hyaluronic acid capsule, and numerous extracellular toxins are produced by most strains, which include streptolysin O, a cholesterol-specific cytolysin, streptolysin S, a cell-associated hemolysin, fibrinogen-binding proteins, streptokinase, numerous pyrogenic exotoxins that act as superantigens, and a cysteine-protease called pyrogenic exotoxin B.

DIAGNOSIS

- Diagnosis of *S. pyogenes* pharyngitis is suspected based on specific clinical criteria and can be substantiated by rapid tests or culture.
- Similarly, impetigo, cellulitis, and erysipelas are suspected based on unique clinical presentations. Cultures of impetiginous lesions will distinguish *Streptococcus* from *Staphylococcus aureus* as the cause. Cultures of lesions associated with cellulitis and erysipelas are useful only 20% of the time, and blood cultures are rarely positive.
- Invasive *S. pyogenes* is more difficult to diagnose early in the course, although blood cultures are positive in more than 50% of cases. In the 50% of patients with necrotizing fasciitis associated with a portal of entry such as surgical incision, postpartum sepsis, or insect bites, cultures of these sites are positive in the vast majority of cases. In the 50% of patients with no portal of entry, infection begins deep in the fascia and muscle, and these patients present with a history of previous nonpenetrating trauma, severe pain, and systemic toxicity. Classic signs of necrotizing infections are not apparent until late in the course at a time that the patient has systemic shock and organ failure.
- Rheumatic fever is diagnosed based on clinical suspicion of patients with an antecedent pharyngitis who present with carditis, Sydenham's chorea, migratory arthritis, and evidence

that the pharyngitis was due to *S. pyogenes* by positive culture or rising anti–streptolysin O titers and using the Jones criteria, which are reviewed elsewhere.

- Poststreptococcal glomerulonephritis is diagnosed based on evidence of renal failure with glomerular damage, as indicated by red blood cell casts and an antecedent streptococcal infection, which can be either pharyngitis or impetigo.

THERAPY

- Penicillin remains the drug of choice for the treatment of all streptococcal infections.
- Most cases of impetigo can be treated with topical bacitracin, mupirocin, or retapamulin, and only in severe cases or in epidemic situations is oral or parenteral administration of penicillin necessary.
- Severe cases of *S. pyogenes* infections, such as necrotizing fasciitis, myonecrosis, and streptococcal toxic shock syndrome, may benefit from clindamycin, which suppresses toxin production and in animal studies and limited human studies is superior to penicillin. Intensive care support, aggressive fluid resuscitation, ventilator support, and surgical intervention are commonly required.

PREVENTION

- Epidemics of streptococcal pharyngitis have been prevented in military recruits by the administration of monthly benzathine penicillin given intramuscularly.
- Rheumatic fever can be prevented by administration of penicillin within 9 days of the onset of streptococcal pharyngitis. Secondary prophylaxis should be considered in patients with rheumatic heart disease based on age, small children in the household, and exposure to cases of streptococcal infection.
- Improved living conditions, improved personal hygiene, and topical treatment of impetiginous lesions can prevent spread to susceptible individuals.
- Prevention of secondary cases should be considered in health care workers and family members with prolonged, intimate contact with patients with necrotizing fasciitis/ streptococcal toxic shock syndrome, particularly those who are immunocompromised, have varicella, have had recent surgery, or have recently given birth. The risk for secondary severe infection is low, but colonization and streptococcal pharyngitis can occur commonly. Oral penicillin for 7 to 10 days is reasonable, although no definitive studies have been done.

131 Nonsuppurative Poststreptococcal Sequelae: Rheumatic Fever and Glomerulonephritis

Stanford T. Shulman and Alan L. Bisno

DEFINITIONS

- Acute rheumatic fever (ARF) and acute poststreptococcal glomerulonephritis (APSGN) are immune-mediated illnesses that develop after some group A streptococcal infections.
- ARF predominantly affects the heart and joints and can lead to chronic rheumatic heart disease, whereas APSGN is an immune-complex nephritis.

EPIDEMIOLOGY

- ARF can follow an untreated group A streptococcal infection of the pharynx in individuals who appear to be genetically susceptible.
- ARF is most frequent in children 5 to 15 years of age and occurs most commonly in winter or spring.
- ARF now is much less common in developed areas of the world, compared with several decades ago. Most cases now occur in developing countries or in minority populations within Australia and New Zealand.
- APSGN can follow group A streptococcal infections of the skin or throat.
- Postpharyngeal APSGN occurs mainly in school-aged children in winter or spring, whereas postpyoderma APSGN is most common in pre–school-aged children in late summer or fall.

MICROBIOLOGY

- Certain M types of group A streptococci (GAS; M-1, M-3, M-5, M-6, M-14, M-18, M-19) are considered rheumatogenic, that is, they have much greater ability to trigger the immune events that result in ARF when compared to nonrheumatogenic types. The molecular basis of rheumatogenicity is unknown.
- Nephritogenic M types of GAS are those with great propensity to lead to APSGN, specifically M-1, M-4, M-12, and M-25 after pharyngitis and M-2, M-9, M-55, M-57, M-59, M-60, and M-61 after pyoderma. The specific antigen(s) involved in this immune-complex nephritis is still somewhat unclear.

DIAGNOSIS

- Diagnosis of ARF is based upon the Jones criteria, comprising five major criteria, four minor criteria, and a requirement for evidence of antecedent group A streptococcal infection.
- The five major Jones criteria are carditis, arthritis, chorea, erythema marginatum, and subcutaneous nodules. The four minor criteria are fever, arthralgia, elevated acute-phase reactants (erythrocyte sedimentation rate, C-reactive protein), and prolonged P-R interval. Diagnosis of ARF requires one major plus at least two minor criteria or two major criteria plus evidence of antecedent group A streptococcal infection.
- The diagnosis of APSGN is generally based upon acute onset of hematuria with hypertension, azotemia, hypocomplementemia, and with evidence of recent streptococcal pharyngitis or pyoderma.

TABLE 131-1 Suggested Schedule of Anti-inflammatory Therapy in Rheumatic Fever

CLINICAL SEVERITY	TREATMENT
Arthralgia or mild arthritis; no carditis	Analgesics only, such as codeine or propoxyphene
Moderate or severe arthritis; no carditis, or carditis *with or without* cardiomegaly, but without failure	Aspirin, 50-70 mg/kg/day for 3 wk, increased if necessary; 25-35 mg/kg/day for the subsequent 6 wk
Carditis with congestive failure, with or without joint manifestations	Prednisone, 2 mg/kg, max 60 mg/day; methylprednisone sodium succinate intravenous in fulminating cases; after 2-3 wk, slow withdrawal to be completed in 3 more wk; aspirin to be continued for 1 mo after discontinuation of prednisone

From Stollerman GH. *Rheumatic Fever and Streptococcal Infection.* New York: Grune & Stratton; 1975.

TABLE 131-2 Secondary Prevention of Rheumatic Fever (Prevention of Recurrent Attacks)

AGENT	DOSE	MODE
Benzathine penicillin G	600,000 U for children ≤27 kg (60 lb), 1.2 million U for those >27 kg (60 lb) every 4 wk*	Intramuscular
Penicillin V	250 mg twice daily	Oral
Sulfadiazine	0.5 g once daily for patients ≤27 kg (60 lb)	Oral
	1.0 g once daily for patients >27 kg (60 lb)	
For Individuals Allergic to Penicillin and Sulfadiazine		
Macrolide or azalide	Variable	Oral

*In high-risk situations, administration every 3 weeks is justified and recommended.
From Gerber MA, Baltimore RS, Eaton CB, et al. Prevention of rheumatic fever and diagnosis and treatment of acute streptococcal pharyngitis. *Circulation.* 2009;191:1541-1551.

THERAPY

- Treatment of ARF includes an anti-inflammatory agent (aspirin for those with arthritis and/or mild carditis; corticosteroids for those with moderate or severe carditis [see Table 131-1]); an agent such as phenobarbital, diazepam, haloperidol, valproate, or risperidone for those with chorea; and a prophylactic antibiotic. A single dose of intramuscular (IM) benzathine penicillin (or an alternative agent for penicillin-allergic individuals) is indicated.
- Treatment of APSGN includes correction of circulatory overload and hypertension by salt and fluid restriction, diuretics as needed, antihypertensives only if severe hypertension or hypertensive encephalopathy is present. Immunosuppressives are not beneficial.

PREVENTION

- Because ARF frequently recurs with subsequent group A streptococcal pharyngitis episodes, long-term prophylaxis is indicated with IM benzathine penicillin every 4 weeks or oral penicillin V twice daily, or for penicillin-allergic individuals with daily sulfadiazine, macrolide, or azalide (see Table 131-2), usually at least until age 21.
- Because APSGN only very rarely recurs, no preventative antibiotic therapy is indicated.

132 Streptococcus pneumoniae

Edward N. Janoff and Daniel M. Musher

EPIDEMIOLOGY

- *Streptococcus pneumoniae* is the leading cause of pneumonia and bacterial meningitis in children younger than 5 years and older adults worldwide.
- The incidence is highest in children younger than 2 years and adults older than 65 years; mortality is highest in older adults.
- Asymptomatic colonization is common and precedes almost all symptomatic clinical infections.
- Large outbreaks are uncommon, but smaller outbreaks occur under crowded conditions (prisons, nursing homes, military training).
- Groups at increased risk for serious pneumococcal disease include individuals at the extremes of age (particularly <2 years and >65 years of age), those with underlying organ dysfunction (asplenia and splenic dysfunction, chronic heart, lung, liver, and kidney disease), and immunocompromising conditions (particularly antibody defects, complement deficiencies, neutropenia, and malignancies).

MICROBIOLOGY

- *Streptococcus pneumoniae* is a gram-positive, α-hemolytic, lancet-shaped diplococcus and is bile soluble and optochin sensitive.
- *Streptococcus pneumoniae* is catalase-negative but produces hydrogen peroxide.
- There are more than 92 capsular polysaccharide serotypes that confer resistance to phagocytosis; serotype is determined by the Quellung reaction.
- Effective phagocytosis and killing typically require antibodies, most often to capsular polysaccharides, complement, and phagocytes (neutrophils and macrophages).
- Pneumolysin is the cholesterol-binding, pore-forming primary toxin that causes both epithelial and endothelial damage and perturbs complement activity.

DIAGNOSIS

- Perform Gram stain and culture of good-quality sputum (<10 epithelial cells, >25 neutrophils/high-power field or >10 neutrophils/epithelial cell) from patients with pneumonia, of cerebrospinal fluid from patients with meningitis, and of middle ear fluid by tympanocentesis from patients with otitis media. Among adults with pneumonia, approximately 10% have positive blood cultures, half of which grow *S. pneumoniae*.
- Perform urine antigen detection in adults ($\approx$70% sensitive in adults with bacteremia; not specific in children).

CLINICAL MANIFESTATIONS

- Otitis media is the most common clinical syndrome, but pneumococcal pneumonia in children and adults underlies most serious infections and death.
- The spectrum of infection ranges from asymptomatic pharyngeal colonization to mucosal disease (otitis media, sinusitis, pneumonia) to invasive disease (bacteria in a normally sterile site; bacteremia, meningitis, empyema, endocarditis, arthritis).

- Most invasive disease results from bacteremic seeding, but meningitis and empyema may also result from extension of local infection.

THERAPY

- A β-lactam antibiotic is the mainstay of therapy for pneumococcal infection. Decreased sensitivity to penicillin derives from structural modifications of penicillin-binding proteins, effects that compromise the efficacy of penicillin in treatment of meningitis and otitis media, but typically not pneumonia.
- Intravenous therapy, particularly ceftriaxone and cefotaxime, are recommended for therapy of bacteremia and most often, with the initial addition of vancomycin, meningitis.
- Respiratory quinolones, linezolid, vancomycin, and macrolides all show clinical activity against *S. pneumoniae*. Combined therapy with a β-lactam and macrolide may improve outcomes.

PREVENTION

- Two vaccines provide protection against invasive pneumococcal disease: a pneumococcal polysaccharide-protein conjugate vaccine (PCV13) with the 13 most common pediatric capsular serotypes for children (>90% protection) and a 23-valent polysaccharide vaccine for adults (PPSV23) (54% to 81% protection). The childhood PCV13 also prevents up to one third of childhood bacterial pneumonia and some proportion of meningitis and otitis media. The efficacy of the 23-valent polysaccharide vaccine against adult pneumonia is less clear. Both PPSV23 and PCV13 are now approved independently for use in older adults. For immunocompromised adults, vaccination with the 13-valent conjugate, followed greater than or equal to 8 weeks later with the 23-valent polysaccharide vaccine, is recommended. Widespread pneumococcal vaccination of children has reduced the overall incidence of invasive disease and hospitalization for pneumonia in all age groups in the United States.

133 Enterococcus Species, Streptococcus gallolyticus Group, and Leuconostoc Species

Cesar A. Arias and Barbara E. Murray

MICROBIOLOGY AND TAXONOMY

- Enterococci are gram-positive facultatively anaerobic bacteria that usually appear oval in shape and can be seen as single cells, pairs, short chains, or even very long chains.
- Enterococci are capable of growing in medium containing 6.5% sodium chloride and at temperatures between 10° and 45° C and are able to hydrolyze esculin in the presence of 40% bile salts.
- *Enterococcus faecalis* and *Enterococcus faecium* are the most clinically relevant species.
- Most clinically relevant species of enterococci produce a leucine aminopeptidase and a pyrrolidonylarylamidase.
- The former *Streptococcus bovis* group is now divided into three main species: *S. gallolyticus*, *S. pasteurianus*, and *S. infantarius*.
- The *Leuconostoc* genus comprises catalase-negative, gram-positive cocci, usually arranged in pairs or chains and are intrinsically resistant to vancomycin.

COLONIZATION, VIRULENCE, AND GENOMICS

- Enterococci are normal commensals of the gastrointestinal tract.
- Enterococci are capable of dominating the gut microbiota of hospitalized patients who receive broad-spectrum antibiotics.
- Specific hospital-associated genetic lineages of *E. faecium* and *E. faecalis* have evolved to become successful in the nosocomial environment.
- The *Streptococcus gallolyticus* group of organisms also carries genes encoding potential cell surface determinants that interact with host proteins.

EPIDEMIOLOGY

- Enterococci are organisms known to cause hospital-associated infections in patients who are critically ill or immunosuppressed.
- Enterococci are among the most common organisms causing infective endocarditis, both hospital- and community-associated.
- Enterococci are able to spread in the hospital usually via the hands of health care workers and the environment.
- Infection control measures are critical to prevent acquisition of these microorganisms.
- Infective endocarditis and bacteremia caused by *S. gallolyticus* is highly associated with gastrointestinal malignancies.

CLINICAL PRESENTATIONS

- Enterococci are capable of causing bloodstream infections, both in community- and hospital-associated clinical settings.
- Infective endocarditis is one of the most serious and life-threatening infections caused by enterococci.
- Enterococci are one of the leading causes of nosocomial urinary tract infections.

- Enterococci have been described in soft tissue infections, intra-abdominal infections and meningitis.
- *S. gallolyticus* group of organisms have been associated with infective endocarditis.
- *Leuconostoc* causes opportunistic infections mainly in immunocompromised patients, although cases in immunocompetent patients have been reported.

THERAPY AND ANTIMICROBIAL RESISTANCE

- Whereas most *E. faecalis* isolates are susceptible to ampicillin and vancomycin, *E. faecium* often exhibit high minimal inhibitory concentrations of ampicillin, and most clinical isolates in the United States are vancomycin-resistant.
- Bactericidal therapy for enterococci often requires the use of a cell wall agent plus an aminoglycoside or ceftriaxone.
- Therapy of choice for severe infections caused by enterococci is the combination of ampicillin plus aminoglycoside (gentamicin and streptomycin).
- Ampicillin plus ceftriaxone is an alternative therapy for *E. faecalis* endocarditis.
- Therapy of severe infections caused by *E. faecium* is challenging, and no reliable therapy is currently available.
- Linezolid and quinupristin-dalfopristin are two U.S. Food and Drug Administration–approved drugs for multidrug resistant *E. faecium,* but these compounds have important limitations because of the lack of bactericidal effect, toxicity, side effects, and emergence of resistance.
- Daptomycin is a lipopeptide antibiotic with in vitro bactericidal activity against enterococci, but development of resistance during therapy seems to be a limitation for the use of this antibiotic.
- Daptomycin combinations (with β-lactams, aminoglycosides, and/or tigecycline) may offer some promise in the future for the treatment of multidrug-resistant enterococcal infections.
- The therapy of choice for endocarditis caused by *S. gallolyticus* group of organisms is a β-lactam in combination with an aminoglycoside for at least part of the therapy.
- Ampicillin or penicillin is the drug of choice for the treatment of *Leuconostoc* infections.

134 *Streptococcus agalactiae* (Group B Streptococcus)

Morven S. Edwards and Carol J. Baker

DEFINITION

- Group B streptococci (GBS) are gram-positive bacteria that cause invasive hematogenous infection in at-risk individuals.

EPIDEMIOLOGY

- GBS asymptomatically colonize the lower gastrointestinal or genital tract in approximately one fourth to one third of adult men and women.
- Distribution is worldwide, but rates vary geographically.
- Invasive infection risk is enhanced in neonates and infants younger than 3 months; pregnant women and adults with diabetes mellitus; and persons with liver or kidney disease, cancer, heart or vascular disease, or neurologic impairment.

MICROBIOLOGY

- β-Hemolytic streptococci exhibit a narrow zone of hemolysis on blood agar.
- GBS have a polysaccharide capsule with pilus-like structures that enhance adherence and invasion.
- GBS grow readily in blood culture media and specimens from cerebrospinal fluid and other sites of infection.

DIAGNOSIS

- In adults, onset is acute, with chills and fever, or acute-on-chronic, with indolent symptoms, especially in association with skin and soft tissue manifestations.
- In infants younger than 3 months, bacteremia without a focus; meningitis; or, less often, other focal infections, such as pneumonia or soft tissue infection, occur.
- Growth of GBS from blood or another normally sterile site is diagnostic.

TREATMENT

- Penicillin is the drug of choice; isolates are uniformly susceptible to β-lactams and meropenem. Isolates are generally susceptible to vancomycin; there have been only a few case reports of resistance.
- The duration of treatment ranges from 10 days for uncomplicated bacteremia to a 4-week minimum treatment course for endocarditis.

PREVENTION

- Intrapartum antibiotic prophylaxis given to colonized parturients during labor prevents early-onset infections in neonates, thus reducing the overall rate of neonatal sepsis (see Table 134-1).
- A glycoconjugate vaccine is in clinical trials and offers the potential for prevention of infections in pregnant women and young infants, as well as invasive infections in nonpregnant adults.

TABLE 134-1 Indications and Nonindications for Intrapartum Antibiotic Prophylaxis to Prevent Early-Onset GBS Disease

INTRAPARTUM GBS PROPHYLAXIS INDICATED	INTRAPARTUM GBS PROPHYLAXIS NOT INDICATED
Previous infant with invasive GBS disease	Colonization with GBS during a previous pregnancy (unless an indication for GBS prophylaxis is present for current pregnancy)
GBS bacteriuria during any trimester of the current pregnancy*	GBS bacteriuria during previous pregnancy (unless an indication for GBS prophylaxis is present for current pregnancy)
Positive GBS vaginal-rectal screening culture in late gestation† during current pregnancy*	Negative vaginal and rectal GBS screening culture in late gestation† during the current pregnancy, regardless of intrapartum risk factors
Unknown GBS status at the onset of labor (culture not done, incomplete, or results unknown) and any of the following: • Delivery at <37 wk gestation • Amniotic membrane rupture ≥18 hr • Intrapartum temperature ≥100.4° F (≥38.0° C)‡ • Intrapartum NAAT§ positive for GBS	Cesarean delivery performed before onset of labor on a woman with intact amniotic membranes, regardless of GBS colonization status or gestational age

GBS, group B streptococci/streptococcal; NAAT, nucleic acid amplification test.

*Intrapartum antibiotic prophylaxis is not indicated in this circumstance if a cesarean delivery is performed before onset of labor on a woman with intact amniotic membranes.

†Optimal timing for prenatal GBS screening is at 35-37 weeks' gestation.

‡If amnionitis is suspected, broad-spectrum antibiotic therapy that includes an agent known to be active against GBS should replace GBS prophylaxis.

§NAAT for GBS is optional and might not be available in all settings. If intrapartum NAAT is negative for GBS but any other intrapartum risk factor (delivery at <37 weeks' gestation, amniotic rupture at ≥18 hours, or temperature ≥100.4° F [≥38.0° C]) is present, then intrapartum antibiotic prophylaxis is indicated.

From Verani JR, McGee L, Schrag SJ; Division of Bacterial Diseases, National Center for Immunization and Respiratory Diseases, Centers for Disease Control and Prevention. Prevention of perinatal group B streptococcal disease—revised guidelines from CDC, 2010. *MMWR Recomm Rep.* 2010;59(RR-10):1-32.

135 Viridans Streptococci, Nutritionally Variant Streptococci, Groups C and G Streptococci, and Other Related Organisms

Scott W. Sinner and Allan R. Tunkel

DEFINITION

- Discussed in this chapter are the major human viridans streptococci, groups C and G streptococci, *Streptococcus iniae* and *Streptococcus suis,* and the genera *Gemella, Abiotrophia, Granulicatella, Rothia,* and *Pediococcus.*

EPIDEMIOLOGY

- Many of these streptococci exist as normal microbiota on various mucosal surfaces of humans, particularly the oral cavity.
- Although generally considered to be bacteria of low virulence, they can cause significant infections, often as a result of weak host defenses, high inocula at the sites of colonization, and vulnerable human tissues that may be prone to infection after transient bacteremia.
- Some species of groups C and G streptococci, along with *S. iniae,* are more often commensals or pathogens of animals but can cause human infection after significant contact of humans with the animals in question.

MICROBIOLOGY

- The viridans streptococci are typically facultatively anaerobic, nonmotile, non–spore-forming gram-positive cocci that are both catalase and coagulase negative and either α- or γ-hemolytic on blood agar.
- The nutritionally variant genera *Abiotrophia* and *Granulicatella* need either supplemental pyridoxal or cysteine for growth on agar.
- Groups C and G streptococci do not always reliably fit into predictable speciation schemes and form relatively large colonies that are often β-hemolytic.

DIAGNOSIS

- Clinical diagnosis of infections caused by these organisms depends on the site of infection and the status of the host.
- Some of the most common or significant syndromes include pharyngitis, soft tissue infections, primary bacteremia in neutropenic hosts, endocarditis, and meningitis.
- Microbiologic diagnosis begins with typical bacterial culture methods in virtually all cases, but these may be supplemented by latex agglutination studies, automated speciation and susceptibility techniques, cultures on nutrient-enriched agar, or molecular techniques such as polymerase chain reaction assay.

THERAPY

- First-line therapy for most infections caused by these organisms is penicillin, if the isolate is susceptible.
- Cephalosporins and vancomycin are the most studied second-line therapies, for use in cases of drug resistance or allergy or intolerance.
- Use and overuse of β-lactams, macrolides, and fluoroquinolones in recent decades has led to a slow but clear increase in drug resistance.

- The route and duration of therapy depend largely on the site of infection and the status of the host.

PREVENTION

- Because most of these organisms are considered part of the normal microbiota of humans, prevention of infection is largely accomplished by maintaining a robust immune system, as well as maintaining healthy mucosal surfaces (e.g., practicing good dental hygiene).
- For the occasional organism that can be acquired from animals, avoidance of specific animal contact is the best prevention.
- Certain groups of patients may enjoy the benefits of the following additional specific preventive strategies: antimicrobial prophylaxis for certain dental procedures in patients at the highest risk for endocarditis, antimicrobial prophylaxis for high-risk neutropenic patients receiving cytotoxic chemotherapy for malignancy, and appropriate surgical prophylaxis at the time of implantation of various foreign bodies.

136 *Streptococcus anginosus* Group

Cathy A. Petti and Charles W. Stratton IV

DEFINITION

- The *Streptococcus anginosus (milleri)* group comprises three distinct species: *S. anginosus*, *S. constellatus*, and *S. intermedius*.

EPIDEMIOLOGY

- The *Streptococcus anginosus* group comprises normal microbiota of the gastrointestinal tract and oropharynx, and when pathogenic, is often associated with abscess formation and endocarditis.

MICROBIOLOGY

- These microorganisms are microaerophilic, catalase-negative, gram-positive cocci and are easily identified by conventional methods. They are generally susceptible to β-lactam antibiotics.

DIAGNOSIS

- Depending on the clinical presentation, infections are usually diagnosed by culturing a specimen from the source of infection.

THERAPY

- β-Lactam antibiotics are generally used; abscesses may require incision and drainage as well as antimicrobial therapy with broader coverage, such as that provided by ampicillin/sulbactam or piperacillin/tazobactam.

PREVENTION

- Not applicable.

137 Corynebacterium diphtheriae (Diphtheria)

Rob Roy MacGregor

DEFINITION

- *Corynebacterium diphtheriae,* a gram-positive bacillus, classically produces epidemic upper respiratory tract infections with high mortality rates in unimmunized subjects.

EPIDEMIOLOGY

- Humans are the only known reservoir, and the disease spreads via air and direct contact. Asymptomatic carriage is important in transmission. Diphtheria is now rare in the West and endemic in the Third World, especially Southeast Asia. Fewer than 5000 annual cases have been reported worldwide since 2000.

MICROBIOLOGY

- The bacillus is nonsporulating, unencapsulated, and nonmotile. It produces brown colonies and halos on tellurite medium and requires lysogenic β-phage to produce toxin responsible for the disease. Four biovars and 86 ribotypes have been identified for tracking. Nontoxigenic strains occasionally cause disease, as do toxin-producing *Corynebacterium ulcerans* strains.

CLINICAL MANIFESTATIONS

- Subacute faucial infection causes low-grade fever, hoarseness, pain, and a necrotic pseudo-membrane that can extend to larynx and cause stridor and fatal obstruction. Circulating toxin causes potentially fatal carditis and motor neuropathy. Cutaneous infection causes indolent ulcers.

DIAGNOSIS

- Diagnosis is presumptive, based on tonsillitis/pharyngitis with necrotic membrane, hoarseness, palatal paralysis, low-grade fever, and recent travel to an endemic area. Confirmation is made by observing brown colonies on tellurite medium, a distinctive Gram stain, and biochemical tests. Polymerase chain reaction shows a toxin gene, which is the key to alert the laboratory for culture.

THERAPY

- Diphtheria antitoxin (DAT), produced in horses and obtained from the Centers for Disease Control and Prevention, must be given intravenously without waiting for diagnosis confirmation. The dose depends on the duration and extent of disease. Test patients first for horse protein hypersensitivity. Consider tracheostomy to protect airway. Cardiographic monitoring is wise because of toxin cardiotoxicity. Antibiotics are given orally or parenterally for 14 days to stop toxin production and eradicate throat carriage. Adults can be given procaine penicillin 600,000 units IM every 12 hours until oral medication is tolerated, followed by penicillin V 250 mg or erythromycin 500 mg every 6 hours.

PREVENTION

- Toxoid immunization consists of TDaP 5 times up to 7 years of age. Td boosters should be given at 10-year intervals. Penicillin or erythromycin should be given for 14 days to carriers to prevent clinical infection or spread. Close contacts of cases should be cultured, given antimicrobial prophylaxis, and, if not fully immunized, vaccinated.

138 Other Coryneform Bacteria and Rhodococci

Rose Kim and Annette C. Reboli

DEFINITION
- Coryneform bacteria encompass several genera, of which *Corynebacterium* is the most frequently encountered in clinical infections.
- Coryneform bacteria are characterized as irregularly shaped, non–spore-forming, aerobic, gram-positive rods.

EPIDEMIOLOGY
- Coryneform bacteria are ubiquitous in the environment (soil and water), commensal colonizers of skin and mucous membranes in humans, and commensals in animals.
- Infections caused by coryneform bacteria are broadly categorized as community acquired or nosocomial; sporadic cases of zoonoses have been reported.
- *Rhodococcus equi* usually occurs in individuals with defective cell-mediated immunity, particularly with human immunodeficiency virus infection, with or without a history of animal exposure.

MICROBIOLOGY
- Coryneform bacteria readily grow on standard culture media. For lipophilic strains, growth is enhanced with addition of Tween 80.
- Species identification and antimicrobial testing of coryneform bacteria is recommended when specimens are collected from normally sterile sites, there is presence of high colony counts with a strong leukocyte reaction, or there is recovery of high colony counts of *Corynebacterium urealyticum* from urine culture.
- Molecular tests, such as 16s ribosomal RNA sequencing, and matrix-assisted laser desorption/ionization time-of-flight mass spectrometry are used for species identification of coryneform bacteria, including *Rhodococcus, Gordonia,* and *Tsukamurella.*

DIAGNOSIS
- Coryneform bacteria are considered clinically significant when patients present with symptoms consistent with infection, along with recovery of bacteria as outlined above ("Microbiology").

THERAPY
- Coryneform bacteria are uniformly susceptible to glycopeptides, such as vancomycin and teicoplanin, and most strains are susceptible to daptomycin and linezolid.
- *Rhodococcus equi* is usually susceptible to vancomycin, teicoplanin, erythromycin, fluoroquinolones, rifampin, carbapenems, aminoglycosides, and linezolid.

PREVENTION
- Prevention of infections caused by coryneform bacteria includes proper skin antisepsis before invasive procedures and caution when handling animals.

139 *Listeria monocytogenes*
Bennett Lorber

DIAGNOSIS
- Clinical settings in which listeriosis should get strong consideration include immunosuppression and pregnancy (see Table 139-1).
- Culture of blood, cerebrospinal fluid, or other normally sterile body fluid or, in the case of gastroenteritis, from stool.
- Serology not useful for invasive disease.

MICROBIOLOGY
- Short, gram-positive rod; grows readily on blood agar; tumbling motility.
- May be mistaken for diphtheroid contaminant.
- Will grow in refrigerated food.

EPIDEMIOLOGY
- Zoonosis, particularly herd animals.
- Human transmission from contaminated food or from pregnant woman to fetus or newborn.
- Highest food risks from delicatessen-style meats and unpasteurized cheeses.
- Most cases occur in neonates, pregnant women, persons 60 years or older, and those with impaired cell-mediated immunity resulting from underlying condition (hematologic malignancy, organ or bone marrow transplantation, acquired immunodeficiency syndrome) or therapy (corticosteroids, antitumor necrosis factor agents). Notify laboratory for special stool cultures if outbreak of febrile gastroenteritis.

CLINICAL SETTINGS
- Neonatal sepsis or meningitis.
- Meningitis or focal central nervous system (CNS) lesions in immunosuppressed patients or those older than 50 years.
- Rhombencephalitis occurs in previously healthy patients who develop fever, cranial nerve palsies, cerebellar signs and hemiparesis, hemisensory deficits, or both.
- Fever in pregnancy, especially third trimester.
- Outbreak of foodborne febrile gastroenteritis.

TREATMENT
- Ampicillin (2 g IV every 4 hours). Add gentamicin (5 mg/kg per day) for CNS infection or endocarditis.
- Trimethoprim-sulfamethoxazole (5/25 mg/kg IV every 8 hours) for penicillin allergic.
  - Add one of the above to vancomycin and ceftriaxone regimen for suspected bacterial meningitis in persons older than 50 years because vancomycin and ceftriaxone are inadequate for listerial meningitis.

TABLE 139-1 Clinical Settings in Which Listeriosis Should Be Considered Strongly in the Differential Diagnosis

- Neonatal sepsis or meningitis
- Meningitis or parenchymal brain infection in:
  - Patients with hematologic malignancies, AIDS, organ transplantation, corticosteroid immunosuppression, and those receiving anti-TNF agents
  - Patients with a subacute presentation of meningitis
  - Adults older than 50 years
- Simultaneous infection of the meninges and brain parenchyma
- Subcortical brain abscess
- Spinal symptoms in the setting of acute bacterial meningitis of uncertain etiology
- Fever during pregnancy, particularly in the third trimester
- Blood, CSF, or other normally sterile specimen reported to have "diphtheroids" on Gram stain or culture
- Foodborne outbreak of febrile gastroenteritis when routine cultures fail to identify a pathogen

AIDS, acquired immunodeficiency syndrome; CSF, cerebrospinal fluid; TNF, tumor necrosis factor.

PREVENTION

- Isolation not necessary.
- Food safety recommendations for those at risk (see Table 139-2).
- *Pneumocystis* prophylaxis with trimethoprim-sulfamethoxazole prevents listeriosis.

TABLE 139-2 Dietary Recommendations for Preventing Foodborne Listeriosis

General Recommendations
Washing and Handling Food

Rinse raw produce thoroughly under running tap water before eating, cutting, or cooking. Even if the produce will be peeled, it should still be washed first.
Scrub firm produce, such as melons and cucumbers, with a clean produce brush.
Dry the produce with a clean cloth or paper towel.

Keep Your Kitchen Cleaner and Safer

Wash hands, knives, countertops, and cutting boards after handling and preparing uncooked foods.
Be aware that *Listeria monocytogenes* can grow in foods in the refrigerator. The refrigerator should be 40° F or lower and the freezer 0° F or lower.
Clean up all spills in your refrigerator right away, especially juices from hot dog and lunch meat packages, raw meat, and raw poultry.

Cook Meat and Poultry Thoroughly

Thoroughly cook raw food from animal sources, such as beef, pork, or poultry to a safe internal temperature.
Use precooked or ready-to-eat food as soon as you can. Do not store the product in the refrigerator beyond the use-by date.
Use leftovers within 3 to 4 days.

Choose Safer Foods

Do not drink *raw (unpasteurized) milk,* and do not eat foods that have unpasteurized milk in them.

Recommendations for Persons at Higher Risk*
Meats

Do not eat hot dogs, luncheon meats, cold cuts, other delicatessen meats (e.g., bologna), or fermented or dry sausages, unless they are heated to an internal temperature of 165° F or until steaming hot just before serving.
Avoid getting fluid from hot dog and lunch meat packages on other foods, utensils, and food preparation surfaces, and wash hands after handling hot dogs, luncheon meats, and delicatessen meats.
Do not eat refrigerated pâté or meat spreads from a delicatessen or meat counter or from the refrigerated section of a store. Foods that do not need refrigeration, such as canned or shelf-stable pâté and meat spreads, are safe to eat. Refrigerate after opening.

Cheeses

Do not eat soft cheese such as feta, queso blanco, queso fresco, brie, Camembert, blue-veined, or panela (queso panela) unless it is labeled as "MADE WITH PASTEURIZED MILK."

Seafood

Do not eat refrigerated smoked seafood, unless it is contained in a cooked dish, such as a casserole, or unless it is a canned or shelf-stable product.
Canned and shelf stable tuna, salmon, and other fish products are safe to eat.

Melons

Wash hands with warm water and soap for at least 20 seconds before and after handling any whole melon.
Scrub the surface of melons with a clean produce brush under running water and dry them with a clean cloth or paper towel before cutting. Be sure that your scrub brush is sanitized after each use.
Promptly consume cut melon or refrigerate promptly. Keep your cut melon refrigerated for no more than 7 days.
Discard cut melons left at room temperature for more than 4 hours.

*Recommendations for persons at higher risk, such as pregnant women, persons with weakened immune systems, and older adults, in addition to the recommendations listed under General Recommendations.

140 *Bacillus anthracis* (Anthrax)

Gregory J. Martin and Arthur M. Friedlander*

EPIDEMIOLOGY AND MICROBIOLOGY

- Sporadic worldwide, anthrax is most common in Africa, the Middle East, and Latin America.
- Naturally acquired human cases are usually associated with animal products.
- Spore-forming gram-positive bacillus grows readily in the laboratory.
- Spores, when protected from ultraviolet light, remain viable for decades or longer.
- Pathogenicity is associated with edema and lethal toxins and a capsule.

CLINICAL MANIFESTATIONS AND DIAGNOSIS

- *Cutaneous anthrax:* 95% of naturally acquired cases are this form. After skin inoculation, a pruritic papule forms in 2 to 5 days. Vesicles rupture, leading to formation of a black eschar at the base of a shallow ulcer. An injectional form has been newly described in injection heroin users and associated with a more aggressive course. Surgical débridement may be required. Gram stain of vesicle fluid, scraping of base of ulcer, or punch biopsy may show gram-positive bacilli and a paucity of polymorphonuclear neutrophils. Culture of material is frequently positive. Direct fluorescent antibody (DFA) test and polymerase chain reaction (PCR) assay also may be used.
- *Inhalational anthrax:* results from handling of animal products, such as wool, hides, or bones or after intentional spore release in bioterrorism. This form has the most dangerous presentation, with near 100% mortality without early antibiotics. It is primarily a mediastinal (not an airspace) process. Blood and pleural fluid cultures are positive. Pleural fluid Gram stain may be positive. DFA test or PCR assay may give most rapid results.
- *Gastrointestinal anthrax:* responsible for approximately 1% of human cases and occurs typically 1 to 5 days after ingestion of contaminated meat. Blood, stool, and ascites should all be obtained for culture, DFA testing, and PCR assay. Gram staining of ascitic fluid may reveal gram-positive bacilli.
- *Anthrax meningitis:* secondary seeding of the meninges occurs during bacteremia in fulminant disease. Death occurs within 24 hours in 75% of cases. Cerebrospinal fluid reveals gram-positive bacilli, and cultures are positive. DFA test and PCR assay may provide the most rapid diagnosis.

THERAPY

- Rapid initiation of antibiotics for all stages is crucial (see Table 140-1).
- For cutaneous anthrax, ciprofloxacin or doxycycline alone is used.
- Inhalational, gastrointestinal, and injectional anthrax and anthrax meningitis should be treated with two bactericidal agents, preferably a quinolone such as ciprofloxacin and a β-lactam such as meropenem, combined with a protein synthesis inhibitor such as linezolid,

---

*The opinions and assertions herein are those of the authors and should not be construed as official or representing the views of the Office of Medical Services of the Department of State, the Department of Defense, or the U.S. government.

TABLE 140-1 Intravenous Triple Therapy[a] for Severe Anthrax[b] with Possible or Confirmed Meningitis

1. A Bactericidal Agent (Fluoroquinolone)	b. Alternatives for Penicillin-Susceptible Strains
Ciprofloxacin 400 mg q8h	
or	Penicillin G 4 million units q4h
Levofloxacin 750 mg q24h	*or*
or	Ampicillin 3 g q6h
Moxifloxacin 400 mg q24h	*plus*
plus	**3. A Protein Synthesis Inhibitor**
2. A Bactericidal Agent (β-Lactam)	**Linezolid[d] 600 mg q12h**
a. For All Strains, Regardless of Penicillin Susceptibility or if Susceptibility Is Unknown	*or*
	Clindamycin 900 mg q8h
Meropenem 2 g q8h	*or*
or	Rifampin[e] 600 mg q12h
Imipenem[c] 1 g q6h	*or*
or	Chloramphenicol[f] 1 g q6-8h
Doripenem 500 mg q8h	**Duration of Therapy**
or	For 2-3 weeks or longer, until clinically stable. Will require prophylaxis to complete an antibiotic course of up to 60 days from onset of illness.

[a]Drug names in **boldface** are preferred agents. Alternative selections are listed in order of preference for therapy for patients who cannot tolerate first-line therapy or if first-line therapy is unavailable.
[b]Severe anthrax includes meningitis; inhalational, injectional, and gastrointestinal; and cutaneous with systemic involvement, extensive edema, or lesions of the head or neck.
[c]Increased risk for seizures associated with imipenem/cilastatin therapy.
[d]Linezolid may exacerbate thrombocytopenia; use for >14 days carries additional hematopoietic toxicity.
[e]Rifampin is not a protein synthesis inhibitor but may be used based on in vitro synergy.
[f]Should only be used if other options are not available, owing to toxicity concerns.
Data from Hendricks KA, Wright ME, Shadomy SV, et al; Workgroup on Anthrax Clinical Guidelines. Centers for Disease Control and Prevention expert panel meetings on prevention and treatment of anthrax in adults. *Emerg Infect Dis.* 2014;20. doi: 10.3201/eid2002.130687.

clindamycin, rifampin, or chloramphenicol. Consider central nervous system penetration of antibiotics for treatment of potential meningitis.
- Immunotherapeutics such as anthrax immune globulin and raxibacumab should be considered in conjunction with antibiotics in severe cases and in some spore exposures.

PREVENTION
- Current vaccines are cell-free supernatants of protective antigen adsorbed to aluminum hydroxide.
- Postexposure vaccination must be done under Centers for Disease Control and Prevention Investigational New Drug protocol (in the United States) at 0, 2, and 4 weeks and administered subcutaneously.

ANTHRAX AS AN AGENT OF BIOTERRORISM
- Anthrax is generally considered the most likely agent for bioterrorism via an aerosol route.
- Gram quantities of stable spores are easy to transport and could cause thousands of cases.
- Early identification of the first cases is difficult owing to the presentation with nonspecific flulike symptoms.
- Nasal swabs are used to identify exposure areas, *not* to determine individual exposures.
- Exposed patients should be given antibiotic prophylaxis with 60 days of ciprofloxacin or doxycycline and anthrax immunization at 0, 2, and 4 weeks.
- Exposed patients should be decontaminated with soap and water. Surfaces may be remediated with a number of different chloride-containing compounds, including household bleach.
- Anthrax is *not* transmissible from patients after they have been decontaminated, and isolation is *not* required.

141 Bacillus Species and Related Genera Other Than *Bacillus anthracis*

Thomas Fekete

DEFINITION
- Gram-positive spore-forming bacilli

EPIDEMIOLOGY
- Worldwide distribution
- Commonly found in soil and water
- Major pathogens of insects
- Infrequent cause of infection in mammals (including humans)
- Normal flora in children and adults

MICROBIOLOGY
- Aerobic or facultatively anaerobic
- Easily cultivated with standard culture technique
- Numerous genera (>56) and species (>545)
- Frequently toxin producing, and toxin contributes to many clinical manifestations of disease
- Susceptibility tests not standardized but can be helpful

DIAGNOSIS
- Culture on routine media at standard temperatures (25° to 37° C)
- Can be challenging to distinguish true pathogen from contaminant
- Characteristic Gram stain properties but can be confused with *Clostridium*
- For food poisoning, can be isolated from food products
- Should be suspected when sterilization of equipment is inadequate
- Infection may follow traumatic injury

THERAPY
- Food poisoning is normally self-limited and requires only supportive treatment
- Deep infection requires antibiotics
- Vancomycin and fluoroquinolones usually active
- May require removal of foreign body such as vascular catheter

PREVENTION
- Optimal management and storage of food
- Careful attention to sterilization techniques
- Early removal of unneeded devices

142 *Erysipelothrix rhusiopathiae*
Annette C. Reboli

DEFINITION
- *Erysipelothrix rhusiopathiae* is a pleomorphic, nonsporulating gram-positive bacillus.
- It causes three major forms of disease in humans: erysipeloid (localized cutaneous infection), diffuse cutaneous infection, and systemic infection (bacteremia with or without endocarditis).

EPIDEMIOLOGY
- A zoonosis, it is widespread in nature and infects wild and domestic animals, including swine, poultry, sheep, and fish.
- Infection in humans is usually due to occupational exposure.
- Portal of entry is usually through abrasions or puncture wounds of the skin, but infection may also follow ingestion of undercooked pork or seafood.

MICROBIOLOGY
- It is an aerobe or facultative anaerobe.
- Most strains produce hydrogen sulfide, a diagnostically important reaction.
- It is sometimes confused with other gram-positive bacilli.
- Vitek 2 and the API Coryne system are reliable for identification.

DIAGNOSIS
- A provisional diagnosis can often be made based on a history of appropriate epidemiologic exposure and, in the case of erysipeloid, characteristic physical findings.
- Definitive diagnosis requires isolation of the organism from blood, other sterile body fluid, or a biopsy specimen.
- Standard methods for culturing blood or biopsy tissue suffice.
- The polymerase chain reaction assay has been used for rapid diagnosis in swine and has been applied successfully to human and environmental samples.

THERAPY
- *E. rhusiopathiae* is highly susceptible to penicillins, cephalosporins, clindamycin, imipenem, linezolid, daptomycin, and ciprofloxacin.
- Most strains are resistant to vancomycin, sulfa drugs, and aminoglycosides.
- Erysipeloid may resolve in the absence of therapy; however, appropriate therapy shortens the illness and reduces the risk for relapse.
- Penicillin is the drug of choice for all forms of infection. When β-lactams are contraindicated, use of fluoroquinolones, daptomycin, linezolid, or clindamycin may be considered.

PREVENTION
- Hand hygiene, use of protective attire such as gloves, and disinfection of contaminated surfaces are essential.
- Commercial vaccines are available for veterinary use.

143 Whipple's Disease

Thomas Marth and Thomas Schneider

DEFINITION

- Whipple's disease (WD) is a rare systemic infectious disorder caused by the actinomycete *Tropheryma whipplei*.

EPIDEMIOLOGY

- Classic WD is rare and is found in middle-aged individuals, approximately three times more often in men than in women.
- *T. whipplei* is found frequently in the stools of children with acute diarrhea.
- *T. whipplei* can cause culture-negative endocarditis.

MICROBIOLOGY AND PATHOGENESIS

- *T. whipplei* is a gram-positive bacterium with high guanine and cytosine content.
- *T. whipplei* is resistant to glutaraldehyde.
- The hallmark of WD is the invasion of the intestinal mucosa with macrophages incompetent to degrade *T. whipplei*.
- An immunologic defect in the pathogenesis of WD is evident and includes macrophages, T cells, and an impaired humoral immune response.

CLINICAL FEATURES AND DIAGNOSIS

- WD occurs as an acute transient disease (presenting, e.g., with fever and diarrhea in children).
- WD occurs in a localized form (e.g., endocarditis or central nervous system disease).
- WD occurs in various clinical manifestations in association with immunosuppression.
- WD occurs as a classic systemic disease with weight loss, arthralgia, diarrhea, and a possible broad spectrum of clinical signs and symptoms.
- Diagnosis is established usually by duodenal biopsy showing typical periodic acid–Schiff positive cells in the lamina propria.
- Diagnosis should be confirmed by polymerase chain reaction assay or immunohistochemistry, which can be performed alternatively from various organ samples or body fluids.

THERAPY

- IV induction therapy with ceftriaxone for 2 to 4 weeks.
- Followed by long-term therapy with oral trimethoprim-sulfamethoxazole for 1 year.
- Close follow-up of treatment success over several years.
- Complications: relapses, neurologic defects, heart valve destruction, immune reconstitution inflammatory syndrome.

PREVENTION

- Ubiquitous bacterial agent, prevention not yet possible.

144 Neisseria meningitidis

David S. Stephens and Michael A. Apicella

DEFINITION

- *Neisseria meningitidis*, the cause of epidemic cerebrospinal fever (first described in 1805), is an obligate human bacterial pathogen most often presenting as acute bacterial meningitis, mild bacteremia to devastating septicemia, and pneumonia.

MICROBIOLOGY

- *N. meningitidis* is a gram-negative diplococcus (0.6×0.8 μm) and member of the bacterial family Neisseriaceae that includes the human pathogen *Neisseria gonorrhoeae*.

BIOLOGY AND PATHOGENESIS

- Meningococcal biology and pathogenesis are defined by (1) *N. meningitidis* colonization and virulence factors, (2) transmission and acquisition among humans, and (3) human susceptibility to invasive meningococcal disease. These factors influence disease incidence and severity and prevention strategies.

EPIDEMIOLOGY

- Disease occurs worldwide, but incidence is variable. Clonal complexes ST-5 and ST-7 (capsular serogroup A); ST-41/44, ST-32, ST-18, ST-269, ST-8, and ST-35 (serogroup B); ST-11 (serogroups C or W-135); ST-23 and ST-167 (serogroup Y); and ST-181 (serogroup X) meningococci currently cause almost all invasive meningococcal disease (see Fig. 144-1).

CLINICAL MANIFESTATIONS AND PATHOPHYSIOLOGY

- Common presentations of invasive meningococcal disease are meningococcemia and acute meningitis. Less common presentations are primary pneumonia (up to 10%, especially with serogroup Y), septic arthritis (2%), purulent pericarditis, chronic meningococcemia, conjunctivitis, epiglottitis, sinusitis, otitis, urethritis, and proctitis.
- *Meningococcemia:* In 20% to 30% of cases, septicemia with shock is the dominant clinical finding with sudden onset of fever, generalized malaise, weakness, cold extremities and skin pallor, leukocytosis or leukopenia, rash, headache and/or drowsiness, and hypotension.
- *Meningitis:* Meningitis is the most common presentation of invasive meningococcal disease and occurs in 40% to 65% of cases, reflecting the meningeal tropism of *N. meningitidis*. Findings include sudden-onset headache, fever, vomiting, myalgias, photophobia, irritability, decreased ability to concentrate, agitation, drowsiness and meningeal signs (neck stiffness, Kernig's or Brudzinski's sign), and cloudy cerebrospinal fluid. Rash may or may not be present.
- *Rash:* Skin lesions are present in 28% to 77% of patients with invasive meningococcal disease on admission but may not always be petechial or purpuric.
- Complement system deficiencies increase risk for meningococcal disease, in particular C5-C9 terminal pathway deficiencies, properdin deficiency, and C3 deficiency.
- Chronic meningococcemia manifests as intermittent fever (often low grade), migratory arthralgias or arthritis, and a nonspecific, often maculopapular rash.

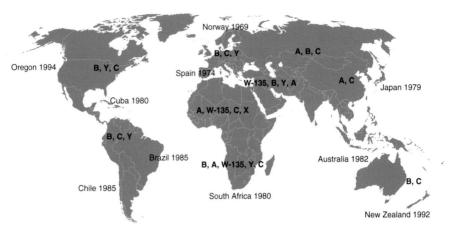

FIGURE 144-1 Epidemiology of meningococcal disease by serogroup. Group B outbreaks are noted by country and year of onset. Clonal complexes ST-5 and ST-7 (serogroup A); ST-41/44, ST-32, ST-18, ST-269, ST-8, and ST-35 (serogroup B); ST-11 (serogroups C or W-135); ST-23 and ST-167 (serogroup Y); and ST-181 (serogroup X) meningococci currently cause almost all invasive meningococcal disease. (Modified from Stephens DS, Greenwood B, Brandtzaeg P. Epidemic meningitis, meningococcaemia, and *Neisseria meningitidis*. Lancet. 2007;369:2196-2210.)

TABLE 144-1 Antibiotic Treatment of Meningococcal Meningitis and Meningococcemia

Ceftriaxone*: in children age >3 mo: 50 mg/kg IV q12h; adults: 1-2 g IV q12h
  or
Cefotaxime 50-75 mg/kg q6-8h, maximum dose 12 g/day
  or
Penicillin G, 50,000 U/kg IV q4h, up to 4 million U q4h
  or
Meropenem, 2 g IV q8h, 6 g/day
If patient is allergic to penicillin and cephalosporins, use chloramphenicol, 25 mg/kg IV q6h up to 1 g q6h.

*Because of concerns in neonates from calcium/ceftriaxone precipitates and displacement of bilirubin from albumin by ceftriaxone, neonates younger than 3 months of age should be started on cefotaxime, 50 mg/kg every 6 to 8 hours.
  Modified from Shin SH, Kwang Kim SK. Treatment of bacterial meningitis: an update. *Exp Opin Pharmacother.* 2012;13:2189-2206.

COMPLICATIONS

• Immune complex–mediated complications may follow meningococcal disease.
• Long-term sequelae occur in 11% to 19% of cases.
• Family and community impact is significant.

DIAGNOSIS

• The definitive diagnosis of invasive meningococcal disease is based on bacteriologic isolation or antigen or DNA identification (by polymerase chain reaction assay) of *N. meningitidis* in a usually sterile body fluid, such as blood, cerebrospinal fluid, synovial fluid, pleural fluid, urine, or pericardial fluid.

TREATMENT

• Invasive meningococcal disease is a medical emergency, and early antibiotic treatment should be the primary goal (see Table 144-1).
• Adjuvant therapy and supportive care should be provided.

TABLE 144-2 Antibiotic Chemoprophylaxis for Household or Intimate Contacts*

ANTIBIOTIC	DOSAGE	COMMENT
Rifampin	Adults: 600 mg q12h for 2 days Children <1 mo: 5 mg/kg q12h for 2 days Children >1 mo: 10 mg/kg q12h (maximum, 600 mg) orally for 2 days	Rifampin can interfere with efficacy of oral contraceptives and some seizure prevention and anticoagulant medications; may stain soft contact lenses. Not recommended for pregnant women.
Ceftriaxone	Children <15 yr: 125 mg, single IM dose Children >15 yr and adults: 250 mg, single IM dose	Ceftriaxone is recommended for prophylaxis in pregnant women.
Ciprofloxacin	Adults: 500 mg, single dose	Not recommended routinely for persons <18 yr, but use in infants and children (20 mg/kg) may be justified after careful assessment of the risks and benefits. Not recommended for pregnant or lactating women. Cases of ciprofloxacin resistance have been reported, and use for prophylaxis should be based on local sensitivity of the meningococcus to the drug.
Azithromycin	10 mg/kg (maximum, 500 mg) single dose	Equivalent to rifampin for eradication of meningococci from nasopharynx, but data are limited.

*Recommended groups for chemoprophylaxis, based on exposure to the index patient in the week before onset of illness:
- Household contacts and persons sharing the same living quarters, particularly young children
- Daycare center, nursery school or child care contacts, frequent playmates of young children
- Close social contacts that were exposed to oral secretions in week before onset, such as by kissing or sharing eating or drinking utensils or toothbrushes
- For airline travel lasting more than 8 hours, passengers who are seated directly next to an infected person should receive prophylaxis.
- Routine prophylaxis is not recommended for health care professionals unless they have had intimate exposure to respiratory secretions of an infected person.
- Because the risk for secondary cases is highest during the first few days after exposure, chemoprophylaxis should be initiated as soon as possible, ideally <24 hours after identification of the index patient.
- If more than 14 days have passed since the last contact with the index patient, chemoprophylaxis is not likely to be of benefit.
- Pharyngeal cultures are not helpful in determining the need for chemoprophylaxis and may unnecessarily delay the use of effective chemoprophylaxis.
- Chemoprophylaxis has also been recommended for patients given penicillin or chloramphenicol for treatment since pharyngeal carriage may not be eliminated with these antibiotics and the patient could remain colonized with a virulent strain.
- Ceftriaxone is recommended for pregnant women.
- May want to avoid ciprofloxacin or azithromycin in individuals at risk of QT-prolongation.

PREVENTION

- Chemoprophylaxis eliminates meningococci from close contacts of confirmed or presumptive cases, protects susceptible individuals, and disrupts the further spread of meningococci. Recommended antibiotics are rifampin, ceftriaxone, ciprofloxacin, and azithromycin (see Table 144-2).
- Meningococcal polysaccharide-conjugate vaccines are licensed for prevention of meningococcal disease (see Table 144-3) and are recommended for adolescents and others at risk for meningococcal disease.

TABLE 144-3   Conjugate Vaccines for *Neisseria meningitidis:* United States, 2015

Menveo (Novartis)	Meningococcal (groups A, C, Y, and W-135) Oligosaccharide Diphtheria CRM197 Conjugate
Menactra (Sanofi Pasteur)	Meningococcal (groups A, C, Y, and W-135) Polysaccharide Diphtheria Toxoid Conjugate Vaccine
MenHibrix (GlaxoSmithKline)	Meningococcal groups C and Y and *Haemophilus b* Tetanus Toxoid Conjugate Vaccine
Bexsero (Novartis)	Meningococcal group B Recombinant Protein Vaccine
Trumenba (Pfizer)	Meningococcal group B Recombinant Protein Vaccine

145 | *Neisseria gonorrhoeae* (Gonorrhea)

Jeanne M. Marrazzo and Michael A. Apicella

DEFINITION

- Gonorrhea is a sexually transmitted infection caused by the organism *Neisseria gonorrhoeae*.

EPIDEMIOLOGY

- Gonorrhea occurs most commonly in adolescents and young adults worldwide.
- Overall, incidence has been declining; however, an exception is among men who have sex with men.
- *N. gonorrhoeae* is the causative agent to consider in evaluation of genital inflammatory syndromes, including cervicitis, urethritis, and pelvic inflammatory disease.
- Most infections, however, involve neither signs nor symptoms; thus, routine screening of young women (≤25 years) or older women with key risk factors is recommended.
- Untreated maternal infection may result in ophthalmia neonatorum, which may be avoided by neonatal prophylaxis.

MICROBIOLOGY

- This gram-negative, intracellular diplococcus is a fastidious microorganism that grows only in vitro in a narrow temperature range (35°C and 38°C) on complex media.
- It has a marked ability to develop resistance to antibiotics; recently there has been the global appearance of strains with increasing resistance to third-generation cephalosporins.
- The gonococcus is naturally competent. This is a factor that has led to the rapid acquisition of antimicrobial resistance.
- *N. gonorrhoeae* is an exclusive human pathogen. It utilizes different pathogenic mechanisms to infect the epithelium of men and women. In men, the asialoglycoprotein receptor present on the urethral epithelia interacts with the terminal galactose of the lipo-oligosaccharide (LOS) to enter human cells. In women, a cooperative interaction occurs between C3b covalently linked to the LOS, gonococcal porin and pilus, and complement receptor 3 (CR3) on the surface of the cervical epithelial cell.

DIAGNOSIS

- Culture or nucleic acid amplification testing are sensitive and specific and can be performed at all potentially infected anatomic sites.

THERAPY

- Options are limited, given widespread resistance to numerous antibiotic classes.
- Parenteral therapy with a third-generation cephalosporin is currently recommended and should be accompanied by treatment with azithromycin or doxycycline for additional coverage (see Table 145-1).
- Sex partners of infected people should be treated presumptively, regardless of diagnostic test results.

TABLE 145-1   Options for the Treatment of Gonorrhea*

Uncomplicated Infection of the Cervix, Urethra, and Rectum

Ceftriaxone, 250 mg IM single dose

Infection of the Pharynx

Ceftriaxone, 250 mg IM single dose

Conjunctivitis (Not Ophthalmia Neonatorum)

Ceftriaxone, 1 g IM single dose

Disseminated Gonococcal Infection

Ceftriaxone, 1 g IM or IV every 24 hr for 24-48 hr[†] after improvement, with switch to oral therapy for completion of 1 wk total antibiotic therapy, including cefixime, 400 mg PO twice daily

Meningitis and Endocarditis

Ceftriaxone, 1-2 g IV every 12 hr for 10-14 days (meningitis) or ≥4 wk (endocarditis)

Ophthalmia Neonatorum

Ceftriaxone, 25-50 mg/kg IV or IM in a single dose, not to exceed 125 mg[‡]

IM, intramuscular; IV, intravenous; PO, orally.

*Treatment of gonorrhea in the adult should always be accompanied by treatment of chlamydial infection, and patients should abstain from sex during treatment. Azithromycin, given as a single oral dose of 1 g, is preferred. Test of cure at 7 days is recommended if the ceftriaxone regimen is not used.

[†]Ceftriaxone administered IM may be reconstituted in 1% lidocaine solution to minimize injection pain. Alternative parenteral regimens include cefotaxime, ceftizoxime, and spectinomycin. See www.cdc.gov/std/treatment for specific regimens.

[‡]Topical antibiotic therapy alone is inadequate for treatment of ophthalmia neonatorum.

Modified from Centers for Disease Control and Prevention. Update to CDC's sexually transmitted diseases treatment guidelines, 2010: oral cephalosporins no longer a recommended treatment for gonococcal infections. *MMWR Morb Mortal Wkly Rep.* 2012;61:590-594; and www.cdc.gov/std/treatment.

- Patients who fail treatment with standard regimens should undergo assessment for reinfection; if reinfection is unlikely, antibiotic resistance should be considered.

PREVENTION

- Because of the asymptomatic nature of most infections, routine screening of young women (≤25 years) and pregnant women is recommended.
- Condoms are very effective in preventing transmission.

146 Moraxella catarrhalis, Kingella, and Other Gram-Negative Cocci

Timothy F. Murphy

DEFINITION

- *Moraxella catarrhalis* is a gram-negative diplococcus that colonizes the upper respiratory tract of children.
- It is a common cause of otitis media in children and exacerbations of chronic obstructive pulmonary disease (COPD) in adults.
- *Kingella kingae* is an increasingly recognized pathogen that causes osteoarticular infections and bacteremia in young children.

EPIDEMIOLOGY

- *M. catarrhalis* is recovered exclusively from humans.
- Nasopharyngeal colonization is common in infancy and childhood and decreases with age.
- *K. kingae* colonizes the oropharynx of children and is more often isolated from those who attend daycare centers. Infections occur sporadically, but occasional clusters are seen.

MICROBIOLOGY

- *M. catarrhalis* is easily overlooked in culture because it is phenotypically identical to *Neisseria* in Gram stain and on culture plates.
- *M. catarrhalis* produces oxidase, catalase, and DNAse, which are used for speciation.

DIAGNOSIS

- An etiologic diagnosis of the most common clinical manifestations of *M. catarrhalis* (otitis media in children and exacerbations of COPD in adults) is not made routinely in clinical practice. Rather, these infections are usually treated empirically, based on a presumptive diagnosis using clinical manifestations.
- A diagnosis of *K. kingae* infections is made by recovering the organism in culture from normally sterile body fluid, including blood and joint fluid aspirate. Polymerase chain reaction–based assays are more sensitive than culture in detecting the organism in joint fluid.

THERAPY

- Most isolates of *M. catarrhalis* produce β-lactamase and are thus resistant to ampicillin. Isolates are susceptible to amoxicillin/clavulanic acid, macrolides, fluoroquinolones, and extended-spectrum cephalosporins.
- Otitis media and exacerbations of COPD are treated with oral antimicrobial agents, with the choice generally guided by expert guidelines.
- *K. kingae* isolates are susceptible to penicillins and cephalosporins.

PREVENTION

- No vaccines are available currently, but research is in progress to develop vaccines to prevent *M. catarrhalis* infections, including otitis media and exacerbations of COPD.

147 Vibrio cholerae

Matthew K. Waldor and Edward T. Ryan

MICROBIOLOGY AND EPIDEMIOLOGY

- *Vibrio cholerae* is a curved motile gram-negative bacillus.
- *V. cholerae* is a noninvasive intestinal pathogen.
- *V. cholerae* O1 and O139 serogroup organisms are the causes of epidemic cholera.
- Non-O1 and non-O139 *V. cholerae* can cause isolated cases of usually mild gastroenteritis.
- Cholera results from secretory diarrhea caused by the actions of cholera toxin (CT) on intestinal epithelial cells.
- CT is an adenosine diphosphate–ribosylating enzyme that leads to chloride, sodium, and water loss from intestinal epithelial cells.
- *V. cholerae* has an aquatic reservoir, particularly in brackish estuarine water.
- The fecal-oral transmission is associated with unsafe water and inadequate sanitation.
- There are an estimated three to five million cholera cases, resulting in approximately 100,000 deaths each year.
- The current cholera global pandemic began in 1961 and represents the seventh in the historical record.
- Cholera is now endemic in more than 50 countries.
- Cholera can lead to explosive epidemics and outbreaks.
- The current pandemic is caused by *V. cholerae* O1 El Tor organisms, with the largest burdens in South Asia, sub-Saharan Africa, and Haiti.

CLINICAL MANIFESTATIONS

- Acute severe watery diarrhea can result in death from dehydration within 6 to 12 hours of onset of clinical symptoms.
- Bowel movements during cholera can become progressively more watery, eventually resembling rice water with a fishy odor.
- Vomiting, ileus, and muscle cramps are common.
- The presence of fever should prompt consideration of additional diagnoses.
- Complications of cholera largely reflect those resulting from hypotension and hypoperfusion and may include acute renal tubular necrosis and stroke, usually in older individuals. Aspiration pneumonia from vomiting may also occur. Death from cholera almost always results from dehydration.

DIAGNOSIS

- Cholera should be considered when an adult or child aged 5 years or older develops severe dehydration or dies of acute watery diarrhea in any area, or when an individual aged 2 years or older develops acute watery diarrhea in an area known to be endemic for cholera.
- Rapid antigen tests are available, including dipstick stool assays.
- Confirmatory microbiologic culturing permits definitive identification and assessment of antimicrobial resistance profiles.

MANAGEMENT

- The cornerstone of management is rapid assessment of the degree of dehydration, followed by prompt fluid restoration (see Table 147-1) as well as vigorous monitoring and matching of ongoing fluid losses.
- Severe dehydration (>10% fluid loss), may require greater than 100 mL/kg of fluid replacement to restore euvolemia, ideally administered within the first 3 to 4 hours of clinical presentation.
- Additional stool losses should be matched at approximately 10 to 20 mL/kg per diarrheal stool or vomiting episode.
- Moderate dehydration (5% to 10% fluid loss) may require 75 to 100 mL/kg of fluid resuscitation within the first 3 to 4 hours of clinical presentation. Individuals with no or mild dehydration may be treated with oral rehydration solution (ORS) alone or liquid ad libitum.
- Intravenous fluids are indicated for severe dehydration and in those unable to ingest adequate ORS. Lactated Ringer's solution supplemented with 5% dextrose (D5LR) (ideally supplemented with additional potassium) is an optimal choice for patients with cholera, although intravenous normal saline or normal saline supplemented with dextrose (and potassium) can also be used.
- Oral rehydration treatment should be encouraged among all individuals able to ingest, regardless of degree of dehydration, and regardless of potential ongoing administration of intravenous fluid.

TABLE 147-1 Composition of Cholera Stools and Therapeutic Fluids for Cholera

		CONCENTRATION (MMOLES/L)					
		Na$^+$	K$^+$	Cl$^-$	HCO$_3^-$	Carbohydrate	Comments
Intravenous fluid	LRS	130	4	109	28	— (278 if D5LR available)	LRS contains potassium and bicarbonate and is preferred over normal saline. Both LRS and NS can be supplemented with dextrose. Dhaka solution more closely approximates losses during cholera, but is not readily available.
	Normal saline	154	0	154	0	—	
	Cholera saline ("Dhaka solution")	133	13	154	48	140	
Oral rehydration therapy	ORS (WHO, 2002)*	75	20	65	10 (citrate)	75 (glucose)	WHO ORS uses glucose as a carbohydrate source. Rice-based ORS formulations have been found in randomized trials to reduce the duration of diarrhea and stool losses in severe cholera. A homemade preparation of ORS could be used in an emergency situation.
	Rice-based ORS (e.g., CeraORS 75)	75	20	65	10 (citrate)	27 g rice syrup solids	
	Homemade ORS: ½ tsp table salt and 6 tsp table sugar in 1 L of safe water	≈75	0	≈75	0	≈75	
Electrolyte losses in stools (composite estimates)	Cholera stool, adult	130	20	100	45	—	Mean maximal rate of purging in severe cholera may exceed 10 mL/kg/hr. Sodium losses in cholera stools exceed those seen in other causes of diarrheal illness.
	Cholera stool, child	100	30	90	30	—	
	Noncholera stool, child (ETEC)	50	35	25	20	—	

Cl$^-$, chloride ion; D5LR, 5% dextrose in lactated Ringer's solution; ETEC, enterotoxigenic *Escherichia coli*; HCO$_3^-$, bicarbonate ion; K$^+$, potassium ion; LRS, lactated Ringer's solution; Na$^+$, sodium ion; NS, normal saline; ORS, oral rehydration solution; WHO, World Health Organization.
*In 2002, the WHO replaced its previous formulation of ORS with the current lower osmolarity formulation to reflect the broad use of ORS for treating dehydration from all-cause gastroenteritis.
Modified from Harris JB, Larocque RC, Qadri F, et al. Cholera. *Lancet.* 2012;379:2466-2476.

TABLE 147-2	Antimicrobial Options for Treating Patients with Cholera			
CLASS	ANTIBIOTIC	PEDIATRIC DOSE*	ADULT DOSE	COMMENTS
Macrolides	Erythromycin	12.5 mg/kg/dose qid × 3 days	250 mg qid × 3 days	Single-dose azithromycin is often the preferred therapy, especially in children, and has been shown to be more effective than ciprofloxacin in randomized trials in regions where reduced susceptibility to fluoroquinolones are common. Rare reports of macrolide resistance.
	Azithromycin	20 mg/kg × single dose	1 g × single dose	
Fluoroquinolones	Ciprofloxacin	15 mg/kg/dose bid × 3 days	500 mg bid × 3 days	In highly susceptible strains, single-dose ciprofloxacin compares favorably against erythromycin and doxycycline in randomized trials. Reduced susceptibility to fluoroquinolones has become common in endemic areas and is associated with treatment failure.
Tetracyclines	Tetracycline	12.5 mg/kg/dose qid × 3 days	500 mg qid × 3 days	Antibiotic resistance to all tetracyclines is common. Empirical use often reserved for outbreaks caused by documented susceptible isolates. Tetracyclines are not recommended for pregnant women or children less than 8 yr.
	Doxycycline	4-6 mg/kg × single dose	300 mg × single dose	

bid, twice a day; qid: four times a day.
*Pediatric doses, based on weight; should not exceed maximum adult dose.
Modified from Harris JB, Larocque RC, Qadri F, et al. Cholera. *Lancet.* 2012;379:2466-2476.

- ORS can be made in resource-limited settings by adding $\frac{1}{2}$ tsp of table salt to 6 tsp of table sugar in 1 L of safe water, ideally supplemented with locally available potassium sources, such as coconut milk, bananas, or orange juice.
- Antibiotics play a secondary role in the treatment of individuals with cholera and usually involve administration of a macrolide or fluoroquinolone antibiotic. Tetracyclines can be used in nonpregnant individuals older than 7 years in areas with confirmed susceptibility (see Table 147-2).
- Antibiotics decrease the duration of diarrhea and may limit secondary transmission.

PREVENTION

- Control primarily focuses on surveillance, case detection, fluid resuscitation and management, vaccination, and provision of safe water and adequate sanitation.
- Two oral killed cholera vaccines are currently commercially available and approved by the World Health Organization (see Table 147-3).
- Additional cholera vaccines are under development.

TABLE 147-3 Internationally Available and WHO Prequalified Oral Killed Cholera Vaccines

VACCINE	DOSES*	DOSING INTERVAL*	DOSING VOLUME*	BOOSTERS*	PROTECTIVE EFFICACY	COMMENTS	REFERENCES
Shanchol (Shantha Biotechnics–Sanofi Pasteur)						Possible longer term protection than that afforded by Dukoral. Does not require buffer to administer vaccine. Currently more affordable than Dukoral. Currently undergoing field studies in Kolkata/Orissa, India, and Dhaka, Bangladesh, and pilot roll out in a number of countries, including Haiti.	82-88
≥1 yr of age	2	14 days (7-42 probably permissible)	1.5 mL	Every 2 yr	60%-70% protective efficacy decreasing to baseline over 36-60 mo in older children and adults; 40% protective efficacy and shorter duration in younger children		
Dukoral† (Crucell)						Licensed in many countries. Has been safely administered to individuals infected with HIV. Provides short-term protection against diarrhea caused by heat-labile toxin expressing strains of ETEC.	89-96
Children 2 to <6 yr of age	3	14 days (7-42 permissible)	3 mL vaccine and 75 mL buffer	Every 6 mo	60%-85% protective efficacy within 6 mo of vaccination, decreasing to baseline over 24-36 mo		
≥6 yr of age	2	14 days (7-42 permissible)	3 mL vaccine and 150 mL buffer	Every 2 yr			

ETEC, enterotoxigenic *Escherichia coli*; HIV, human immunodeficiency virus; WHO, World Health Organization.
*Per manufacturer.
†Field studies have involved both the current preparation of WC-rBS vaccine, supplemented with recombinant cholera toxin B subunit (rBS), and an initial preparation of WC-BS containing nonrecombinant B subunit (BS).
Modified from Harris JB, Larocque RC, Qadri F, et al. Cholera. *Lancet.* 2012;379:2466-2476.

148 Other Pathogenic Vibrios

Marguerite A. Neill and Charles C. J. Carpenter

DEFINITION

- Vibrios are gram-negative rods whose environmental niche is primarily marine and estuarine waters.
- They may also be found in freshwater sources.
- The halophilic vibrios require higher concentrations of salt for growth.

EPIDEMIOLOGY

- The most common *Vibrio* species causing human illness are *Vibrio parahemolyticus* and *Vibrio vulnificus.*
- The incidence of vibriosis in the United States has been increasing in the past 15 years, indicating that current prevention efforts are not effective.
- Illness is more common in the warmer summer months when *Vibrio* populations are higher and there is increased human exposure from shellfish consumption and recreational water exposure.
- *Vibrio* species primarily cause diarrhea of varying severity, soft tissue infection, and/or bacteremia.
- *V. vulnificus* causes a distinct soft tissue infection with rapidly developing hemorrhagic bullae.
- *Vibrio* infections are more severe and more often fatal in people with cirrhosis or underlying liver disease.

MICROBIOLOGY

- The major pathogenic vibrios grow well in blood culture media and common nonselective media used for wound cultures.
- Selective media such as thiosulfate citrate bile salts sucrose facilitates identification from fecal specimens.

DIAGNOSIS

- *Vibrio* infection should be suspected in people with diarrhea, sepsis, or wound infection after seafood consumption or marine water exposure.

THERAPY

- Rapid recognition of possible *V. vulnificus* infection is key to improving survival and requires antimicrobial treatment as well as surgical débridement
- Survival is improved in *V. vulnificus* infection when a third-generation cephalosporin is added to doxycycline or a quinolone, provided débridement of necrotic tissue is done.

- Treatment with doxycycline or a quinolone can decrease symptoms and fecal shedding in people with diarrhea continuing for 5 days.

PREVENTION

- No vaccine is available for the noncholera vibrios.
- Thorough cooking of seafood with prompt consumption or refrigeration is needed to decrease the risk for *Vibrio* infection.

149 Campylobacter jejuni and Related Species

Ban Mishu Allos, Nicole M. Iovine, and Martin J. Blaser

DEFINITION

- *Campylobacter* spp. are small, curved, gram-negative rods that cause acute gastrointestinal illness that typically lasts from 1 to 7 days. The diarrhea is frequently bloody and is associated with abdominal pain. *C. jejuni* is the most common human clinical isolate, but many other *Campylobacter* spp. have been identified.

EPIDEMIOLOGY

- *Campylobacter* spp. are found in a variety of animals and are a common cause of human diarrheal disease worldwide. In developed nations, the incidence peaks in late summer and fall, but infections occur year-round in developing countries. Transmission to humans occurs most commonly from consumption or handling of poultry.

MICROBIOLOGY

- Many, but not all, *Campylobacter* spp. thrive at 42° C. The organisms are quite small (0.3 to 0.6 μm in diameter) and motile. They are microaerophilic and grow best at an oxygen concentration of 5% to 10%.

DIAGNOSIS

- The gold standard for diagnosis is via isolation of the organism from a stool or occasionally a blood culture.

THERAPY

- The most important tenet of treatment is to replace fluid and electrolytes to prevent dehydration. Antibiotics may shorten the duration of symptoms. Erythromycin, 250 mg four times per day for 5 to 7 days, will treat most infections. Extended-spectrum macrolides are equally efficacious.

PREVENTION

- The best way to prevent infection is by thoroughly cooking poultry and other foods of animal origin before consuming them. Meticulous attention to avoid cross-contamination during food preparation may also prevent some infections. No effective vaccine is currently available.

150 Helicobacter pylori and Other Gastric Helicobacter Species

Timothy L. Cover and Martin J. Blaser

DEFINITION

- *Helicobacter pylori* is a gram-negative bacterium that persistently colonizes the human stomach.
- Most *H. pylori*–colonized persons remain asymptomatic, but the presence of *H. pylori* is associated with an increased risk of peptic ulceration and gastric cancer.

EPIDEMIOLOGY

- *H. pylori* is present in humans throughout the world, but the prevalence is variable and depends on age and geography.
- The prevalence of *H. pylori* in developed countries has been declining over the past several decades.

MICROBIOLOGY

- *H. pylori* is a urease-positive, gram-negative, spiral-shaped bacterium.

DIAGNOSIS

- Noninvasive approaches are serology, urea breath test, and stool antigen test.
- Invasive approaches are endoscopy and analysis of gastric tissue.

THERAPY

- Treatment is not indicated except in patients with peptic ulceration or patients considered to have a high relative risk of gastric cancer.

PREVENTION

- Prevention of *H. pylori* acquisition by immunization is not routinely practiced.

151 Enterobacteriaceae

Michael S. Donnenberg

DEFINITION

- Family of gram-negative, non–spore-forming facultative anaerobes that ferment glucose, reduce nitrate to nitrite, and produce catalase

EPIDEMIOLOGY

- Cause a wide variety of diseases in humans of all ages, the spectrum of which varies by organism and subtype

MICROBIOLOGY

- Includes *Escherichia coli, Proteus* spp., *Klebsiella* spp., and *Citrobacter* spp. among others
- *Salmonella* spp., *Shigella* spp., *Yersinia* spp. (see discussions in other chapters)

DIAGNOSIS

- Standard culture techniques
- Specific subtypes identified by immunoassays for toxin production or polymerase chain reaction assay for virulence genes
- Pulsed-field gel electrophoresis helpful in identifying outbreaks

THERAPY

- Varies by organism, site, and susceptibility pattern and can include a range from antimicrobial agents being contraindicated to being untreatable with currently available antimicrobial agents

PREVENTION

- Strict adherence to infection control measures for nosocomial spread of highly resistant strains
- Reduce risk for foodborne infections by observing good food hygiene
- No currently licensed vaccine

152 Pseudomonas aeruginosa and Other Pseudomonas Species

Erika D'Agata

EPIDEMIOLOGY

- *Pseudomonas* species are gram-negative bacteria that inhabit diverse environments, including soil, water, plants, insects, and animals.
- *P. aeruginosa* is the most important *Pseudomonas* species affecting humans, causing serious infections associated with substantial morbidity and mortality.
- Other *Pseudomonas* species, including *P. fluorescens, P. luteola, P. putida,* and *P. stutzeri,* are less virulent but are still implicated in a wide variety of infections, primarily occurring among immunocompromised patients.
- *P. aeruginosa* has many virulence factors, including pili, flagella, enzyme secretion systems, and quorum-sensing molecules.
- *P. aeruginosa* is one of the most frequent pathogens implicated in hospital-acquired infections, including ventilator-associated pneumonia and catheter-associated urinary tract infections. Long-term acute care hospitals have very high rates of infections caused by *P. aeruginosa*
- Characteristic infections caused by *P. aeruginosa* include ecthyma gangrenosum, malignant otitis externa, hot hand-foot syndrome, and hot tub folliculitis.
- Resistance to single and multiple antimicrobial agents is rising rapidly.

MICROBIOLOGY OF *P. AERUGINOSA*

- *P. aeruginosa* is an aerobic rod-shaped bacteria.
- Growth occurs in a variety of culture media forming smooth round colonies, with a characteristic grapelike or "corn-taco" odor, and a green-blue coloration.
- Identification is based on colony morphology, coloration, oxidase positivity, and growth at 42° C.

THERAPY

- The efficacy of treatment with two antipseudomonal antimicrobial agents versus monotherapy has not been definitively answered.
- The majority of evidence suggests that empirical treatment with combination therapy is indicated if antimicrobial resistance rates are high.
- Streamlining to a single antimicrobial agent, once antimicrobial susceptibility profiles are available, should then be considered.

Stenotrophomonas maltophilia and *Burkholderia cepacia*

Amar Safdar

MICROBIOLOGY AND EPIDEMIOLOGY

- *Stenotrophomonas maltophilia* and *Burkholderia cepacia* are gram-negative bacteria that acquire motility via multitrichous polar flagella. They do not ferment glucose, and many clinical isolates tend to give a weak oxidase reaction.
- Slow-growing morphotypes, known as small-colony variants of *B. cepacia* and *S. maltophilia*, may appear and exhibit a high degree of resistance to antibiotics and may go undetected in routine cultures.
- These free-living organisms are present in most aquatic and humid environments, including hospital drinking water.
- *Burkholderia cenocepacia* and *Burkholderia multivorans* are the prominent bacterial strains isolated from patients with cystic fibrosis. Patient-to-patient transmission is believed to contribute to colonization.
- Community-acquired *S. maltophilia* pneumonia has emerged as a serious concern in patients with no known risk factors, such as critical unit stay; mechanical ventilation or prolonged treatment-induced neutropenia; recent carbapenem, higher-generation cephalosporin, or fluoroquinolone therapy; or extended hospital stays.

CLINICAL MANIFESTATIONS

- *S. maltophilia* may involve any organ. Lungs are frequent sites of infection. Pulmonary infection is often preceded by respiratory tract colonization. Lobular or lobar consolidation is common, whereas pleural effusions are seldom noted.
- Most *S. maltophilia* bloodstream infections arise from infected indwelling intravascular devices. Non–catheter-related bacteremia is often seen in patients with prolonged neutropenia.
- *S. maltophilia* wound infections in burn patients are being reported as the second most common gram-negative bacterial infections after those caused by *Aeromonas hydrophila*. Skin lesions in mostly neutropenic patients are difficult to distinguish from pyoderma gangrenosum, leukemia cutis, vasculitis, and disseminated *Pseudomonas*, *Fusarium*, *Candida*, and rapidly growing mycobacterial infections.
- In patients with cystic fibrosis, after initial *B. cepacia* infection, 50% of patients with *B. multivorans* may develop chronic asymptomatic bacterial colonization, whereas nearly all (94%) patients with *B. cenocepacia* retain bacterial presence after the initial infection episode.

COMPLICATIONS

- Lack of acute inflammation may underwhelm initial clinical presentation of *S. maltophilia* pneumonia in the immunosuppressed patient. Patients may present with serious pulmonary hemorrhage at the time of diagnosis owing to high propensity for tissue necrosis and hemorrhage.
- Non–catheter-related *S. maltophilia* bacteremia is a serious complication associated with high rate of treatment failure and death. Patients often have profound neutropenia lasting longer than 10 days; and in nearly 70% of patients, hematogenous dissemination arises from

lung or soft tissue infection. Indicators for poor outcome in cancer patients include neutropenia more than 10 days, bacteremic pneumonia, shock syndrome, severe thrombocytopenia, and delay in appropriate therapy.

- *B. cenocepacia* is associated with prolonged respiratory tract colonization, and the risk for death with invasive disease is more than fivefold higher compared with infections due to the other eight *B. cepacia* complex genomovars.
- *B. cepacia* complex infection in patients with cystic fibrosis with diminished forced expiratory volume in 1 second has steadily been associated with poor prognosis. Infection in critically ill patients, presence of septic shock, and advanced underlying conditions also herald higher mortality.

DIAGNOSIS

- Early diagnosis requires a high level of suspicion for *S. maltophilia* lung infection.
- Up to 36% of *Burkholderia* species may be misidentified by automated systems as other nonfermentative bacteria, such as *Achromobacter* or *Ralstonia.*
- Swift and accurate molecular methods using 16S or 23S ribosomal RNA gene sequencing may replace conventional methods.
- Whole-cell matrix-assisted laser desorption/ionization time-of-flight mass spectrometry holds promise as a rapid, accurate identification method for *B. cepacia* and *S. maltophilia.*

THERAPY

- Monotherapy is not recommended, owing to high frequency of treatment failure and infection relapse.
- Trimethoprim-sulfamethoxazole (TMP/SMX) has the most potent and reliable in vitro activity against clinical isolates of *S. maltophilia;* however, drug resistance has increased among 30% to 40% of disease-associated isolates worldwide.
- The newer fluoroquinolones, such as moxifloxacin, show improved activity against *S. maltophilia.* However, resistance has developed after single-drug therapy, which can be prevented by drug combinations including ticarcillin-clavulanic acid and/or TMP/SMX.
- Carbapenems, TMP/SMX, chloramphenicol, and tetracycline are active against most *B. cepacia* complex isolates. Treatment pending susceptibility testing will depend on experience of the institution.
- Most active drugs against *B. cepacia* include minocycline (38%), meropenem (26%), and ceftazidime (23%). Ceftazidime, tobramycin, and ciprofloxacin retain antimicrobial activity against planktonic and biofilm-embedded organisms.

PREVENTION

- Nosocomial outbreaks underscore the current practice of strict infection prevention measures with main emphasis on decreasing transmission on health care workers' hands and cohort segregation of infected or colonized hospitalized patients with multidrug-resistant bacteria.
- Continued surveillance of hospital water supply remains critical in preventing iatrogenic and hospital-related acquisition of these free living, nearly ubiquitous bacteria.
- Immunization: preclinical experiments using outer membrane protein immunogenic epitopes against *B. multivorans* and *B. cenocepacia* appear promising.
- Immunotherapy: various strategies to boost innate local immune response against gram-negative bacteria are being investigated.

154 Burkholderia pseudomallei and Burkholderia mallei: Melioidosis and Glanders

Bart J. Currie

DEFINITION

- Melioidosis is a disease of humans and animals resulting from infection with the soil and water bacterium *Burkholderia pseudomallei.*
- Glanders is a disease primarily of horses resulting from infection with *Burkholderia mallei.*

EPIDEMIOLOGY: MELIOIDOSIS

- The major endemic regions for melioidosis are Southeast Asia and northern Australia.
- Cases have occurred in other tropical and subtropical locations, such as the Indian subcontinent, China, Africa, the Caribbean, and Central and South America.
- Most cases occur during the rainy season, and clusters can follow severe weather events.
- Exposure occurs through percutaneous inoculation, inhalation, and ingestion (more common with glanders).
- Zoonotic and nosocomial infections are exceedingly rare with melioidosis (more common with glanders).
- Disease and outcomes are tightly linked to risk factors, especially diabetes (see Table 154-1).

MICROBIOLOGY

- *B. pseudomallei* is a small, gram-negative, oxidase-positive, motile, aerobic bacillus.
- *B. mallei* is a small, gram-negative, oxidase-positive, nonmotile aerobic bacillus.
- *B. mallei* does not persist in the environment outside its equine host, and genetic studies suggest that *B. mallei* evolved in animals from the environmental pathogen *B. pseudomallei.*

DIAGNOSIS: MELIOIDOSIS

- Most infections with *B. pseudomallei* are asymptomatic.
- Eighty-five percent of cases are acute illness after recent infection; 11% are chronic infections (sick more than 2 months), and activation from latency is rare (longest is 62 years after infection).
- Over half are bacteremic, and up to one quarter present with septic shock with high mortality.
- Presentation is pneumonia in about half of cases, but there are diverse other presentations (see Table 154-2).
- Culture is required for diagnosis by using blood, sputum, urine, pus, and it is facilitated by inoculating swabs from pus, throat, and rectum directly onto selective medium.
- Identification of *B. pseudomallei* and *B. mallei* by various methods can be problematic.
- Locally developed antigen and DNA detection techniques are available in some locations. Serology has poor specificity because of background positivity in endemic regions.

TABLE 154-1 Risk Factors for Melioidosis

RISK FACTOR*	THAILAND (% OF CASES)	AUSTRALIA (% OF CASES)
Diabetes	23-60	37
Alcohol excess	12	39
Renal disease	20-27	10
Chronic lung disease	NR	27
Thalassemia	7	0
No risk factors	24-36	20

NR, not reported.
Australia data from Currie BJ, Fisher DA, Howard DM, et al. Endemic melioidosis in tropical northern Australia: a 10-year prospective study and review of the literature. Clin Infect Dis. 2000;31:981-986.
*Not listed: malignancy, steroid therapy, iron overload, cardiac failure.
Thailand data from Punyagupta S. Melioidosis: review of 686 cases and presentation of a new clinical classification. In: Punyagupta S, Sirisanthana T, Stapatayavong B, eds. *Melioidosis.* Bangkok: Bangkok Medical; 1989:217-229; Chaowagul W, White NJ, Dance DA, et al. Melioidosis: a major cause of community-acquired septicemia in northeastern Thailand. *J Infect Dis.* 1989;159:890-899; Suputtamongkol Y, Chaowagul W, Chetchotisakd P, et al. Risk factors for melioidosis and bacteremic melioidosis. *Clin Infect Dis.* 1999;29:408-413; and Limmathurotsakul D, Chaowagul W, Chierakul W, et al. Risk factors for recurrent melioidosis in northeast Thailand. *Clin Infect Dis.* 2006;43:979-986.

TABLE 154-2 Clinical Presentations and Outcomes of Melioidosis in Northern Australia

	TOTAL		BACTEREMIC		NONBACTEREMIC	
	Number	Deaths (Mortality)	Number	Deaths (Mortality)	Number	Deaths (Mortality)
Septic Shock Present	116 (21%)	58 (50%)	103	48 (47%)	13	10 (77%)
Pneumonia	88	43 (49%)	78	35 (45%)	10*	8 (80%)
No evident focus	13	8 (62%)	12	7 (58%)	1†	1 (100%)
Genitourinary	10	5 (50%)	9	4 (44%)	1‡	1 (100%)
Osteomyelitis/septic arthritis	4	2 (50%)	4	2 (50%)	0	0 (0%)
Soft tissue abscess	1	0 (0%)	0	0	1	0 (0%)
Not Septic Shock	424 (79%)	19 (4%)	195	13 (7%)	229	6 (3%)
Pneumonia	190	12 (6%)	89	9 (10%)	101	3 (3%)
Skin infection	68	0 (0%)	1	0 (0%)	67	0 (0%)
Genitourinary	66	2 (3%)	41	2 (5%)	25	0 (0%)
No evident focus	52	2 (4%)	47	2 (4%)	5	0 (0%)
Soft tissue abscess(es)	18	0 (0%)	4	0 (0%)	14	0 (0%)
Osteomyelitis/septic arthritis	16	0 (0%)	10	0 (0%)	6	0 (0%)
Neurologic	14	3 (21%)	3	0 (0%)	11	3 (27%)
Total	540	77 (14%)	298 (55%)	61 (20%)	242 (45%)	16 (7%)

*Seven blood cultures not done; three blood cultures negative.
†Culture was positive for *Burkholderia pseudomallei* only from rectal swab, although fatal septic shock.
‡Blood culture not done.
From Currie BJ, Ward L, Cheng AC. The epidemiology and clinical spectrum of melioidosis: 540 cases from the 20-year Darwin prospective study. *PLoS Negl Trop Dis.* 2010;4:e900.

TABLE 154-3 Antibiotic Therapy for Melioidosis

Initial Intensive Therapy (Minimum of 10-14 Days)

Ceftazidime (50 mg/kg, up to 2 g) q6h
or
Meropenem (25 mg/kg, up to 1 g) q8h
or
Imipenem (25 mg/kg, up to 1 g) q6h
Any one of the three may be combined with TMP-SMX (6/30 mg/kg, up to 320/1600 mg) q12h
(recommended for neurologic, cutaneous, bone, joint, and prostatic melioidosis)

Eradication Therapy (Minimum of 3 Months)

TMP-SMX (6/30 mg/kg, up to 320/1600 mg) q12h

TMP-SMX, trimethoprim-sulfamethoxazole.

TABLE 154-4 Duration of Antibiotic Therapy for Melioidosis

ANTIBIOTIC DURATION-DETERMINING FOCUS		MINIMUM INTENSIVE PHASE DURATION (WK)*	ERADICATION PHASE DURATION (MO)
Skin abscess		2	3
Bacteremia with no focus		2	3
Pneumonia	Without lymphadenopathy† or ICU admission	2	3
	With either lymphadenopathy† or ICU admission	4	3
Deep-seated collection‡		4§	3
Osteomyelitis		6	6
Central nervous system (CNS) infection		8	6
Arterial infection‖		8§	6

CNS, central nervous system; ICU, intensive care unit.
*Clinical judgement to guide prolongation of intensive phase if improvement is slow or if blood cultures remain positive at 7 days.
†Defined as enlargement of any hilar or mediastinal lymph node to greater than 10-mm diameter.
‡Defined as abscess anywhere other than skin, lungs, bone, CNS, or vasculature; septic arthritis is considered a deep-seated collection.
§Intensive phase duration is timed from date of most recent drainage or resection where culture of the drainage specimen or resected material grew *Burkholderia pseudomallei* or where no specimen was sent for culture; clock is not reset if specimen is culture-negative.
‖Most commonly presenting as mycotic aneurysm.

THERAPY

- Ceftazidime or a carbapenem ± trimethoprim-sulfamethoxazole (TMP-SMX) is given initially, followed by TMP-SMX (see Tables 154-3 and 154-4).
- Therapy of glanders is as for melioidosis, although gentamicin, azithromycin, or clarithromycin may have a role.

PREVENTION

- Melioidosis: Education is needed in endemic areas about minimizing exposure to wet season soils, surface water, and potential aerosols during windy monsoonal rains, especially for diabetics.
- Cystic fibrosis patients should consider avoiding travel to high-risk areas.
- Glanders: Control of glanders in the equine species and strict precautions to prevent laboratory-acquired infection are crucial.
- Vaccines are under development for both melioidosis and glanders.

155 *Acinetobacter* Species

Michael Phillips

DEFINITION AND EPIDEMIOLOGY

- *Acinetobacter* species are associated with specific ecologic niches.
- *A. baumannii* and the closely related and phenotypically indistinguishable *A. pittii* and *A. nosocomialis* cause the bulk of human infections and are typically acquired in the health care setting.
- *Acinetobacter* species readily incorporate multiple resistance mechanisms, and pan-resistant strains have emerged.

THERAPY

- Antimicrobial treatment is based on antimicrobial susceptibility testing. Potential options, with adult dosage for normal renal function, include the following:
  - Cefepime, 2 g IV every 8 hours
  - Imipenem, 1 g IV every 6 hours
  - Meropenem, 1 g IV every 8 hours
  - Ampicillin/sulbactam, 3 g/1.5 g every 6 hours (sulbactam is the active component)
  - Tigecycline, 100 mg IV loading dose, then 50 mg IV every 12 hours
  - Colistin (colistimethate sodium), 5 mg/kg loading dose, then 2.5 mg/kg every 12 hours
  - Polymyxin B, 2.5 mg/kg on day 1, then either 2.5 mg/kg daily or 1.25 mg/kg every 12 hours (polymyxin B 1 mg = 10,000 units)

PREVENTION

- Prevention of *Acinetobacter* transmission in health care settings requires a multifactorial approach, with environmental disinfection and hand hygiene as the cornerstone.
- The emergence of *A. baumannii* strains resistant to essentially all potent antimicrobial agents, coupled with a dearth of antibiotics in development, constitutes a significant public health threat.

156 *Salmonella* Species

David A. Pegues and Samuel I. Miller

DEFINITION

- Salmonellosis includes gastroenteritis and other infections caused by nontyphoidal *Salmonella* (NTS).

EPIDEMIOLOGY

- There are approximately 1 million cases of NTS infection annually in the United States.
- Nontyphoidal salmonellosis is associated with diverse reservoirs, including fresh and prepared food items and other animal sources.

MICROBIOLOGY

- There are more than 2500 *Salmonella* serotypes.
- Strains with multidrug resistance and decreased susceptibility to fluoroquinolones are increasingly prevalent.

DIAGNOSIS

- Freshly passed stool should be plated directly on MacConkey agar or more selective media.
- Obtain blood cultures for patients suspected of bacteremia or vascular infection.
- Serogrouping is performed with commercially available antisera.

THERAPY

- Antimicrobial therapy is not indicated for uncomplicated *Salmonella* gastroenteritis and prolongs the duration of fecal carriage.
- Ceftriaxone or fluoroquinolones should be administered empirically for treatment of severe gastroenteritis or when occurring in high-risk patients and for directed therapy of bacteremia or focal infections with NTS.

PREVENTION

- Control of foodborne outbreaks of NTS depend on a coordinated public health response and identification of controllable hazards from the farm to the table.

157 Bacillary Dysentery: *Shigella* and Enteroinvasive *Escherichia coli*

Herbert L. DuPont

DEFINITION
- Diarrhea illness caused by strains of invasive forms of *Shigella* or invasive *Escherichia coli* comprises bacillary dysentery.

EPIDEMIOLOGY
- Shigellosis is the most infectious (communicable from person to person) of the bacterial enteropathogens.

MICROBIOLOGY
- *Shigella* spp. are small gram-negative rods in the family Enterobacteriaceae.
- Similar to strains of *Shigella,* enteroinvasive *E. coli* possesses somatic antigens and a plasmid that controls invasiveness.

DIAGNOSIS
- Patients passing bloody stools or those associated with other cases of shigellosis should have stools processed for *Shigella.*
- The sooner a stool specimen is cultured, the higher the yield for *Shigella.*
- Once specimens are plated on gram-negative media at 37°C and incubated overnight, lactose-negative colonies are tested biochemically and serologically for *Shigella.*

THERAPY
- Antibiotics are useful in the management of shigellosis and can be livesaving for infection caused by the Shiga bacillus (*S. dysenteriae* 1).
- The treatment of choice for adults is a fluoroquinolone antibiotic given for 3 days.
- For children, cephalosporin, ciprofloxacin, or azithromycin may be used.

PREVENTION
- Because person-to-person spread is so important in *Shigella* infection, hand washing and other hygienic methods should be used to prevent spread.
- Vaccines are in development to prevent *Shigella* infection.

158 Haemophilus Species, Including *H. influenzae* and *H. ducreyi* (Chancroid)

Timothy F. Murphy

DEFINITION

- Gram-negative coccobacillus with fastidious growth requirements.
- Nontypeable (nonencapsulated) *Haemophilus influenzae* is a common cause of otitis media in children and exacerbations of chronic obstructive pulmonary disease (COPD) in adults.
- Encapsulated *H. influenzae* type b causes invasive infections, including meningitis and epiglottitis, in children younger than 6 years.
- *Haemophilus ducreyi* causes chancroid, a genital ulcer disease that facilitates human immunodeficiency virus transmission.
- Other *Haemophilus* species are unusual causes of human disease.

EPIDEMIOLOGY

- The ecologic niche is the human respiratory tract.
- Colonization of the nasopharynx by nontypeable *H. influenzae* begins in infancy, is common during childhood, and persists at a lower rate in adults.
- Invasive *H. influenzae* type b infections are rare in regions of the world where *H. influenzae* type b conjugate vaccines are used widely but are prevalent in regions where the vaccine is not used.
- The prevalence of chancroid appears to be decreasing, based on the number of reported cases, but the difficulty in diagnosis may result in underestimates of prevalence.

MICROBIOLOGY

- Many members of the genus *Haemophilus* are part of the normal bacterial flora of the human upper respiratory tract.
- Fastidious growth requirements are used to distinguish the species in the laboratory.

DIAGNOSIS

- An etiologic diagnosis of most common clinical manifestations of nontypeable strains (otitis media in children and exacerbations of COPD in adults) is not made routinely in clinical practice. Rather, these infections are usually treated empirically, based on a presumptive diagnosis by using clinical manifestations.
- Invasive infections caused by *H. influenzae* type b are established by isolating the organism or detecting capsular antigen from normally sterile body fluids, including cerebrospinal fluid or blood.

THERAPY

- Otitis media and exacerbations of COPD are treated with oral antimicrobial agents, with the choice generally guided by expert guidelines.
- *H. influenzae* type b meningitis: ceftriaxone, 75 to 100 mg/kg divided into 12 hourly doses or cefotaxime, 200 mg/kg/day, divided into six hourly doses. Also administer dexamethasone, 0.6 mg/kg/day IV in four divided doses for 4 days to children older than 2 months.
- Chancroid: azithromycin, 1 g orally (single dose) or ceftriaxone, 250 mg IM (single dose).

PREVENTION

- All children should receive the *H. influenzae* type b conjugate vaccine series beginning at 2 months as part of routine childhood vaccination.
- Incompletely immunized household contacts of cases of meningitis should receive rifampin prophylaxis (20 mg/kg once daily [600 mg maximum] for 4 days).
- Sexual contacts of patients with chancroid should be treated, even if asymptomatic.

159 Brucellosis (*Brucella* Species)

H. Cem Gul and Hakan Erdem

DIAGNOSIS
- Brucellosis is diagnosed by isolation of *Brucella* from blood, bone marrow, or tissue or by serology, although the polymerase chain reaction assay is available in a few laboratories. The preferred serology is the tube agglutination test with a titer of at least 1 : 160. The Rose-Bengal card agglutination test is useful for screening. *Brucella canis* requires a separate serology.

MICROBIOLOGY
- *Brucella melitensis, Brucella suis, Brucella abortus,* and, rarely, *B. canis* cause brucellosis and are nonmotile gram-negative coccobacilli.

EPIDEMIOLOGY
- Although uncommon in the United States, brucellosis is a worldwide zoonosis of wild and domestic animals, principally cattle, swine, goats, and sheep. Infection is acquired by contact with infected animals, their tissues, or ingestion of unpasteurized milk or dairy products from infected cows, goats, and sheep.

CLINICAL SETTINGS
- Fever, sweating, myalgia, weight loss, headache, and malaise without localizing symptoms are evident. Lymphadenopathy or hepatosplenomegaly may occur. Onset can be acute or insidious and persist for weeks or months if untreated.
- Focal infections include osteomyelitis (particularly spondylitis or sacroiliitis), epididymo-orchitis, endocarditis, meningitis, meningoencephalitis, and myeloradiculitis.

TREATMENT
- Doxycycline with streptomycin is the standard regimen. For alternatives and treatment of neurobrucellosis, see Table 159-1.

TABLE 159-1	Treatment of Brucellosis	
CLINICAL FORM	**PREFERRED REGIMEN**	**ALTERNATIVE REGIMEN**
Uncomplicated	Doxycycline 100 mg PO twice daily for at least 6 wk	Doxycycline 100 mg PO twice daily for at least 6 wk
	plus	*plus*
	Streptomycin 1 g IM daily for 2-3 wk	Gentamicin 5 mg/kg IM daily for 1 wk
		or
		Doxycycline 100 mg PO twice daily for at least 6 wk
		plus
		Rifampin 600-900 mg (15 mg/kg) once daily for at least 6 wk
Neurobrucellosis	Ceftriaxone 2 mg IV twice daily for at least 1 mo	Trimethoprim-sulfamethoxazole 160/800 mg PO twice daily for 5-6 mo
	plus	*plus*
	Doxycycline 100 mg PO twice daily; for 4-5 mo	Doxycycline 100 mg PO twice daily; for 5-6 mo
	plus	*plus*
	Rifampin 600-900 mg (15 mg/kg) PO once daily for 4-5 mo	Rifampin 600-900 mg (15 mg/kg) PO once daily for 5-6 mo

160 *Francisella tularensis* (Tularemia)

Robert L. Penn

DEFINITION

- Tularemia is the zoonotic disease caused by *Francisella tularensis.*

EPIDEMIOLOGY

- Tularemia is widely distributed but is primarily a disease of the Northern Hemisphere.
- In the United States the majority of cases reported in 2010 occurred in Arkansas, Missouri, Kansas, South Dakota, California, and Oklahoma.
- Tularemia peaks in the late spring and summer in the United States.
- Lagomorphs and rodents are important animal reservoirs.
- Major vectors of transmission include ticks and biting flies in the United States and mosquitoes in Europe.
- Other routes of transmission include aerosol droplets, contaminated mud or water, and animal bites.
- Occupations that have an increased risk for tularemia include laboratory worker, farmer, landscaper, veterinarian, sheep worker, hunter or trapper, and cook or meat handler.
- Tularemia spread by aerosol is a potential bioterrorist weapon.

MICROBIOLOGY

- *Francisella* organisms are small, aerobic, pleomorphic gram-negative coccobacilli.
- *F. tularensis* requires cysteine or cystine (or another sulfhydryl source) for growth and therefore will not grow well on most routine solid media.
- Although there are three species in the genus *Francisella* and four *F. tularensis* subspecies (see Table 160-1), only *F. tularensis* subsp. *tularensis* and *F. tularensis* subsp. *holarctica* are relatively common.
- Infections caused by *F. tularensis* subsp. *tularensis* are generally more severe than those caused by *F. tularensis* subsp. *holarctica.*
- The infectious dose in humans is 10 to 50 organisms when injected intradermally or when inhaled.
- *F. tularensis* is a facultative intracellular pathogen that survives within host macrophages by impairing phagosome-lysosome fusion, and it is capable of suppressing or avoiding many other humoral and cellular host defenses.
- Recovery from infection depends on development of host cell-mediated immunity.

CLINICAL MANIFESTATIONS

- Tularemia starts abruptly with fever, chills, headache, anorexia, and fatigue after an average incubation period of 3 to 5 days.
- There are six major patterns of illness: ulceroglandular (see Fig. 160-1), glandular, oculoglandular, pharyngeal, typhoidal, and pneumonic (see Fig. 160-2); pneumonic and typhoidal tularemia are expected to be the primary forms resulting from a bioterrorism event.
- Secondary rashes are relatively common.

TABLE 160-1 Characterization of *Francisella* Species

FEATURE	*F. TULARENSIS* SUBSPECIES			*F. PHILOMIRAGIA*	*F. HISPANIENSIS*
	tularensis	*holarctica*	*novicida*		
Cysteine growth requirement	+	+	−	−	−
Growth in broth plus 6% NaCl	−	−	+*	+†	NA
Motility	−	−	−	−	NA
Oxidase	−	−	−	+†	+
Nitrate reduction	−	−	−	−	NA
Acid from:					
Glucose	+*	+*	+*	+*	+
Glycerol	+	−	+	+	+
Gelatin hydrolysis	−	−	−	*	NA
Relative virulence					
Humans	High	Intermediate	Low	Low	Low
Rabbits	High	Low	Low	NA	NA

NA, not available; NaCl, sodium chloride.
*Variable or delayed.
†Using Kovacs test; negative using cytochrome-oxidase test.
Data from Huber B, Escudero R, Busse HJ, et al. Description of *Francisella hispaniensis* sp. nov., isolated from human blood, reclassification of *Francisella novicida* (Larson et al. 1955) Olsufiev et al. 1959 as *Francisella tularensis* subsp. *novicida* comb. nov. and emended description of the genus *Francisella*. *Int J Syst Evol Microbiol.* 2010;60(pt 8):1887-1896; Petersen JM, Schriefer ME, Araj GF. *Francisella* and *Brucella*. In: Versalovic J, Carroll KC, Funke G, et al, eds. *Manual of Clinical Microbiology.* Vol 1. 10th ed. Washington, DC: ASM Press; 2011:751-769; Sjöstedt AB. *Francisella*. In: Brenner DJ, Krieg NR, Staley JT, et al, eds. *Bergey's Manual of Systematic Bacteriology.* Vol 2. 2nd ed. New York: Springer-Verlag; 2005:200-210; and Escudero R, Elia M, Saez-Nieto JA, et al. A possible novel *Francisella* genomic species isolated from blood and urine of a patient with severe illness. *Clin Microbiol Infect.* 2010;16:1026-1030.

- The most common complications of tularemia are lymph node suppuration and persistent debility.

DIAGNOSIS

- Diagnosis rests on clinical suspicion, and because of its potential danger, laboratory personnel should be notified whenever tularemia is suspected.
- *F. tularensis* is a Tier 1 select agent, and its possession and shipment are tightly restricted.
- Routine cultures and smears are often negative, and the diagnosis is usually confirmed serologically; direct fluorescent antibody and polymerase chain reaction tests for rapid diagnosis are available in specialized laboratories.

THERAPY

- Streptomycin and gentamicin are the drugs of choice for all forms of tularemia except meningitis (see Table 160-2).
- Selected adults and children with mild to moderate disease may be treated with oral agents (see Table 160-2).
- Surgical therapy is limited to drainage of suppurated nodes or of empyemas.

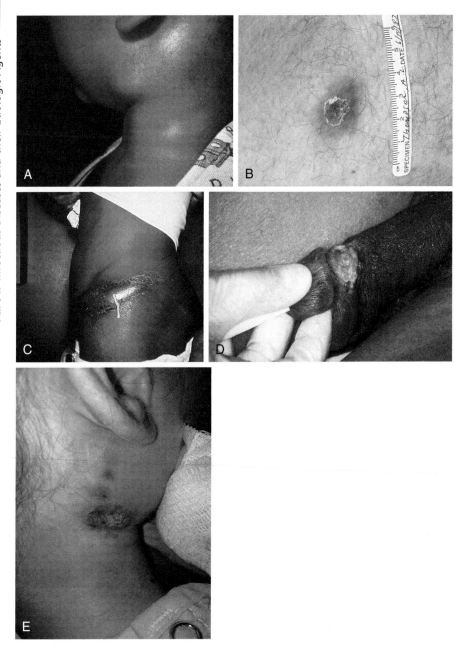

FIGURE 160-1   Examples of primary lesions seen in ulceroglandular tularemia. A, Large cervical and submandibular lymph nodes in a young child; an ulcer was found under the hairline on her forehead at the site of a tick bite. B, Papule undergoing central necrosis with desquamation on the thigh of a middle-aged man. C, Inguinal adenopathy and suppurative mass in a young hunter who had carried a dead hare at his side. D, Penile ulcer that was suspected of being syphilis or another sexually transmitted disease until the history of a recent tick bite was obtained by the infectious diseases consultant. E, Cervical ulcer and nodular adenopathy with a sporotrichoid appearance in a 6-year-old girl who had a tick removed from the area of the ulcer 2 weeks before presentation. The nodes coalesced, suppurated, and required drainage after 3 days of gentamicin therapy. Cultures of the ulcer and node drainage both grew *F. tularensis*. (A and C courtesy Dr. Joseph A. Bocchini, Louisiana State University Health Sciences Center, Shreveport, LA; D courtesy Dr. John W. King, Louisiana State University Health Sciences Center, Shreveport, LA; and E courtesy Dr. Robin Trotman, CoxHealth Infectious Diseases Specialty Clinic, Springfield, MO.)

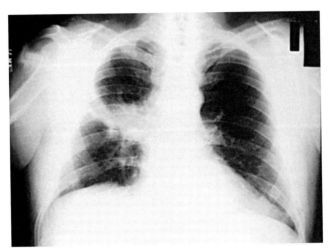

FIGURE 160-2   Chest radiograph of untreated tularemia pneumonia. This patient remained symptomatic for more than 3 months. The diagnosis was established serologically when poorly developed granulomas were found in a transbronchial biopsy specimen, other causes were excluded, and the exposure history was finally obtained. (From Penn RL, Kinasewitz GT. Factors associated with a poor outcome in tularemia. *Arch Intern Med.* 1987;147:265-268.)

PREVENTION

- The best prevention is avoiding exposure to the organism; a vaccine for tularemia is not available.
- Patients with tularemia do not need special isolation because person-to-person spread does not occur. Standard precautions for handling contaminated secretions are adequate.
- Antibiotic prophylaxis after potential exposures of unknown risk such as tick bites is not recommended.
- Either ciprofloxacin, 500 mg, or doxycycline, 100 mg, given orally twice daily for 14 days is recommended for adults with suspected or proven high-risk exposure to *F. tularensis*.
- Observation without prophylactic antibiotics is appropriate for exposed children (except during a bioterrorist event) and for adults with lower risk exposures.

TABLE 160-2 Antibiotic Therapy for Tularemia

INDICATION AND PATIENT GROUP	RECOMMENDED ANTIBIOTICS AND DOSAGES
Moderate to Serious Disease	
Adults	Streptomycin,* 10 mg/kg IM q12h for 7-10 days (not to exceed 2 g/day), or Gentamicin,* 5 mg/kg/day IM or IV divided q8h for 7-10 days
Children	Streptomycin,* 15 mg/kg IM q12h for 7-10 days (not to exceed 2 g/day), or Gentamicin,* 2.5 mg/kg IM or IV q8-12h for 7-10 days
Mild Disease	
Adults	Ciprofloxacin,† 500 mg orally twice daily for 14 days, or Doxycycline, 100 mg orally twice daily for 14 days
Children	Doxycycline,‡ 2-4 mg/kg/day orally divided q12h or once daily for 14 days (not to exceed 200 mg/day)
Meningitis	
Adults	Streptomycin or gentamicin in the doses given for moderate to serious disease plus either chloramphenicol, 15-25 mg/kg IV q6h (not to exceed 4 g/day), or doxycycline, 100 mg IV twice daily for 14-21 days
Children	Streptomycin or gentamicin in the doses for moderate to serious disease plus either chloramphenicol, 15 mg/kg IV q6h (not to exceed 4 g/day), or doxycycline, 2-4 mg/kg/day IV divided q12h or once daily (not to exceed 200 mg/day) for 14-21 days

*The streptomycin and gentamicin doses listed are for patients with normal renal function, and they need to be adjusted for renal impairment. In adults with normal renal function, once-daily administration of gentamicin also is acceptable.
†A ciprofloxacin dose of 750 mg twice daily also has been used in some reports.
‡Doxycycline should be used in patients younger than 8 years of age only if the risks are outweighed by the benefits.

161 *Pasteurella* Species

John J. Zurlo

DEFINITION

- Frequent cause of skin and soft tissue infections following an animal bite or scratch
- Often part of a mixed bacterial infection
- Complications include septic arthritis and osteomyelitis
- Less frequently causes pneumonia in patients with underlying lung disease
- Other deep-seated complications are uncommon but carry high morbidity and mortality

EPIDEMIOLOGY

- Worldwide distribution
- Principal reservoir is animals
- Infection most often occurs following bites or scratches from dogs and especially cats
- Infections have been reported following bites or scratches from a large number of other animals
- Infections also occur in individuals with animal exposure without bites or scratches

MICROBIOLOGY

- Nonmotile, facultatively anaerobic, gram-negative coccobacilli
- Grows best on sheep blood and chocolate agar, not usually on MacConkey agar
- Somewhat fastidious
- Can be difficult to isolate from nonsterile specimens, especially sputum
- *P. multocida* with three subspecies: *multocida, septica, gallicida* (least common) (see Table 161-1)
- Several other related species of genus *Pasteurella* cause human disease

DIAGNOSIS

- Progressive skin and soft tissue inflammation following an animal bite injury, especially following puncture wounds
- Isolation of the organism from wound/tissue culture, often as part of a mixed bacterial infection
- Sputum or pleural fluid isolates from patients with underlying lung conditions presenting with lower respiratory tract infections

THERAPY

- Treat infected bite wounds empirically with broad-spectrum antibiotics until microbiology is established: ampicillin/sulbactam 3 g IV q6h or piperacillin/tazobactam 3.375 g IV q6h
- For patients with β-lactam allergy, use a fluoroquinolone, doxycycline, or trimethoprim/sulfamethoxazole along with anaerobic coverage (metronidazole or clindamycin)
- Once defined as *Pasteurella* species, penicillin is the agent of choice
- β-lactam resistance is rare, mostly described in respiratory isolates
- Aggressive surgical débridement of soft tissue infections

TABLE 161-1   *Pasteurella* Species

Pasteurella sensu stricto

P. multocida
    Subspecies *multocida*
    Subspecies *septicum*
    Subspecies *gallicida*
P. canis
P. dagmatis
P. stomatis

Pasteurella-related Species

P. aerogenes
P. bettyae
P. caballi
P. pneumotropica

Data from Versalovic J, Carroll KC, Jorgensen JH, et al, eds. *Manual of Clinical Microbiology*, 10th ed. Washington, DC: ASM Press; 2011:574-587.

PREVENTION

- Antimicrobial prophylaxis for selected bite wounds, usually with amoxicillin/clavulanic acid 875 mg orally twice daily for 5 days

162 *Yersinia* Species (Including Plague)
Paul S. Mead

DEFINITION
- Three human pathogens: Yersinia enterocolitica, Y. pseudotuberculosis, Y. pestis
- Zoonoses with multiple animal hosts, widespread in environment
- All have tropism for lymph nodes, but clinical illness and ecology differ

EPIDEMIOLOGY
- Globally distributed but *Y. pestis* usually found within distinct ecologic foci
- *Y. enterocolitica, Y. pseudotuberculosis:* fecal-oral transmission, enteric pathogens, more common in children, illness often self-limited
- *Y. pestis:* vector borne, highly invasive, all ages, frequently fatal, potential bioterrorism agent

MICROBIOLOGY
- Aerobic, gram-negative members of Enterobacteriaceae
- Growth at 37° C on MacConkey agar, sheep blood *(Y. pestis, Y. pseudotuberculosis), Salmonella-Shigella* media *(Y. enterocolitica),* and brain-heart infusion
- Automated identification systems may misidentify

CLINICAL MANIFESTATIONS AND DIAGNOSIS
- Regional suppurative lymphadenitis, sepsis, or fulminant pneumonia with plague
- Bioterrorism mass exposure: fulminant pneumonia
- Enteritis and pseudoappendicitis with *Y. enterocolitica, Y. pseudotuberculosis*
- Reactive arthritis or erythema nodosum may follow diarrhea; HLA-B27 predisposes
- Culture of blood, stool, bubo, or sputum
- Acute and convalescent serology

THERAPY
- Immediate use of antimicrobial agents: lifesaving for plague or *Yersinia* bacteremia
- Plague: streptomycin, 1 g twice daily; gentamicin, 5 mg/kg once daily; or levofloxacin, 500 to 750 mg once daily, preferred (see Table 162-1 for options)
- *Y. enterocolitica, Y. pseudotuberculosis* (aminoglycosides, tetracycline, fluoroquinolones)
- Antimicrobial agents generally unnecessary for enteritis or mesenteric lymphadenitis

PREVENTION
- Safe handling and preparation of pork products
- Avoid unpasteurized milk and dairy products
- Reduce rodent harborage; control fleas on pets
- Avoid contact with rodents and sick animals
- Bioterrorism exposure: doxycycline 100 mg twice daily or levofloxacin 500 mg, once daily

TABLE 162-1 Working Group on Civilian Biodefense Recommendations for Treatment of Adult Patients with Pneumonic Plague

Contained Casualty Setting
Preferred Choices

Streptomycin, 1 g IM twice daily

Gentamicin, 5 mg/kg IM or IV once daily or 2 mg/kg loading dose followed by 1.7 mg/kg IM or IV three times daily

Alternative Choices

Doxycycline, 100 mg IV twice daily or 200 mg IV once daily*

Ciprofloxacin, 400 mg IV twice daily[†]

Chloramphenicol, 25 mg/kg IV four times daily

Mass Casualty Setting or Postexposure Prophylaxis
Preferred Choices

Doxycycline, 100 mg orally twice daily*

Ciprofloxacin, 500 mg orally twice daily[†]

Alternative Choice

Chloramphenicol, 25 mg/kg orally four times daily

*Doxycycline and ciprofloxacin are pregnancy categories D and C, respectively.

[†]Ciprofloxacin has not been approved by the U.S. Food and Drug Administration (FDA) for this indication. Since the publication of the Working Group Recommendations, levofloxacin has been approved by FDA treatment of plague. Therefore, levofloxacin, at adult dosages of 500 to 750 mg once daily, should be considered the fluoroquinolone of choice for treatment and prophylaxis of plague.

Modified from Inglesby TV, Dennis DT, Henderson DA, et al. Plague as a biological weapon: medical and public health management. Working Group on Civilian Biodefense. *JAMA.* 2000;283:2281-2290.

163 *Bordetella pertussis*

Valerie Waters and Scott A. Halperin

DEFINITION

- Pertussis, infection with *Bordetella pertussis*, is divided in three stages:
  - Catarrhal stage: rhinorrhea, nonpurulent conjunctivitis, occasional cough, low-grade fever
  - Paroxysmal stage: paroxysms or fits of coughing, inspiratory whoop
  - Convalescent stage: gradually diminishing cough lasting up to 8 weeks
- Clinical case definition: cough greater than or equal to 14 days and one or more of the following: paroxysmal cough, inspiratory whoop, or post-tussive vomiting

EPIDEMIOLOGY

- With introduction of whole-cell pertussis vaccine in 1940s, pertussis rates dropped dramatically.
- Peaks of disease continue to occur every 3 to 5 years.
- Most cases, hospitalizations, and deaths occur in unimmunized infants younger than 6 months of age.
- Outbreaks in children with high vaccine rates may be partly due to waning immunity from acellular pertussis vaccine.

MICROBIOLOGY

- *Bordetella* species are small gram-negative coccobacilli; growth is fastidious.
- Filamentous hemagglutinin and fimbriae are two major adhesins.
- Pertussis toxin (PT) helps organism evade host defenses and causes systemic manifestations; it also acts as an adhesin.

DIAGNOSIS

- Diagnosis is traditionally made by culture from nasopharyngeal swabs or aspirates; specific swabs, transport media, and growth media should be used to enhance recovery.
- Newer polymerase chain reaction assays are more sensitive for detection of *B. pertussis* and are the procedure of choice.
- Antibodies to *B. pertussis* PT can be used for diagnosis.
- Direct fluorescent antibody is available but not recommended.

THERAPY

- Erythromycin, 40 to 50 mg/kg/day in four divided doses, is recommended for children (maximum 2 g/day) or clarithromycin, 15 mg/kg/day in two divided doses (maximum 1 g/day) for 7 to 14 days. Azithromycin is recommended for infants younger than 1 month of age. Five days of azithromycin is probably effective for treatment or prophylaxis in adults (500 mg first day, then 250 mg daily) and is better tolerated and has fewer serious drug interactions than erythromycin, 500 mg four times daily for 14 days.
- Supportive care is paramount in management of pertussis, especially in infants.

PREVENTION

- Immunization is the single most effective means of preventing pertussis.
- Pertussis immunization schedule in the United States and Canada for children and adolescents: DTaP (diphtheria toxoid, tetanus toxoid, acellular pertussis vaccine, pediatric formulation) 2, 4, 6, and 18 months, with booster at 4 to 6 years; and Tdap (tetanus toxoid, diphtheria toxoid, acellular pertussis vaccine, adult formulation [reduced doses of "d" and "ap" components]) for preadolescents/adolescents.
- In the United States and Canada, all adults age 19 years and older are recommended to receive a single dose of Tdap. The exception is pregnant women who, in the United States, are recommended to receive Tdap for each pregnancy, ideally in the 27th to 36th week of pregnancy, to protect their newborns from pertussis.
- All health care workers with patient contact should be given a single dose of Tdap if they have not been vaccinated as an adult, irrespective of when they received the last dose of tetanus toxoid.
- Prophylaxis can be considered for close contacts exposed within 21 days of onset of cough in the index case. Adults and adolescents are given erythromycin 500 mg four times daily for 7 to 14 days, azithromycin 500 mg the first day and 250 mg daily for 4 additional days, or clarithromycin 500 mg twice daily for 7 days.

164 Rat-Bite Fever: *Streptobacillus moniliformis* and *Spirillum minus*

Ronald G. Washburn

DEFINITION

- Rat-bite fever is an acute febrile illness characterized by rash and relapsing fever.

EPIDEMIOLOGY

- The infection is transmitted by bites or scratches from rodents or carnivores that prey on rodents or by ingestion of contaminated milk or water. Rat-bite fever is not generally reportable, and the incidence is probably higher than the literature reflects.

MICROBIOLOGY

- In the United States and Europe, rat-bite fever is caused by *Streptobacillus moniliformis*, a fastidious gram-negative bacillus. In Asia, the causative organism is *Spirillum minus*, a spirochete that has never been grown in culture.

DIAGNOSIS

- *S. moniliformis* is diagnosed by clinical presentation plus culture in enriched media or polymerase chain reaction. *S. minus* is diagnosed by clinical presentation plus direct visualization or xenodiagnosis.

THERAPY

- Penicillin is the treatment of choice for both types of rat-bite fever.

PREVENTION

- Preventive measures include eradication of rats, avoidance of nonpasteurized milk and water, and use of gloves by laboratory workers when handling rats.

165 Legionnaires' Disease and Pontiac Fever

Paul H. Edelstein and Craig R. Roy

DEFINITION

- Legionnaires' disease is a noncontagious type of bacterial pneumonia caused by *Legionella* spp. bacteria, most commonly *L. pneumophila*.
- Pontiac fever is a several day–long, nonpneumonic, febrile, influenza-like illness associated with exposure to *Legionella* spp. that resolves spontaneously.
- Legionellosis includes Legionnaires' disease, Pontiac fever, and extrapulmonary *Legionella* spp. infection not associated with pneumonia.

EPIDEMIOLOGY

- Legionnaires' disease is acquired by inhaling a water aerosol containing *Legionella* spp. bacteria, and possibly by microaspirating *Legionella* spp.–containing water.
- About 20 to 80 cases annually per million population occur in most developed countries, with the elderly, males, cigarette smokers, and immunosuppressed patients most at risk.
- About 1% to 5% of patients hospitalized for community-acquired pneumonia have Legionnaires' disease.
- Pontiac fever is associated with inhalation of *Legionella* spp.–containing water but not necessarily caused by the bacterium. It occurs in sporadic and epidemic form at apparently low incidence but may be more common than is reported.

MICROBIOLOGY

- Constituted of more than 58 known species, the *Legionella* bacteria are ubiquitous in the aqueous environment and probably moist soils.
- Optimal bacterial growth requires specialized media that contain cysteine and iron.
- The bacteria are facultative intracellular parasites of free-living amebas and human monocytes and macrophages that use hostlike proteins to masquerade as host and to avail themselves of intracellular resources.

DIAGNOSIS

- Clinical and roentgenographic differentiation of Legionnaires' disease from common causes of pneumonia is not generally possible.
- Specific and specialized laboratory testing can be helpful for disease diagnosis but is not highly sensitive in all settings. Urine antigen testing, the most commonly used test, is about 70% and 30% sensitive in community-acquired and nosocomial disease, respectively.

THERAPY

- Macrolides, tetracyclines, and quinolone antimicrobials can all be used to successfully treat the disease, with azithromycin and levofloxacin being the most active.

- For cure, 3 to 14 days' therapy is required, depending on disease severity, host factors, and type of therapy used.

PREVENTION
- No vaccine is available.
- Proper environmental design and maintenance reduce disease risk.

166 Capnocytophaga

J. Michael Janda

DEFINITION

- Endogenous or zoonotic-associated infections have been reported, depending on the species of *Capnocytophaga* involved.
- Symptoms range from sepsis (most often) with and without central nervous system involvement to ocular disease, illnesses associated with pregnancy, and those involving bone, joints, and soft tissues.

EPIDEMIOLOGY

- Endogenous infections arise in children or adults with blood dyscrasias and significant neutropenia.
- Sepsis arises from human species seeding into the circulatory system through abraded or damaged gums or gingival pockets in the oral cavity.
- Mortality rate is low (<5%) with appropriate treatment.
- Zoonotic infections arise primarily in males from a dog bite or intimate contact with dogs.
- Persons most at risk include dog owners, breeders, veterinarians, kennel workers, or hunters.
- Individuals at highest risk for developing serious life-threatening infections with disseminated intravascular coagulation include splenectomized persons or functionally asplenic patients and those with ethanol abuse or immunosuppression.
- Reported mortality rates range from 20% to 33%.

MICROBIOLOGY

- Bacilli are gram negative with tapered ends.
- They are slow growing and fastidious, requiring 3 to 10 days of incubation on supportive media.
- No standardized method of determining drug susceptibilities exists, but testing should be attempted, if possible.

DIAGNOSIS

- Is history compatible with *Capnocytophaga* infection (dog bite)?
- Does Gram or Wright-Giemsa stain of blood or other sterile specimens show bacilli with tapered ends sometimes within polymorphonuclear leukocytes?
- Conventional tests that include catalase, oxidase, and arginine dihydrolase are slow but reliable.
- Rapid molecular tests include 16S rRNA gene sequencing for rapid diagnosis on specimens or identification of isolated organisms and matrix-assisted laser desorption/ionization time-of-flight (MALDI-TOF) mass spectrometry for future organism characterization.

THERAPY

- Infection is broadly susceptible to many antimicrobial agents.
- Penicillin/β-lactamase inhibitor combination or extended-spectrum cephalosporin is drug of first choice.
- Acquired drug resistance has been reported in some isolates.

PREVENTION

- Clinicians must be made aware of these organisms, the diseases they cause, and the patients at risk.
- Laboratories may require extra incubation time, a specialized incubation atmosphere, and richer media to isolate these organisms.
- Use rapid testing methods to decrease time to diagnosis.

167 Bartonella, Including Cat-Scratch Disease

Tejal N. Gandhi, Leonard N. Slater, David F. Welch, and Jane E. Koehler

EPIDEMIOLOGY AND MICROBIOLOGY

- Fastidious, facultatively intracellular, pleomorphic gram-negative bacilli
- Transmission via feces of arthropod vectors or by direct inoculation into nonintact skin
- *Bartonella bacilliformis:* endemic only in the Andes mountains; reservoir—humans, and possibly, an animal reservoir
- *Bartonella henselae:* globally endemic; reservoir—cats; vector—cat flea; transmitted to humans usually via cat scratch
- *Bartonella quintana:* sporadic outbreaks worldwide; associated with homelessness and other conditions of poor sanitation; reservoir—humans; vector—human body louse

CLINICAL FEATURES

- Chronic bloodstream infections (for months) is a hallmark of *Bartonella* infections
- *B. bacilliformis:* biphasic illness; Oroya fever (acute phase) characterized by fever, hemolytic anemia, and high fatality rate when untreated; verruga peruana (late phase) characterized by crops of angioproliferative skin lesions with an evolution of stages
- *B. henselae:* cat-scratch disease (CSD): self-limited regional lymphadenopathy
- *B. henselae:* bacillary angiomatosis (BA): vascular proliferative disorder observed in patients with advanced human immunodeficiency virus (HIV) infection and other immunocompromising conditions; cutaneous BA, hepatic, and splenic bacillary peliosis (BP)
- *B. henselae:* blood culture–negative endocarditis, usually in patients with preexisting valvular lesions
- *B. henselae:* cause of fever of unknown origin (FUO) in immunocompetent children, and in immunocompromised patients (HIV-infected and transplant recipients)
- *B. quintana:* trench fever: usually a self-limited febrile illness
- *B. quintana:* blood culture–negative endocarditis; can occur in patients with normal heart valves
- *B. quintana:* bacillary angiomatosis (cutaneous, subcutaneous, osseous)
- *B. quintana:* cause of FUO in HIV-infected patients

DIAGNOSIS

- Difficult to culture
- Serology: mainstay for diagnosis, but cross-reactivity among *Bartonella* species common
- Histopathology: CSD—granulomatous inflammation; BA—vascular proliferation; Warthin-Starry or Steiner stain demonstrates *Bartonella* bacilli in tissue
- Polymerase chain reaction testing on tissue or blood

THERAPY

- CSD: no treatment (self-limited); possibly azithromycin for severe CSD
- Endocarditis: doxycycline for 6 weeks and gentamicin for first 2 weeks; renal insufficiency common in *Bartonella* endocarditis, thus rifampin can be substituted for gentamicin in the setting of renal insufficiency

- Bacteremia: doxycycline for 4 weeks and gentamicin for first 2 weeks
- BA/BP: doxycycline is first choice and erythromycin or azithromycin is second choice; in HIV-infected and transplant recipients, doxycycline is preferred due to tolerability issues and drug-drug interaction potential with erythromycin; duration of 3 months or longer for cutaneous disease and 6 months or longer for severe *Bartonella* infection (e.g., BP, central nervous system)
- Neuroretinitis: doxycycline and rifampin for 4 to 6 weeks

PREVENTION

- Avoid arthropod vectors; eradicate body lice to reduce risk of *B. quintana*
- Avoid cat scratches, bites, licks, and cat fleas to reduce risk of *B. henselae;* control of cat flea infestation is important

168 Klebsiella granulomatis (Donovanosis, Granuloma Inguinale)

Ronald C. Ballard

DEFINITION

- Donovanosis is an ulcerative sexually transmitted infection caused by an intracellular bacterium, *Klebsiella granulomatis*.

EPIDEMIOLOGY

- Donovanosis is largely confined to discrete geographic areas of the tropics.
- Donovanosis is sexually transmitted but of low infectivity.

MICROBIOLOGY

- *Klebsiella granulomatis* is a gram-negative, encapsulated, intracellular bacterium exhibiting bipolar densities.

DIAGNOSIS

- For microscopic examination, biopsies or smears are obtained from the margin of active lesions for "Donovan bodies."

THERAPY

- The treatment of choice is azithromycin, 1 g weekly for up to 4 to 6 weeks.
- Treatment should be continued until complete epithelialization has occurred.

169 Other Gram-Negative and Gram-Variable Bacilli

James P. Steinberg and Eileen M. Burd

SHORT VIEW SUMMARY

Definition

- Gram-negative and gram-variable aerobic bacilli that are less commonly encountered as causes of infection and are not discussed in other chapters are considered here.
- The taxonomy of many of these organisms has been and continues to be in a state of flux.
- The organisms considered are broadly divided into those that ferment glucose and those that weakly ferment or do not ferment glucose. Specific genera considered include *Aggregatibacter, Aeromonas, Cardiobacterium, Chromobacterium, Dysgonomonas, Plesiomonas, Achromobacter, Alcaligenes, Chryseobacterium, Elizabethkingia, Comamonas, Delftia, Eikenella, Flavobacterium, Myroides, Ochrobactrum, Oligella,* less common species of *Pseudomonas, Ralstonia, Cupriavidus, Rhizobium, Roseomonas, Shewanella, Sphingobacterium, Sphingomonas, Bergeyella, Weeksella, Gardnerella, Mobiluncus,* uncommon *Neisseria* species, and Centers for Disease Control and Prevention Groups NO-1, WO-1, WO-2, O-1, O-2, and O-3.

Epidemiology

- Some of these gram-negative bacilli are ubiquitous in the environment.
- Many are generally considered to be of low virulence but may be opportunistic pathogens under certain circumstances.
- Some infections have been linked to hospital sources, particularly unclean water sources, nonsterile environmental surfaces, or contaminated solutions.

Microbiology

- Many of these organisms are fastidious and difficult to grow.
- Identification of glucose nonfermenting gram-negative bacilli poses a challenge to clinical laboratories because conventional biochemical systems frequently fail to provide accurate identification. Accurate identification, especially to species level, often requires cell wall fatty acid analysis, 16S rRNA gene sequencing–based technologies, or matrix-assisted laser desorption/ionization-time of flight mass spectrometry.

Diagnosis

- The types of infections caused by these organisms are quite varied and are diagnosed by analysis of cultures of samples taken from the infection site.
- Because these organisms are infrequently encountered and are often of low virulence, interpretation of culture results must be correlated with clinical findings.

Therapy

- The small number of patients reported and the variety of antibiotic regimens used do not permit identification of the optimal therapeutic regimen for most of these organisms.

- Methods for antibiotic susceptibility testing for many of these organisms are not standardized and Clinical and Laboratory Standards Institute breakpoints for interpretation may not be available.
- Some of the environmental bacteria are of concern because they carry resistance genes on transferable genetic elements and could serve as reservoirs of resistance genes when introduced into the clinical setting.
- Some of these infections may be difficult to eradicate when the causative bacteria exist in well-developed biofilms.

Prevention

- Attention should be given to practices to prevent device-related infections, particularly in immunocompromised individuals.
- Hospital-based programs of surveillance and methods for prevention and control to eliminate health care–associated infections should be implemented.

170 Syphilis *(Treponema pallidum)*

Justin D. Radolf, Edmund C. Tramont, and Juan C. Salazar

DEFINITION

- Syphilis is a chronic, multistage sexually transmitted disease caused by the spirochete *Treponema pallidum.*

EPIDEMIOLOGY

- According to the World Health Organization, 11 million new cases of venereal syphilis occur globally each year.
- Globally, 1.5 million pregnant women are estimated to be infected each year; approximately one third of these infections will result in stillbirths or other adverse outcomes of pregnancy.
- In developing countries, transmission is largely heterosexual, while transmission among men who have sex with men predominates in industrialized nations.
- Genital ulcers caused by syphilis are a major cofactor for bidirectional transmission of human immunodeficiency virus (HIV).

MICROBIOLOGY

- *T. pallidum* subspecies *pallidum, pertenue,* and *endemicum* cause venereal syphilis, yaws, and endemic syphilis, respectively. *Treponema carateum* causes pinta.
- All pathogenic treponemes are noncultivable and indistinguishable by routine clinical laboratory tests.
- Humans are the only natural hosts for *T. pallidum* subsp. *pallidum.*
- *T. pallidum* possesses both inner and outer membranes; its outer membrane lacks lipopolysaccharide and contains a paucity of integral membrane proteins and surface-exposed lipoproteins, hence its designation as "the stealth pathogen."
- *T. pallidum* must acquire essentially all nutrients from its obligate human host and generates adenosine triphosphate primarily by glycolysis.
- *T. pallidum* disseminates early during the course of infection and invades the central nervous system in a substantial percentage of persons with early syphilis.

DIAGNOSIS

- Because *T. pallidum* cannot be cultivated in vitro, diagnosis of syphilis depends on direct demonstration of treponemes in clinical samples or reactivity in serologic tests, or both.
- Darkfield microscopy and polymerase chain reaction are useful for detecting treponemes in exudative lesions, principally chancres.
- Serodiagnosis of syphilis involves two types of serologic tests: nontreponemal and treponemal. The former detects antibodies against lipoidal antigens (primarily cardiolipin), whereas the latter detects antibodies against *T. pallidum* proteins.
- Nontreponemal antibody tests are used as indicators of disease activity; nontreponemal titers tend to decline with therapy. Treponemal tests remain reactive for life.
- Treponemal tests are used to confirm that reactivity in nontreponemal tests is due to syphilis as opposed to being a biologic false positive.

THERAPY

- Penicillin G is the preferred form of therapy for all stages and types of infection.
- 2.4 million units of IM benzathine penicillin is the Centers for Disease Control and Prevention–recommended regimen for early syphilis *regardless* of HIV status.
- Doxycycline is the preferred alternative for nonpregnant, penicillin-allergic patients.
- Penicillin-allergic pregnant females should be desensitized.

PREVENTION

- Prophylactic treatment is indicated for partners exposed to known active cases within the past 90 days regardless of whether lesions are present or serologies are reactive.
- Early identification and treatment of gestational syphilis prevents congenital infection.

171 Endemic Treponematoses

Edward W. Hook III

DEFINITION

- The endemic treponematoses include yaws, endemic syphilis, and pinta. All are cutaneous diseases most common in children and caused by treponemes closely related to *Treponema pallidum*, the causative agent of syphilis.

EPIDEMIOLOGY

- The endemic treponematoses are spread only from human to human by direct contact. The infections are most common in children but if untreated may progress to cause chronic skin and bone disease. Over the past 2 decades, yaws rates have increased worldwide. Endemic syphilis and pinta remain very uncommon.

MICROBIOLOGY

- The treponemal species that cause the endemic treponematoses cannot be easily cultured for diagnosis. Microbiologic diagnosis is most often based on nontreponemal and treponemal serologic reactivity in tests designed for syphilis diagnosis.

DIAGNOSIS

- The diagnosis of endemic treponematoses is based on clinical recognition of compatible skin lesions, confirmed by serologic testing.

THERAPY

- Until recently, benzathine penicillin was the mainstay of therapy of the endemic treponematoses. Recently, azithromycin has been proven as an easy-to-administer alternative to penicillin injections for therapy of yaws.

PREVENTION

- Yaws appears to be amenable to mass therapy as a control and prevention measure. In 2012, the World Health Organization announced plans to embark on mass therapy initiatives designed to eliminate yaws by 2020.

172 *Leptospira* Species (Leptospirosis)

David A. Haake and Paul N. Levett

DEFINITION

- Leptospirosis is caused by infection with pathogenic spirochetes of the genus *Leptospira*.

EPIDEMIOLOGY

- Leptospirosis is a zoonosis of global distribution.
- Leptospirosis is maintained in nature by chronic renal infection of carrier animals, especially rodents.
- Infections typically occur following occupational or recreational exposure to water or soil contaminated with rodent urine.
- In developing countries with poor housing standards, leptospirosis outbreaks occur regularly in urban settings after heavy rainfall and flooding.

MICROBIOLOGY

- Twenty-one named leptospiral species have been described, of which 11 are known to be pathogenic (see Table 172-1).

DIAGNOSIS

- Clinical diagnosis requires a high index of suspicion based on epidemiologic exposure.
- Serologic tests are helpful when positive but may have poor sensitivity during the first week of illness.
- The signs and symptoms of early leptospirosis are nonspecific.

THERAPY

- Antibiotic therapy (see Table 172-2) should be initiated as early in the course of the disease as suspicion allows. For mild disease, doxycycline, amoxicillin, or oral ampicillin is recommended. For more severe disease, intravenous ceftriaxone, ampicillin, or penicillin is used.
- Patients with early renal disease with high-output renal dysfunction and hypokalemia should receive aggressive volume repletion and potassium supplementation.
- Patients who progress to oliguric renal failure should undergo rapid initiation of hemodialysis or peritoneal dialysis, which is typically required on only a short-term basis.

PREVENTION

- The most effective preventive strategy is to reduce direct contact with potentially infected animals and indirect contact with urine-contaminated soil and water.
- Chemoprophylaxis with doxycycline 200 mg once a week is recommended for individuals who will be unavoidably exposed to endemic environments.

TABLE 172-1 Species of *Leptospira* and Some Pathogenic Serovars

SPECIES	SELECTED PATHOGENIC SEROVARS
L. interrogans	Icterohaemorrhagiae, Copenhageni, Canicola, Pomona, Australis, Autumnalis, Pyrogenes, Bratislava, Lai
L. noguchii	Panama, Pomona
L. borgpetersenii	Ballum, Hardjo, Javanica
L. santarosai	Bataviae
L. kirschneri	Bim, Bulgarica, Grippotyphosa, Cynopteri
L. weilii	Celledoni, Sarmin
L. alexanderi	Manhao 3
L. alstonii	Sichuan
L. meyeri	Sofia
L. wolffii	Khorat
L. kmetyi	Manilae
L. wolbachii	Nonpathogen
L. biflexa	Nonpathogen
L. vanthielii	Nonpathogen
L. terpstrae	Nonpathogen
L. yanagawae	Nonpathogen
L. idonii	Nonpathogen
L. inadai	Indeterminate
L. fainei	Indeterminate
L. broomii	Indeterminate
L. licerasiae	Indeterminate

TABLE 172-2 Antimicrobial Agents Recommended for Treatment and Chemoprophylaxis of Leptospirosis

INDICATION	COMPOUND	DOSAGE
Chemoprophylaxis	Doxycycline	200 mg PO orally once per week
Treatment of mild leptospirosis	Doxycycline	100 mg bid PO
	Ampicillin	500-750 mg q6h PO
	Amoxicillin	500 mg q6h PO
Treatment of moderate to severe leptospirosis	Penicillin	1.5 MU IV q6h
	Ceftriaxone	1 g IV q24h
	Ampicillin	0.5-1 g IV q6h

173 Relapsing Fever Caused by *Borrelia* Species

James M. Horton

DEFINITION
- Relapsing fever is caused by spirochetes of the *Borrelia* genus.
- The illness is characterized by relapsing fevers with spirochetes evident on a blood smear.

ORGANISM
- *Borrelia* species are divided between *B. burgdorferi,* which causes Lyme disease, and the *Borrelia* species that cause relapsing fever.
- The relapsing fever species are divided between the louse-borne and tick-borne species.

EPIDEMIOLOGY
- Tick-borne relapsing fever occurs on almost every continent, but in the United States it is endemic in the Rocky Mountains.

PATHOPHYSIOLOGY
- The spirochete changes surface antigens about every 7 days, causing the cyclic, relapsing fever.

CLINICAL MANIFESTATIONS
- The patient presents with fever for 3 days alternating with afebrile periods lasting about 7 days.

DIAGNOSIS
- Spirochetes can be seen on the peripheral blood smear during febrile periods.

THERAPY
- Doxycycline or penicillin is effective treatment.
- Jarisch-Herxheimer reactions are common, and the patient should be observed in a clinic or hospital for about 3 hours after starting antibiotic therapy.

PREVENTION
- Postexposure therapy with doxycycline is preventive.

174 Lyme Disease (Lyme Borreliosis) Due to *Borrelia burgdorferi*

Allen C. Steere

DEFINITION

- A tick-borne infection caused by the spirochete *Borrelia burgdorferi* sensu lato leading to a multisystem illness primarily in the skin, joints, nervous system, heart, or a combination of these.

EPIDEMIOLOGY

- The vectors of Lyme disease are 14 closely related ixodid tick species that are part of the *Ixodes ricinus* complex.
- The disease occurs in parts of North America, Europe, and Asia.
- The disorder in the United States occurs primarily in three distinct foci: in the Northeast from Maine to North Carolina; in the Midwest in Wisconsin, Minnesota, and Michigan; and in the West, primarily in northern California.
- The peak onset of early infection is in the summer months.
- About 30,000 cases are reported yearly in the United States, mostly from the northeastern United States.

MICROBIOLOGY

- The genus *Borrelia* currently includes 13 closely related species known collectively as *Borrelia burgdorferi* sensu lato (*B. burgdorferi* in the general sense).
- The human infection is caused primarily by three pathogenic species: *B. burgdorferi* sensu stricto (*B. burgdorferi* in the strict sense) is the sole cause in the United States, whereas *Borrelia afzelii* and *Borrelia garinii* are the primary causes of the infection in Europe.

DIAGNOSIS

- Culture of *B. burgdorferi* in Barbour-Stoenner-Kelly (BSK) medium permits definitive diagnosis but has been possible reliably only from biopsies of erythema migrans skin lesions, an early disease manifestation.
- Diagnosis is usually based on characteristic clinical findings and a positive IgG serologic test result, using a two-test approach of enzyme-linked immunosorbent assay and Western blot.

THERAPY

- For early infection, appropriate oral antibiotic therapy (usually doxycycline, 100 mg twice daily or amoxicillin, 500 mg three times daily) for 14 to 21 days is usually successful.
- For neurologic involvement or some cases of arthritis, intravenous antibiotic therapy (often ceftriaxone, 2 g daily) for 28 days may be necessary.

PREVENTION

- Personal protection methods to avoid tick bites and tick checks after exposure in endemic areas are the major prevention strategies.
- A vaccine for Lyme disease consisting of recombinant OspA with adjuvant was shown to be safe and effective, but the vaccine is not now available.

175 *Clostridium difficile* Infection

Dale N. Gerding and Vincent B. Young

DEFINITION

- *Clostridium difficile* infection (CDI) is acute diarrhea and colitis that is most often preceded by antimicrobial use and is caused by an anaerobic spore-forming, toxin-producing bacterium.

EPIDEMIOLOGY

- *C. difficile* is found in water, soil, meats, and vegetables and is particularly common in health care environments, where the spores are difficult to eradicate. Patients are exposed to and ingest *C. difficile* spores in the health care setting from contact with the environment or health care workers who do not practice good hand hygiene.
- If the patient has taken antibiotics recently, the normal microbiota is likely to be disrupted; and in this disrupted microbiota, the ingested spores, which are resistant to stomach acid, can germinate and proliferate in the colon, producing two major toxins: TcdA and TcdB.
- The two toxins produce a marked neutrophilic inflammatory response in the colon, resulting in diarrhea, erosion of the mucosa, and formation of pseudomembranes composed of necrotic cells and proteinaceous material that extend over the mucosal surface.
- Recurrence of diarrhea after treatment occurs in 25% of patients and requires re-treatment.

MICROBIOLOGY

- *C. difficile* is an obligate gram-positive anaerobic bacterium that can survive in environments under aerobic conditions by forming spores.
- The majority of strains produce both toxins A and B. A third toxin, binary toxin, is produced by recent epidemic strains that have caused outbreaks with increased severity and mortality.
- Some strains of *C. difficile* lack the genes for toxin production and are nontoxigenic and not believed to cause CDI.

DIAGNOSIS

- Diagnosis of CDI is based on the presence of clinical symptoms (usually defined as more than three watery, loose or unformed stools within ≤24 hours) coupled with a diagnostic test (usually of a stool specimen) that either detects the presence of the *C. difficile* organism or its toxin genes or detects *C. difficile* toxin using an enzyme immunoassay or cell cytotoxin assay.

THERAPY

- The first steps in effective treatment are to stop any therapy with the offending antibiotic and provide fluid and electrolyte support, if needed.
- Specific treatment consists of metronidazole or vancomycin orally for mild-to-moderate disease, vancomycin orally for severe disease (white blood cell count >15,000/mL or creatinine concentration >1.5 times baseline), and vancomycin orally or by nasogastric tube plus

intravenous metronidazole for severe complicated (also called fulminant) CDI that presents as hypotension, shock, ileus, or megacolon.
- Patients with recurrent CDI may benefit from fidaxomicin treatment, and multiple CDI recurrences are effectively treated by fecal microbiota transplant (FMT).

PREVENTION

- Prevention in the health care environment is focused on preventing patient exposure to spores of *C. difficile* by utilizing isolation, cohorting, gloves and gowns, and hand washing (alcohol rubs are ineffective against spores). Bleach is used in the environment to eradicate spores.
- It is exceedingly difficult to prevent spore exposure, so antimicrobial stewardship programs to reduce unnecessary antimicrobial use are extremely effective in limiting the number of susceptible patients.
- A number of new preventive approaches are undergoing clinical investigation, including vaccines to induce antibodies to toxins A and B, monoclonal antibodies to provide passive immunity, and biotherapeutics that are live bacterial organisms such as FMT or spores of nontoxigenic *C. difficile*.

176 Tetanus *(Clostridium tetani)*

Aimee Hodowanec and Thomas P. Bleck

DEFINITION

- Tetanus is a nervous system disease caused by a toxin (tetanospasmin) produced by *Clostridium tetani.*
- Tetanus is divided into four clinical types: *generalized, localized, cephalic,* and *neonatal.*

EPIDEMIOLOGY

- Acute injury and injection drug use are risk factors for tetanus.
- Tetanus is rare in developed countries due to the availability of effective vaccines.
- In developing countries, neonatal tetanus can occur when there is failure of aseptic technique and mothers are inadequately immunized.
- In the United States, tetanus is more common in people older than 60 years, likely due to waning immunity.

MICROBIOLOGY

- *C. tetani* is an obligately anaerobic bacillus.
- Tetanus produces two toxins: tetanospasmin and tetanolysin.
- It develops a terminal spore that is extremely stable in the environment, retaining the ability to germinate and cause disease indefinitely.

DIAGNOSIS

- Diagnosis of tetanus relies on history and examination findings.
- Culturing *C. tetani* is difficult and not helpful.

THERAPY

- The airway must be secured at the time of presentation.
- Benzodiazepines provide the mainstay of symptomatic therapy.
- Passive immunization with human tetanus immune globulin (HTIG) shortens the disease course and may lessen disease severity.
- Antibiotic therapy with metronidazole (Flagyl) may improve outcomes.

PREVENTION

- All children should be vaccinated against tetanus through DTaP vaccine series.
- Adults should receive a tetanus booster (Td) every 10 years. One of the Td doses should be replaced with Tdap.
- Wound management of minor, clean wounds should include completion of tetanus immunization if incomplete, or a booster dose of vaccine (Td), if the last dose was given more than 10 years before. Patients with serious contaminated wounds should also receive HTIG.

177 Botulism *(Clostridium botulinum)*

Aimee Hodowanec and Thomas P. Bleck

DEFINITION

- Botulism is a toxin-mediated paralytic illness caused by *Clostridium botulinum*. It is classified as foodborne botulism, infant botulism, wound botulism, iatrogenic botulism, botulism of undetermined etiology, or inhalational botulism.

EPIDEMIOLOGY

- Foodborne botulism occurs in outbreaks, whereas other forms are sporadic.
- Foodborne botulism is associated with home-canned or fermented foods.
- Infant botulism historically is associated with honey ingestion.
- Wound botulism is associated with injection drug use of "black-tar" heroin.
- Botulinum toxins A and B are used for therapeutic and cosmetic purposes and may cause iatrogenic botulism.
- Botulism is a potential bioterrorism agent deployed by aerosol or ingestion.

MICROBIOLOGY

- *C. botulinum* is a gram-positive, strictly anaerobic bacillus that forms a subterminal spore.
- *C. botulinum* produces seven distinct toxins, designated types A through G.

DIAGNOSIS

- Presumptive diagnosis based on clinical presentation: acute, bilateral cranial neuropathies with symmetrical descending weakness.
- Mouse bioassay is the gold standard for botulinum toxin.
- Culture of serum, stool, and environmental samples requires strict anaerobic conditions and is low yield.
- Characteristic electrophysiologic study findings are suggestive of botulism.

THERAPY

- Supportive care remains the mainstay of botulism treatment.
- Heptavalent botulinum antitoxin is available for noninfant botulism in the United States.
- Human botulinum immune globulin (BabyBIG) is available for the treatment of infant (younger than 1 year) botulism. To obtain, contact the California Department of Health Services, Infant Botulism Treatment and Prevention Program (510-540-2646; www.infantbotulism.org).

PREVENTION

- Proper food preparation prevents foodborne botulism.
- There is no currently available vaccine.

178 Gas Gangrene and Other *Clostridium*-Associated Diseases

Andrew B. Onderdonk and Wendy S. Garrett

CHARACTERISTICS OF *CLOSTRIDIUM* SPP.

- Member of the phylum Firmicutes
- Anaerobic gram-positive rods capable of forming endospores
- Ubiquitous in nature
- Phenotypic classification methods include carbohydrate fermentation, detection of short-chain fatty acid end products of fermentation, Gram-stain morphology, colony morphology, and detection of specific toxins
- Various species associated with human disease (see Table 178-1)

CLOSTRIDIUM PERFRINGENS AND CLOSTRIDIAL MYONECROSIS (GAS GANGRENE)

- *C. perfringens* produces a variety of toxins (see Table 178-2)
- Most common following traumatic crushing injuries that result in lowered tissue oxygen levels, penetrating trauma involving foreign bodies contaminated with soil, gastrointestinal or biliary tract surgery, and septic abortion
- Diagnosis: Initial symptoms include severe pain, redness at the wound site followed by rapidly spreading brown to purple discoloration, edema and gas, and serosanguineous discharge with a characteristic "mousy" odor. Full-blown sepsis with hypotension, renal failure, and metabolic acidosis occurs rapidly.
- Treatment involves prompt surgical débridement of infected tissues, including amputation for extremities, or hysterectomy in uterine gas gangrene. Antibiotic treatment is also important, and most strains are sensitive to penicillin, metronidazole, clindamycin, and the carbapenems.

FOOD POISONING CAUSED BY *CLOSTRIDIUM PERFRINGENS*

- *C. perfringens* type A involved in most cases
- Involves the ingestion of at least 10^8 viable enterotoxin-producing cells
- Period of incubation is 7 to 15 hours; cases resolve spontaneously within 24 to 48 hours

OTHER CLOSTRIDIAL INFECTIONS

- Bacteremia—clostridia account for 1% of all positive blood cultures. Risk factors include hemodialysis, intestinal malignancy, and inflammatory bowel disease.
- Biliary tract infections—clostridia can be isolated from more than 20% of diseased gallbladders, and *C. perfringens* accounts for 50%.
- Female genital tract infections—clostridia are present in up to 20% of non–sexually transmitted disease genital infections and may be present as part of bacterial vaginosis. *C. perfringens* and *C. sordellii* can be isolated from postpartum and postabortion infections.
- Pleuropulmonary infections—clostridia are recovered from up to 10% of pulmonary infections with *C. perfringens* accounting for the majority.

TABLE 178-1 Clostridial Species Commonly Associated with Human Disease

SPECIES	SPORE LOCATION	LECITHINASE PRODUCED	LIPASE	ENTEROTOXINS PRODUCED	HISTOTOXINS, HEMOLYSINS, PROTEASES	NEUROTOXINS PRODUCED
Tissue Infections						
C. perfringens	ST, C	+	–	Yes	Yes	No
C. ramosum	T	–	–	No	Yes	No
C. septicum	ST	–	–	No	Yes	No
C. sordellii	ST	+	–	No	Yes	No
C. bifermentans	ST	+	–	No	Yes	No
C. tertium	T	–	–	No	Yes	No
C. sphenoides	ST	–	–	No	Yes	No
C. baratii	ST	–	–	No	Yes	No
C. novyi	ST	+	+	No	Yes	No
C. histolyticum	ST	–	–	No	Yes	No
Intoxications						
C. difficile	ST	–	–	Yes	Yes	No
C. botulinum	ST, T	–	+	No	Yes	Yes
C. tetani	T	–	–	No	Yes	Yes

C, centrally; ST, subterminally; T, terminally.

TABLE 178-2 Toxins Produced by *Clostridium perfringens*

TOXIN	STRAIN TYPES	BIOLOGIC ACTIVITY
α	All strains	Lecithinase
β	B and C	Necrotoxin, necrosis of the bowel
ε	B and D	Lethal, hemorrhagic
ι	E	Adenosine diphosphate ribosylating; lethal
cpe enterotoxin	A, C, and D	Cytopathic
Neuraminidase	All strains	Hydrolyzes *N*-acetylneuraminic acid
δ	B and C	Hemolysins
κ	All strains	Collagenase
λ	B, D, and E	Protease
μ	All strains	Hyaluronidase
ν	All strains	DNAase

179 Bacteroides, Prevotella, Porphyromonas, and Fusobacterium Species (and Other Medically Important Anaerobic Gram-Negative Bacilli)

Wendy S. Garrett and Andrew B. Onderdonk

DEFINITION

- *Bacteroides*, *Porphyromonas*, *Prevotella*, and *Fusobacterium* spp. account for the majority of infections caused by anaerobic gram-negative rods. *Bilophila* and *Sutterella* spp. also cause human infections, although they are less frequently encountered.

EPIDEMIOLOGY

- These organisms are part of the normal human microbiome and can be isolated from the oral cavity, gastrointestinal tract, and vaginal vault of humans.

MICROBIOLOGY

- The organisms are obligately anaerobic, gram-negative, non–spore-forming rods. Members of this group can be proteolytic, saccharolytic, or both. Some species produce catalase and superoxide dismutase in low concentrations. Some species have capsular polysaccharides that have been shown to be potent immunomodulators, whereas other species produce abundant proteases that can degrade tissue.

DIAGNOSIS

- Identification in the clinical laboratory includes colony morphology, Gram stain, pigment production visualized in natural light and as fluorescence emission after exposure to ultraviolet light, and numerous biochemical tests (e.g., Vitek).

THERAPY

- Treatment is directed by culture and sensitivity test results (see Table 179-1).

TABLE 179-1 Antibiotic Sensitivities of Medically Important Gram-Negative Anaerobic Rods

	PENICILLIN	β-LACTAM	PIPERACILLIN/ TAZOBACTAM	AMOXICILLIN/ CLAVULANIC ACID	CLINDAMYCIN	CARBAPENEM	METRONIDAZOLE	MOXIFLOXACIN
Bacteroides fragilis group	R	V	S	S	V	S	S	S
Prevotella	R	V	S	S	S	S	S	S
Porphyromonas	R	V	S	S	S	S	S	S
Fusobacterium	S	V	S	S	S	S	S	S

R, resistant >30%; S, sensitive <5%; V, variable >5%.

180 Mycobacterium tuberculosis

Daniel W. Fitzgerald, Timothy R. Sterling, and David W. Haas

MICROBIOLOGY

- Humans are the only reservoir for *Mycobacterium tuberculosis*.
- The organism is an acid-fast, aerobic bacillus with a high cell wall content of high-molecular-weight lipids.
- Visible growth takes 3 to 8 weeks on solid media.
- An estimated 10,000 organisms/mL are required for sputum smear positivity.
- Incomplete necrosis produces cheesy, acellular material (i.e., caseous necrosis).
- Pulmonary cavities contain huge numbers of organisms.

EPIDEMIOLOGY

- *M. tuberculosis* infects one third of the world's population, with 8.7 million new cases reported each year.
- Almost all infections are due to inhalation of droplet nuclei.
- Key determinants of infection of tuberculin-negative persons are closeness of contact and infectiousness of the source.
- The strongest risk factor for progression to active tuberculosis is acquired immunodeficiency syndrome (AIDS).
- Greatest case rates are in countries heavily affected by AIDS.
- Drug resistance can be primary or secondary.
- Multidrug-resistant tuberculosis (MDR-TB) indicates resistance to both isoniazid and rifampin.
- Extensively drug-resistant tuberculosis (XDR-TB) indicates resistance to isoniazid, rifampin, a fluoroquinolone, and a second-line injectable drug.
- Transmission of XDR-TB is of immense concern.

IMMUNOLOGY AND PATHOGENESIS

- Infection requires a cellular immune response.
- Airborne droplet nuclei reach the terminal air-spaces where they are ingested by alveolar macrophages and then carried by lymphatics to regional lymph nodes.
- Occult preallergic lymphohematogenous dissemination occurs to the lung apices and elsewhere.
- Granulomas form when antigen load is small and tissue hypersensitivity is high.
- Age influences likelihood and pattern of disease.
- Tuberculosis in advanced AIDS is characterized by middle or lower lung field location, absence of cavitation, increased extrapulmonary disease, and a negative tuberculin test.

TUBERCULIN SKIN TESTING AND INTERFERON-γ RELEASE ASSAYS

- To detect latent *M. tuberculosis* infection, a positive skin test is defined by induration.
- Skin testing is recommended for persons at high risk for developing tuberculosis and those with possible latent infection who can be treated if the test is positive.

365

- The skin test is negative in at least 20% of active tuberculosis cases.
- Interferon-γ release assays may be used instead of skin testing.

DIAGNOSIS

- Culture is the gold standard.
- Liquid broth cultures require 1 to 3 weeks to detect organisms.
- Nucleic acid amplification tests have sensitivities and specificities that approach culture.
- Three sputum specimens increase sensitivity.
- A radiograph showing a patchy or nodular infiltrate in the lung apices is highly suggestive, especially if the infiltrate is cavitary.
- Pulmonary tuberculosis can occur in persons with normal chest radiographs.

THERAPY (SEE TABLES 180-1 AND 180-2)

- Multidrug regimens, typically starting with at least four active drugs, are recommended.
- At least 6 months of therapy is usually required.
- Isoniazid (INH) is the cornerstone of therapy; rifampin, the second major antituberculous agent, causes many drug-drug interactions; pyrazinamide is essential for 6-month regimens.
- Adjustment of doses of antiretroviral agents during treatment of tuberculosis with rifampin and rifabutin is discussed in *Mandell, Douglas, and Bennett's Principles and Practice of Infectious Diseases*, 8th Edition, Chapter 38.
- Directly observed therapy is crucial.
- Susceptibility testing is important to guide therapy.
- With appropriate chemotherapy, patients become noninfectious within 2 weeks.
- Treatment of XDR-TB is usually associated with poor outcomes.
- Bedaquiline is a recently approved drug for MDR-TB.

THERAPY FOR LATENT INFECTION

- In the United States, 9 months of INH is widely prescribed for latent infection.
- Twelve weeks of directly observed, once-weekly INH plus rifapentine is as effective as 9 months of INH. For adults weighing more than 50 kg, the dose of both drugs is 900 mg once a week.

PREVENTION

- Case finding and treatment is the most effective method of tuberculosis control.
- Hospitalized human immunodeficiency virus–positive patients with respiratory symptoms should be admitted to negative-pressure isolation rooms. N95 masks are used for health care workers.
- Childhood bacillus Calmette-Guérin vaccination in high-burden countries decreases incident tuberculosis.

TABLE 180-1 Drug Regimens for Culture-Positive Pulmonary Tuberculosis Caused by Drug-Susceptible Organisms

		INITIAL PHASE			CONTINUATION PHASE		
Regimen	Drugs	Interval and Doses* (Minimal Duration)	Regimen	Drugs	Interval and Doses*† (Minimal Duration)	Range of Total Doses (Minimal Duration)
1	INH RIF PZA EMB	7 days/wk for 56 doses (8 wk) or 5 days/wk for 40 doses (8 wk)‡	1a	INH/RIF	7 days/wk for 126 doses (18 wk) or 5 days/wk for 90 doses (18 wk)‡	182-130 (26 wk)
			1b	INH/RIF	Twice weekly for 36 doses (18 wk)§	92-76 (26 wk)
			1c‖	INH/RPT	Once weekly for 18 doses (18 wk)	74-58 (26 wk)
2	INH RIF PZA EMB	7 days/wk for 14 doses (2 wk), then twice weekly for 12 doses (6 wk) or 5 days/wk for 10 doses (2 wk),‡ then twice weekly for 12 doses (6 wk)	2a	INH/RIF	Twice weekly for 36 doses (18 wk)§	62-58 (26 wk)
			2b‖	INH/RPT	Once weekly for 18 doses (18 wk)	44-40 (26 wk)
3	INH RIF PZA EMB	Three times weekly for 24 doses (8 wk)	3a	INH/RIF	Three times weekly for 54 doses (18 wk)	78 (26 wk)
4	INH RIF EMB	7 days/wk for 56 doses (8 wk) or 5 days/wk for 40 doses (8 wk)§	4a	INH/RIF	7 days/wk for 217 doses (31 wk) or 5 days/wk for 155 doses (31 wk)§	273-195 (39 wk)
			4b	INH/RIF	Twice weekly for 62 doses (31 wk)§	118-102 (39 wk)

EMB, ethambutol; INH, isoniazid; PZA, pyrazinamide; RIF, rifampin; RPT, rifapentine.

*When directly observed therapy is used, drugs may be given 5 days/wk and the necessary number of doses adjusted accordingly. Although there are no studies that compare five with seven daily doses, extensive experience indicates this would be an effective practice.

†Patients with cavitation on an initial chest radiograph and positive cultures at completion of 2 months of therapy should receive a 7-month (31 weeks; either 217 doses [daily] or 62 doses [twice weekly]) continuation phase.

‡Five-day-a-week administration is always given by directly observed therapy.

§Not recommended for HIV-infected patients with CD4+ cell counts <100 cells/mm³.

‖Options 1c and 2b should be used only in HIV-negative patients who have negative sputum smears at the time of completion of 2 months of therapy and who do not have cavitation on an initial chest radiograph. For patients started on this regimen and found to have a positive culture from the 2-month specimen, treatment should be extended an extra 3 months.

Modified from Centers for Disease Control and Prevention. Treatment of tuberculosis. American Thoracic Society, CDC and Infectious Diseases Society of America. *MMWR Recomm Rep.* 2003;52(RR-11):1-88.

TABLE 180-2 First-Line Tuberculosis Medications*

DRUG DOSE (MAXIMUM)	MAJOR ADVERSE REACTIONS	RECOMMENDED MONITORING	DOSAGE FORMS	COMMENTS
Isoniazid* (INH)				
Daily C: 10-15 mg/kg (300 mg) A: 5 mg/kg (300 mg) *Once weekly* C: Not recommended A: 15 mg/kg (900 mg) *Twice weekly* C: 20-30 mg/kg (900 mg) A: 15 mg/kg (900 mg) *Three times weekly* C: Not recommended A: 15 mg/kg (900 mg)	Hepatic enzyme elevation, peripheral neuropathy, hepatitis, rash, CNS effects, increased phenytoin, (Dilantin), and disulfiram (Antabuse) levels	Baseline hepatic enzymes. Repeat monthly if baseline abnormal, risk factors for hepatitis, or symptoms of adverse reactions.	*Scored tablets:* 50 mg, 100 mg, and 300 mg *Syrup:* 50 mg/5 mL *Aqueous solution (IV/IM):* scarce and may not be available	Hepatitis risk increases with age and alcohol consumption. Overdose may be fatal. Aluminum-containing antacids reduce absorption. Pyridoxine (vitamin B_6) may decrease peripheral neuritis and CNS effects.
Rifampin* (RIF)				
Daily C: 10-20 mg/kg (600 mg) A: 10 mg/kg (600 mg) *Once weekly* C: Not recommended A: Not recommended *Twice weekly* C: 10-20 mg/kg (600 mg) A: 10 mg/kg (600 mg) *Three times weekly* C: Not recommended A: 10 mg/kg (600 mg)	Hepatitis, fever, thrombocytopenia, flulike syndrome, rash, gastrointestinal upset, renal failure. Reduces levels of many drugs, including methadone, warfarin (Coumadin), birth control pills, theophylline, dapsone, ketoconazole, PIs, and some NNRTIs. Orange discoloration of secretions (sputum, urine, sweat, tears) and may permanently stain soft contact lenses.	CDC no longer recommends routine monitoring tests. However, many clinicians continue to order baseline CBC, platelets, hepatic enzymes. Repeat if baseline abnormal, risk factors for hepatitis or symptoms of adverse reactions.	*Capsules:* 150 mg and 300 mg *Syrup:* can be formulated from capsules by pharmacy *Aqueous solution (IV/IM):* scarce and may not be available	Patients on methadone will need an increased dose of methadone (average 50%) to avoid opiate withdrawal. Interaction with many drugs leads to decreased levels of one or both. May make glucose control more difficult in diabetics. Contraindicated for patients taking PIs and some NNRTIs. Women on birth control pills need a barrier method while on rifampin.

Pyrazinamide (PZA)

Dosage	Adverse Reactions	Preparation	Monitoring	Comments
Daily C: 15-30 mg/kg (2 g) A: 15-30 mg/kg (2 g) *Once weekly* C: Not recommended A: Not recommended *Twice weekly* C: 50 mg/kg (2 g) A: 50-70 mg/kg (4 g) *Three times weekly* C: Not recommended A: 50-70 mg/kg (3 g)	Gastrointestinal upset, hepatotoxicity, hyperuricemia, arthralgias, rash, gout (rare)	Scored tablets: 500 mg		May complicate management of diabetes mellitus. Treat increased uric acid only if symptomatic. Most common reason for TB patients experiencing GI upset.

Ethambutol† (EMB)

Dosage	Adverse Reactions	Preparation	Monitoring	Comments
Daily C: 15-20 mg/kg (1000 mg) A: 15-25 mg/kg (1600 mg) *Once weekly* C: Not recommended A: Not recommended *Twice weekly* C: 50 mg/kg (2.5 g) A: 50 mg/kg (4 g) *Three times weekly* C: Not recommended A: 25-30 mg/kg (2400 mg)	Decreased red-green color discrimination, decreased visual acuity (optic neuritis), rash	Tablets: 100 mg and 400 mg	Baseline tests of visual acuity and color vision. Monthly testing for patients taking >15-25 mg/kg, for those taking EMB for >2 mo, and for patients with renal insufficiency.	Optic neuritis may be unilateral; check each eye separately. Not recommended for children too young to monitor vision unless drug resistant. Use lowest possible dose in range (except for drug-resistant patients). EMB should be discontinued immediately and permanently for any signs of visual toxicity.

Rifabutin (RBT)

Dosage	Adverse Reactions	Preparation	Monitoring	Comments
Daily C: Not recommended A: 5 mg/kg (300 mg) *Once weekly* C: Not recommended A: Not recommended *Twice weekly* C: Not recommended A: 5 mg/kg (300 mg) *Three times weekly* C: Not recommended A: 5 mg/kg (300 mg)	Hepatitis fever, thrombocytopenia, neutropenia, leukopenia, flulike symptoms, hyperuricemia. Orange discoloration of secretions (sputum, urine, sweat, tears) and may permanently stain soft contact lenses. Reduces levels of many drugs, including methadone, warfarin (Coumadin), birth control pills, theophylline, dapsone, ketoconazole, PIs, and NNRTIs. With increased rifabutin levels, severe arthralgias, uveitis, leukopenia occur.	Capsules: 150 mg	Baseline hepatic enzymes. Repeat if baseline values abnormal, risk factors for hepatitis, or symptoms of adverse reactions.	Patients on methadone may need an increased dose to avoid opiate withdrawal. Interaction with many drugs leads to decreased levels of one or both. May make glucose control more difficult in diabetics. Women on birth control pills need to use a barrier method while on rifabutin. In combination with NNRTIs or PIs, dosages change significantly.

Continued

Chapter 180 *Mycobacterium tuberculosis*

TABLE 180-2 First-Line Tuberculosis Medications—cont'd

DRUG DOSE (MAXIMUM)	MAJOR ADVERSE REACTIONS	RECOMMENDED MONITORING	DOSAGE FORMS	COMMENTS
Rifapentine (RPT) *Once weekly only* C: Not approved for use in children A: 10 mg/kg (600 mg) *(Data indicate that 900 mg of RPT is well-tolerated and CDC is recommending this higher dose for latent tuberculosis.)*	Hepatitis, thrombocytopenia, neutropenia, leukopenia, hyperuricemia, flulike syndrome. Reduces levels of many drugs, including methadone, warfarin (Coumadin), birth control pills, theophylline, dapsone, ketoconazole, PIs, and NNRTIs. Orange discoloration of secretions (sputum, urine, sweat, tears) and may permanently stain soft contact lenses.	Baseline hepatic enzymes, CBC, and platelets. Repeat if baseline values are abnormal, risk factors for hepatitis are present, or there are symptoms of adverse reactions.	Tablets *(film-coated):* 150 mg *Indications:* Pulmonary TB patients who are HIV negative, noncavitary, not pregnant, with organisms pan-sensitive and culture negative at 2 months (two consecutive negative cultures). Administered once weekly with INH during the continuation phase of treatment.	See drug interactions with rifampin.

A, adult; C, child; CBC, complete blood cell count; CDC, Centers for Disease Control and Prevention; CNS, central nervous system; HIV, human immunodeficiency virus; IM, intramuscular; IV, intravenous; NNRTIs, non-nucleoside reverse-transcriptase inhibitors; PIs, protease inhibitors; PO, orally.

*Combination drugs are recommended in the rare instance in which a patient is placed on self-administered therapy: IsonaRif contains INH, 150 mg, RIF, 300 mg; Rifamate contains INH, 150 mg, RIF, 300 mg; Rifater contains INH, 50 mg, RIF, 120 mg, and PZA, 300 mg.

†In 2003, the CDC recommended dosing based on weight ranges for PZA and EMB. After reviewing available data, the Maryland TB Expert panel recommended that the previously recommended dosage ranges be utilized, advising use of the lowest possible dose in the dose range.

Modified from the 2007 Maryland Guidelines for Prevention and Treatment of Tuberculosis. Available at http://phpa.dhmh.maryland.gov/OIDPCS/CTBCP/CTBCPDocuments/tbguidelines.pdf.

181 Mycobacterium leprae (Leprosy)

Cybèle A. Renault and Joel D. Ernst

MICROBIOLOGY AND EPIDEMIOLOGY

- Acid-fast– and Gram stain–positive *Mycobacterium leprae* cannot be cultured in vitro.
- Predominant mode of transmission is likely through respiratory droplets or nasal secretions, although transmission may also occur through skin contact, transplacentally, via breast milk, and after zoonotic (particularly armadillo) exposure.
- Risk factors for clinical disease include age (bimodal distribution: adolescents and adults older than 30 years are at highest risk), gender (no differences noted in children, although adult men have double the risk compared with adult women), and degree of contact (individuals in contact with patients with multibacillary disease are at highest risk).
- Estimates of leprosy incidence and prevalence are underestimated owing to difficulty in diagnosing subclinical disease (the majority of those infected) and in light of the associated stigmatization of infected individuals.

CLINICAL MANIFESTATIONS AND IMMUNOLOGIC SPECTRUM OF DISEASE

- Clinical and pathologic manifestations arise in a distinct and well-characterized spectrum based on host immune response to the organism. Spectrum ranges from tuberculoid leprosy (small number of skin lesions, few bacilli in lesions, and a robust T-lymphocyte response) to lepromatous leprosy (larger number of skin lesions, clinically apparent infiltration of peripheral nerves, large number of bacilli, and a low T-lymphocyte response).
- Clinical manifestations vary significantly, depending on the subtype of disease. There are two clinical classification systems: World Health Organization (WHO) (used in resource-limited settings) and Ridley-Jopling (used when histopathology is available).
- Skin lesions are hypopigmented, erythematous, or infiltrative with or without neurologic signs or symptoms, including hypoesthesia, weakness, autonomic dysfunction, or peripheral nerve thickening.
- Peripheral sensory nerve damage (mediated directly by *M. leprae* or by the immune response to the organism) is the leading cause of functional morbidity and is seen throughout the disease spectrum.
- Reactions include reversal reactions, which present most often as increased erythema of preexisting skin lesions and progressive peripheral neuropathy, and erythema nodosum leprosum (ENL), which presents as systemic signs and painful erythematous skin nodules.

DIAGNOSIS

- Leprosy is diagnosed using a combination of clinical examination and skin slit smears or skin biopsy.
- Skin slit smear: Heat fixation and Ziehl-Neelsen or Fite staining are used to evaluate bacillary load and typically done in six sites.
- Skin biopsy: Histopathology is the gold standard for establishing a definitive diagnosis and for accurately classifying the subtype of disease but is often not available in endemic countries.

Part II Infectious Diseases and their Etiologic Agents

TABLE 181-1	Recommended Regimens to Treat Leprosy in Adults					
		WHO RECOMMENDATIONS		U.S. (NHDP) RECOMMENDATIONS		
Disease Stage	Agent	Dose	Duration	Dose	Duration	
Paucibacillary or "tuberculoid" disease (TT, BT)	Dapsone	100 mg/day	6 mo	100 mg/day	12 mo	
	Rifampin	600 mg/mo		600 mg/day		
Multibacillary or "lepromatous" disease (BB, BL, LL)	Dapsone	100 mg/day	12 mo	100 mg/day	24 mo	
	Rifampin	600 mg/ mo		600 mg/day		
	Clofazimine	50 mg/day, 300 mg/mo		50 mg/day		

BB, mid-borderline; BL, borderline lepromatous; BT, borderline tuberculoid; LL, lepromatous leprosy; NHDP, National Hansen's Disease Program; TT, tuberculoid; WHO, World Health Organization.

- *M. leprae* polymerase chain reaction assay is not currently available for commercial use but can be performed in specialized centers (e.g., National Hansen's Disease Program [NHDP]) to identify the organism in skin specimens that stain positive for acid-fast organisms but where culture results are negative.

THERAPY (SEE TABLE 181-1)

- Dapsone, rifampin, and clofazimine are the three established antimicrobial agents. Alternative agents include ofloxacin, minocycline, and clarithromycin. Standard therapy uses multiple drugs to increase cure rate and prevent emergence of drug resistance and treatment failure.
- Recommended treatment courses vary based on subtype of disease and resources available. Although both the WHO and NHDP recommend multiple drug therapy, the U.S. recommendations include daily rifampin (in contrast to monthly dosing) and recommend longer durations of therapy compared with WHO recommendations.
- Choice of therapy for reversal reactions should be made based on the severity of disease. Treatment of choice for both reversal and ENL reactions, particularly in the setting of acute neuritis, is corticosteroids. Thalidomide (for ENL only) and clofazimine are corticosteroid-sparing agents that can be used in chronic cases. Multiple drug therapy should always be continued in patients presenting with reactions.

182 *Mycobacterium avium* Complex
Fred M. Gordin and C. Robert Horsburgh, Jr.

MICROBIOLOGY AND EPIDEMIOLOGY

- *Mycobacterium avium* and *Mycobacterium intracellulare* are closely related in a complex (MAC).
- MAC is found in water, soil, and animals but not spread from person to person.
- The source from which patients acquire the disease is usually unknown.
- MAC causes pulmonary disease, lymphadenitis, and disseminated disease.
- Pulmonary disease occurs in older patients with chronic obstructive pulmonary disease, prior pneumonia, cystic fibrosis, and steroid use, as well as older women with no predisposing factors.
- Lymphadenitis is mostly in children younger than 5 years of age.
- Disseminated disease occurs mostly in patients with acquired immunodeficiency syndrome and a CD4$^+$ cell count less than 50/mm^3.

CLINICAL MANIFESTATIONS AND DIAGNOSIS

- Pulmonary disease can be infiltrative with or without cavities, nodular (solitary or multinodular), pleural, or as a hypersensitivity pneumonitis. It can closely mimic tuberculosis. Diagnosis requires a triad of clinical symptoms, radiographic abnormalities, and culture.
- Lymphadenitis is usually cervicofacial, unilateral, and painless. Diagnosis is via lymph node aspiration or excision.
- Disseminated disease is usually accompanied by fever, weight loss, and night sweats. Diagnosis is made in more than 90% of patients by blood cultures for *M. avium* complex (MAC).

TREATMENT (SEE TABLES 182-1 AND 182-2)

- For pulmonary disease:
    - Start treatment for pulmonary disease with clarithromycin or azithromycin, plus ethambutol and either rifampin or rifabutin. More advanced disease may require the addition of aminoglycosides, usually amikacin.
    - Treat pulmonary disease until cultures have been negative for at least 12 months; the usual total duration is 18 to 24 months.
    - Hypersensitivity pneumonitis may be treated with avoidance of exposure or short-term inhaled steroids, or both.
- Lymphadenitis can be treated with surgical excision or clarithromycin plus ethambutol until the node resolves.
- Human immunodeficiency virus (HIV)-infected patients with disseminated disease should be treated with clarithromycin plus ethambutol and possibly rifabutin or rifampin. These individuals should have antiretroviral therapy initiated after 2 to 4 weeks. Antibiotic therapy for disseminated MAC should be continued for 1 year and may then be discontinued if the CD4$^+$ cell count is greater than 100/mm^3. Immune reconstitution inflammatory syndrome may complicate recovery.

PREVENTION

- HIV-infected persons with fewer than 50 CD4$^+$ cells/mm^3 should be given azithromycin 1200 mg once weekly to prevent disseminated MAC. This can be stopped once sustained CD4$^+$ cell counts above 100/mm^3 have occurred.

TABLE 182-1 Drugs Employed in the Treatment of *Mycobacterium avium* Complex Disease

DRUG	USUAL DAILY DOSE*	USUAL INTERMITTENT DOSE	COMMON ADVERSE EFFECTS
Clarithromycin	500 mg bid	1 g tiw	GI distress, bitter taste, rash, hearing loss, drug interactions
Azithromycin	250 mg qd	500-600 mg tiw	GI distress, hearing loss
Ethambutol	15 mg/kg qd	25 mg/kg tiw	At high doses: optic neuritis, GI distress
Rifabutin	300 mg qd	300 mg tiw	GI distress, hepatitis, neutropenia, drug interactions; at high doses: uveitis, arthralgias
Rifampin	600 mg qd	600 mg tiw	GI distress, hepatitis, neutropenia, drug interactions
Amikacin	Not recommended	15 mg/kg IV tiw	Vestibular and auditory abnormalities, renal toxicity
Streptomycin	Not recommended	15 mg/kg IM (maximum tiw 1 g)	Vestibular and auditory abnormalities, renal toxicity

GI, gastrointestinal; tiw, three times weekly; IM, intramuscularly; IV, intravenously.
*Oral dosing unless otherwise indicated.

TABLE 182-2 Regimens for Pulmonary *Mycobacterium avium* Complex

INITIAL THERAPY FOR NODULAR/ BRONCHIECTATIC DISEASE	INITIAL THERAPY FOR CAVITARY DISEASE	ADVANCED (SEVERE) OR PREVIOUSLY TREATED DISEASE
Clarithromycin 1000 mg tiw *or* Azithromycin 500-600 mg tiw *plus*	Clarithromycin 500-1000 mg/day *or* Azithromycin 250-300 mg/day *plus*	Clarithromycin 500-1000 mg/day *or* Azithromycin 250-300 mg/day *plus*
Ethambutol 25 mg/kg tiw *plus*	Ethambutol 15 mg/kg/day *plus*	Ethambutol 15 mg/kg/day *plus*
Rifampin 600 mg tiw	Rifampin 600 mg/day *with or without*	Rifabutin 300 mg/day *or* Rifampin 600 mg/day *plus*
	Streptomycin *or* Amikacin	Streptomycin *or* Amikacin

tiw, three times weekly.
Modified from An official ATS/IDSA statement: diagnosis, treatment, and prevention of nontuberculous myco-bacterial diseases. *Am J Respir Crit Care Med.* 2007;175:367-416.

183 Infections Caused by Nontuberculous Mycobacteria Other Than *Mycobacterium Avium* Complex

Barbara A. Brown-Elliott and Richard J. Wallace, Jr.

DEFINITION

- Composed of species other than *Mycobacterium tuberculosis* complex (MTBC)
- Previously known as "atypical mycobacteria" or "mycobacteria other than *M. tuberculosis*"
- More than 150 species of nontuberculous mycobacteria (NTM)
- Divided into rapidly, intermediate, and slowly growing species

EPIDEMIOLOGY

- Most species are worldwide and ubiquitous in the environment, including household water, potting soil, vegetable matter, animals, and birds.
- NTM include pathogens and nonpathogens.
- Cases in chronic (e.g., pulmonary) infections involve patients with underlying disease such as bronchiectasis and cystic fibrosis.
- Other cases involve extrapulmonary sites, including skin and soft tissue, bones, joints, bursae, tendon sheaths, lymph nodes, eyes, ears, blood, brain, and cerebrospinal fluid.

MICROBIOLOGY

- Acid-fast bacilli (AFB) stain poorly with Gram staining.
- Identification of definitive species level is only accomplished by molecular or proteomic methods at present.

Rapidly Growing Mycobacteria

- Rapidly growing mycobacteria (RGM) produce mature colonies on solid media within 7 days.
- Routine culture media such as blood agar, chocolate agar, trypticase soy agar, most MTBC media (Middlebrook 7H10 or 7H11 agar and Lowenstein-Jensen agar), and various broths, including rapid broth detection systems, support the growth of most species.
- Preference is for 28° to 30°C incubation for some species, although many species also grow at 35°C.
- Some RGM, especially *Mycobacterium abscessus*, are adversely affected by harsh decontamination methods that are used for isolation of MTBC.
- Currently six groups of pathogenic species are defined based on presence or absence of pigment and genetic relatedness.

Intermediately Growing Mycobacteria

- Most MTBC media including Middlebrook 7H10 or 7H11 agar and Lowenstein-Jensen agar support growth of species.
- They require 7 to 10 days to reach mature growth.
- Primarily two pigmented species are involved:
  - *Mycobacterium marinum* (pathogen) grows optimally at 28° to 30°C and is associated with marine water and marine animals.

- *Mycobacterium gordonae* (nonpathogen) grows optimally at 35° to 37° C and is a common tap water contaminant.

Slowly Growing Mycobacteria

- Produce mature colonies in more than 7 days on solid media
- Most MTBC media, including Middlebrook 7H10 or 7H11 agar, Lowenstein-Jensen agar, Middlebrook broth, and rapid detection broth systems, support growth of species, except for fastidious species such as *Mycobacterium haemophilum* (requires hemin or iron) and *Mycobacterium genavense* (requires Mycobactin J).
- Most species except *M. haemophilum* (28° to 30° C), *Mycobacterium xenopi* (42° to 45° C), and some environmental species grow optimally at 35° to 37° C.

DIAGNOSIS
Pulmonary

- Signs and symptoms of NTM lung disease are variable and nonspecific.
- Patients often present with chronic cough or throat clearing, with or without sputum production and severe fatigue. Less frequently malaise, dyspnea, fever, hemoptysis, and weight loss may occur.
- Clinical diagnosis depends on multiple positive microbiologic cultures of respiratory samples for AFB.
- Follow the American Thoracic Society guidelines for diagnosis.
- High-resolution chest computed tomography is useful.
- Routine chest radiographs are recommended.
- Single positive sputum cultures are not definitive for NTM disease.
- Expert consultation is required for patients with infrequently encountered species of NTM.

Extrapulmonary

- Infection may involve fever, drainage, bacteremia, granulomatous systemic infections, necrosis, etc. depending on the site of infection.
- Clinical diagnosis depends on positive microbiologic smears and cultures for mycobacteria of drainage, biopsy tissue, or body fluid, leading to isolation of specific NTM.

THERAPY
Rapidly Growing Mycobacteria

- *Pulmonary disease*
  - Most pulmonary disease is caused by *M. abscessus* or *M. abscessus* subsp. *massiliense*.
  - Antimicrobial therapy alone is generally unsuccessful for microbiologic eradication of *M. abscessus*.
  - Rifampin, rifabutin, ethambutol, isoniazid, streptomycin, and pyrazinamide are not effective.
  - Multidrug regimens of macrolides (azithromycin or clarithromycin), high-dose IV cefoxitin (8 to 12 g/day in divided doses) or imipenem (1 g twice daily), and low-dose parenteral amikacin (peaks in the 20 to 25 µg/mL range on once-daily dosing) probably optimal for *M. abscessus*. Daily IV tigecycline often included; dosage adjustment is usually necessary for clinical improvement, not cure. The role of inhaled amikacin is not yet established.
  - Patients with *M. abscessus* are treated for several months until clinically improved and may require several courses of treatment.
  - Macrolides may not be useful for isolates of *M. abscessus* (but not *M. massiliense*), *Mycobacterium fortuitum*, and *Mycobacterium smegmatis* that contain functional inducible *erm* genes.
  - Other antimicrobials are often useful for species other than *M. abscessus* (minocycline, doxycycline, trimethoprim/sulfamethoxazole [TMP-SMX], quinolones, linezolid, and, for *Mycobacterium chelonae*, tobramycin).
- *Extrapulmonary disease*

- Generally clinicians prescribe a multidrug regimen based on in vitro susceptibility testing, including a macrolide (except in case of *erm*-positive species).
- Rifampin, rifabutin, ethambutol, and isoniazid are not effective.
- Patients with significant disease are treated for 6 months, depending on the severity of infection.
- Other antimicrobials often useful for species of the *M. fortuitum* group are minocycline, doxycycline, TMP-SMX, quinolones, linezolid, and, for *M. chelonae,* tobramycin.

Intermediately Growing Mycobacteria
- *M. marinum* is found on skin and in soft tissue infections (usually hands).
- Treatment options include macrolides, rifampin, TMP-SMX, or a combination of rifampin and ethambutol.

Slowly Growing Mycobacteria
- *Pulmonary disease*
  - Antibiotic treatment generally follows the regimen for *Mycobacterium avium* complex: rifampin, ethambutol, and a macrolide (clarithromycin or azithromycin) with adjustments depending on in vitro antimicrobial susceptibility testing.
  - Patients are generally treated for 12 months of culture negativity.
- *Extrapulmonary disease*
  - Treatment is the same as for pulmonary disease except that it is usually for 6 months depending on the severity of infection.

PREVENTION
- No evidence of person-to-person spread of NTM exists.
- Tap (household) water is considered the major reservoir for most common NTM species.
- Biofilms may render NTM less susceptible to disinfectants and antimicrobials.
- Public health concerns are increasing.

184 *Nocardia* Species

Tania C. Sorrell, David H. Mitchell, Jonathan R. Iredell, and Sharon C-A. Chen

DEFINITION

- Nocardiosis results from infection by members of the genus *Nocardia,* which are ubiquitous environmental saprophytes that cause localized or disseminated disease in humans and animals.

MICROBIOLOGY AND EPIDEMIOLOGY

- Microscopically, *Nocardia* appear as gram-positive, beaded, weakly acid-fast, branching rods.
- Molecular speciation has revolutionized taxonomy by identifying several new species and reassigning species, especially from the commonest pathogenic group, the former *N. asteroides* complex.
- Infection arises by direct inoculation through the skin or by inhalation.
- Mycetomas from *Nocardia* species, most often caused by *N. brasiliensis,* affect immunocompetent hosts in tropical countries.
- Immunocompromise, alcoholism, and certain lung diseases predispose patients to pulmonary and disseminated nocardiosis, most often due to *N. cyriacigeorgica, N. nova,* or *N. farcinica.*

CLINICAL MANIFESTATIONS

- Primary skin infection can cause sporotrichoid lesions and lead to pyogenic abscesses or to chronically progressive, destructive disease with sinus tract formation (mycetoma) usually on a distal limb.
- Presentation of lung disease may be subacute or chronic with productive or nonproductive cough, dyspnea, hemoptysis, and fever and other systemic symptoms. Cavity formation within the pneumonia or spread to the central nervous system (CNS), or both, are suggestive of nocardiosis. Isolated CNS lesions also occur and their presentation can be insidious.

DIAGNOSIS

- Cerebral imaging, preferably magnetic resonance imaging, should be performed in all cases of pulmonary and disseminated nocardiosis to rule out insidious CNS disease.
- The microbiology laboratory should be informed of suspected nocardiosis because it may not be detected by routine laboratory methods. Respiratory secretions, skin biopsies, or aspirates from deep collections are the most useful and are typically positive on Gram stain. Modified acid-fast stain of sputum or pus is helpful in suggesting the diagnosis. Growth of *Nocardia* species may take 48 hours to several weeks but usually 3 to 5 days.
- Species identification is predictive of antimicrobial susceptibility; it requires molecular identification tests based on nucleic acid technology (NAT).
- Recently mass spectrometry analysis using matrix-assisted laser desorption/ionization time-of-flight mass spectrometry has been reported to be a reliable and more rapid alternative to NAT.

THERAPY AND FOLLOW-UP

- Trimethoprim-sulfamethoxazole (TMP-SMX) is the mainstay of treatment, and monotherapy is usually successful in patients with isolated skin infection or mycetomas that are not extensive (see Table 184-1).
- In systemic disease, speciation and/or susceptibility testing results should guide definitive combination therapy.
- Empirical therapy with amikacin and imipenem or meropenem or amikacin and TMP-SMX are recommended in immunocompromised patients or those with disseminated disease but no brain involvement.
- For isolated cerebral disease, empirical TMP-SMX plus imipenem or meropenem are suitable.
- When additional sites are involved or the patient has life-threatening disease, empirical three-drug regimens such as TMP-SMX, imipenem or meropenem, and amikacin (or ceftriaxone, in patients with renal failure) are preferred. Initial adjunctive therapy with linezolid is an option, especially if one of these classes of drug is contraindicated.
- Clinical improvement is generally evident within 3 to 5 days or, at the most, 7 to 10 days after initiation of appropriate therapy.
- Prolonged therapy is necessary to prevent relapse.
- Surgical excision may be required depending on the extent and site of the lesions or the response to medical therapy, or both.
- Patients with deep-seated infection should be monitored clinically and radiologically during and for up to 12 months after cessation of therapy.

TABLE 184-1 Antimicrobial Susceptibility of Selected *Nocardia* Species

	N. cyriacigeorgica	*N. farcinica*	*N. nova complex*	*N. transvalensis complex*	*N. brasiliensis*
Trimethoprim-sulfamethoxazole	S	R	S	S	S
Amoxicillin clavulanate	R	V	R	V	S
Ceftriaxone	S	R	S	S	R
Imipenem	S	S	S	S	R
Amikacin	S	S	S	R	S
Linezolid	S	S	S	S	S
Moxifloxacin	V	S	R	ND	R
Clarithromycin	R	R	R	S	R
Minocycline	V	R	V	R	R
Tigecycline	V	R	V	ND	S

ND, no data; R, generally inactive; S, generally active (some isolates may be resistant); V, may be active but resistance common.
Data taken from multiple published sources.

185 Agents of Actinomycosis

Thomas A. Russo

DEFINITION

- Indolent infection
- Chronicity, crosses tissue boundaries, masslike features
- Mimics malignancy
- Sinus tract(s) may develop, resolve, and recur
- Refractory or relapsing infection may occur after a short course of therapy

MICROBIOLOGY

- Primarily caused by *Actinomyces* spp.
- Gram-positive, primarily filamentous bacteria
- Most are anaerobes, few are microaerophilic
- "Companion organisms" are usually present

EPIDEMIOLOGY/PATHOGENESIS

- Human commensal of oral, gastrointestinal, pelvic mucosa
- Disruption of mucosal surface initiating factor
- All ages and normal hosts infected
- Association with intrauterine devices and bisphosphonates

CLINICAL MANIFESTATIONS

- All organs and sites could be involved
- Orocervicofacial most common
- Classic presentation as painless mass at angle of the jaw
- Alternative presentations are myriad

DIAGNOSIS

- Challenging, often missed, mistaken for cancer
- Sulfur granules
- Inform laboratory
- Prior antibiotics can inhibit growth on culture
- Increasing role for polymerase chain reaction
- Often made via pathology after potentially unnecessary surgery

THERAPY

- Based on clinical experience, individualized
- High dose and prolonged course of antibiotics
- Standard 2 to 6 weeks intravenously, followed by 6 to 12 months orally
- Imaging helpful in defining duration
- Penicillin, tetracyclines, erythromycin, and clindamycin have greatest experience
- A short course of treatment directed against "companion organisms" may be warranted
- Medical therapy usually curative, even with extensive disease
- Interventional radiology for drainage of accessible abscess
- Surgery reserved for critical sites (e.g., central nervous system) and refractory disease

186 *Aspergillus* Species

Thomas F. Patterson

DEFINITION

- Aspergillosis is caused by species of the mold *Aspergillus.*
- Syndromes range from colonization; fungus ball due to *Aspergillus* (aspergilloma); allergic responses to *Aspergillus,* including allergic bronchopulmonary aspergillosis; to semi-invasive or invasive infections, from chronic necrotizing pneumonia to invasive pulmonary aspergillosis and other invasive syndromes.

EPIDEMIOLOGY

- The highest incidence of infection occurs in patients undergoing hematopoietic stem cell transplantation or solid-organ transplantation (see Table 186-1).
- Infection is more likely in patients with extensive immunosuppression or in those with relapse or recurrence of underlying malignancy.
- Improved survival has been noted with early diagnosis and newer therapies, but mortality rates in severely or persistently immunosuppressed patients are substantial.

MICROBIOLOGY

- Culture-based diagnosis is useful to establish the specific diagnosis.
- *Aspergillus* species complexes exhibit distinct antifungal susceptibilities so that culture-based diagnosis is clinically relevant (see Table 186-2).
- Molecular analysis is required to establish species-level identity.
- Increasing rates of antifungal resistance are reported in some settings with a global clone of antifungal-resistant species.

DIAGNOSIS

- Proven infection is established by culture of the organism.
- Biomarkers such as galactomannan, β-D-glucan, and polymerase chain reaction assay are useful for establishing probable diagnosis.
- Serial assessment of biomarkers may be useful for measuring response to therapy.

THERAPY

- Voriconazole is recommended for primary therapy in most patients (see Table 186-3).
- Liposomal amphotericin B can be used as primary therapy in patients in whom voriconazole is not tolerated or contraindicated because of drug interactions or other reasons.
- Alternative agents for salvage therapy include amphotericin B lipid complex, the echinocandins (caspofungin, micafungin, or anidulafungin), posaconazole, or itraconazole.
- Combination therapy is not recommended for routine use, but some subgroups of patients (e.g., those with early diagnosis of infection based on detection of galactomannan or those with failure of primary therapy with a single agent) may benefit from such an approach.

TABLE 186-1   Incidence and Mortality of Invasive Aspergillosis in Transplantation

Type of Transplant	INCIDENCE (%)		12-Week Mortality (%)
	Range	Mean	
Allogeneic stem cell	2.3-11	7	40-75
Autologous stem cell	0.5-2	1	50
Lung	2.4-9	6	5-21
Liver	1-8	4	45-59
Heart	0.3-6	2	15-21
Kidney	0.1-2	0.5	25-48

Data from the following sources:

Kontoyiannis DP, Marr KA, Park BJ, et al. Prospective surveillance for invasive fungal infections in hematopoietic stem cell transplant recipients, 2001-2006: overview of the Transplant-Associated Infection Surveillance Network (TRANSNET) Database. Clin Infect Dis. 2010;50:1091-1100.

Neofytos D, Treadway S, Ostrander D, et al. Epidemiology, outcomes, and mortality predictors of invasive mold infections among transplant recipients: a 10-year, single-center experience. Transpl Infect Dis. 2013;15: 233-242.

Steinbach WJ, Marr KA, Anaissie EJ, et al. Clinical epidemiology of 960 patients with invasive aspergillosis from the PATH Alliance registry. J Infect. 2012;65:453-464.

Pappas PG, Alexander BD, Andes DR, et al. Invasive fungal infections among organ transplant recipients: results of the Transplant-Associated Infection Surveillance Network (TRANSNET). Clin Infect Dis. 2010;50: 1101-1111.

Singh N, Paterson DL. Aspergillus infections in transplant recipients. Clin Microbiol Rev. 2005;18:44-69.

Neofytos D, Fishman JA, Horn D, et al. Epidemiology and outcome of invasive fungal infections in solid organ transplant recipients. Transpl Infect Dis. 2010;12:220-229.

Baddley JW, Andes DR, Marr KA, et al. Factors associated with mortality in transplant patients with invasive aspergillosis. Clin Infect Dis. 2010;50:1559-1567.

PREVENTION

- Antifungal prophylaxis with posaconazole or possibly voriconazole is recommended in high-risk patients.
- The risk-benefit ratio of prophylaxis in individual patients at risk should be considered.
- Infection control is important to reduce risk in hospitalized patients, but long duration of risk (>180 days) in high-risk hematopoietic stem cell transplant or solid-organ transplant patients makes community-acquired infection likely.

TABLE 186-2 Characteristics of *Aspergillus* Species Associated with Invasive Infection

ASPERGILLUS SPECIES	FREQUENCY OF SPECIES COMPLEX ISOLATED IN CLINICAL INFECTION (%)	COLONY CHARACTERISTICS	MICROSCOPIC FEATURES	CLINICAL SIGNIFICANCE
A. fumigatus	50-67	Smoky gray-green; may have pale yellow or lavender reverse; grows at 50°C	Columnar; uniseriate; smooth to finely roughened conidia 2-3.5 μm	Most common invasive species; most pathogenic
A. flavus	8-14	Olive to lime green	Radiate to loosely columnar; uniseriate or biseriate; rough conidiophore; conidia 3-6 μm	Sinusitis; skin infection; produces aflatoxin
A. terreus	3-5	Beige to cinnamon buff	Columnar; biseriate; globose; small 2-2.5 μm conidia; globose accessory conidia along hyphae	Increasingly detected; resistant to amphotericin B; more susceptible to newer azoles
A. niger	5-9	Initially white, rapidly turning black with yellow reverse	Radiate; biseriate; globose, black, very rough conidia 4-5 μm	Uncommon in invasive infections; superficial agent of otic disease; colonization

Data from the following references:

Patterson TF, Kirkpatrick WR, White M, et al. Invasive aspergillosis: disease spectrum, treatment practices, and outcomes. I3 Aspergillus Study Group. Medicine (Baltimore). 2000;79:250-260.

Alastruey-Izquierdo A, Mellado E, Cuenca-Estrella M. Current section and species complex concepts in Aspergillus: recommendations for routine daily practice. Ann N Y Acad Sci. 2012;1273:18-24.

Balajee SA, Kano R, Baddley JW, et al. Molecular identification of Aspergillus species collected for the Transplant-Associated Infection Surveillance Network. J Clin Microbiol. 2009;47:3138-3141.

Sutton DA, Fothergill AW, Rinaldi MG, eds. Guide to Clinically Significant Fungi. Baltimore: Williams & Wilkins; 1998.

TABLE 186-3 Antifungal Agents for Invasive Aspergillosis

AGENT	CLASS	ROUTE OF ADMINISTRATION	DOSE	COMMENTS
Primary Therapy				
Voriconazole	Azole	IV/ oral	6 mg/kg (IV) q12h × 2 doses, followed by 4 mg/kg (IV) q12h or 200 mg (PO) q12h. Some experts advise oral dosing as 4 mg/kg (PO) q12h.	Recommended for primary therapy in most patients due to randomized trial demonstrating improved survival as compared with amphotericin B deoxycholate; caution for use in patients with potential liver toxicity and for drug interactions; measurement of serum levels advocated for efficacy and avoidance of toxicity (controversial)
Alternative Primary Therapy				
Liposomal amphotericin B	Polyene	IV	3 mg/kg/day	Well tolerated; minimal infusion reactions or nephrotoxicity; initial doses of 10 mg/kg/day more toxic and not more effective
Other Agents				
Amphotericin B	Polyene	IV	1-1.5 mg/kg/day	Previous gold standard; significant toxicity in higher doses; limited efficacy in high-risk patients
Amphotericin B lipid complex	Polyene	IV	5 mg/kg/day	Indicated for patients intolerant or refractory to standard therapy; case-controlled data suggest better efficacy than amphotericin B deoxycholate
Amphotericin B colloidal dispersion	Polyene	IV	3-6 mg/kg/day	More infusion-related toxicity than other lipid formulations; efficacy similar to amphotericin B in primary treatment
Posaconazole	Azole	Oral	Investigational in United States for *Aspergillus* treatment: 400 mg (PO) bid; prophylaxis 200 mg (PO) tid	Oral formulation; efficacy in salvage therapy and prophylaxis
Itraconazole	Azole	Oral	200 mg bid (PO)	Erratic bioavailability improved with oral solution; serious cardiac adverse events with higher doses, drug interactions common; intravenous formulation not currently available
Caspofungin	Echinocandin	IV	50-70 mg/day	Approved for refractory infection and intolerance to standard therapy; well tolerated; limited efficacy as monotherapy for primary infection; preclinical and anecdotal data showing improved efficacy in combination with azoles
Micafungin	Echinocandin	IV	Investigational in United States for *Aspergillus* treatment (50-100 mg/day)	Efficacy for prevention and salvage treatment of aspergillosis
Anidulafungin	Echinocandin	IV	Investigational for *Aspergillus* (100 mg/day)	Combination trial data showing improved outcomes in patients with galactomannan diagnosis of invasive pulmonary aspergillosis

187 Agents of Mucormycosis and Entomophthoramycosis

Dimitrios P. Kontoyiannis and Russell E. Lewis

DEFINITION

- Mucormycosis is an aggressive, angioinvasive fungal infection caused by filamentous fungi in the subphylum Mucormycotina, which afflict immunocompromised or severely hyperglycemic patients. Skin and soft tissue infections in immunocompetent patients may be encountered in patients with severe soft tissue trauma (e.g., tornadoes, combat injuries).
- Entomophthoramycosis is a rare infection of the paranasal sinuses, subcutaneous tissues, or gastrointestinal tract caused by filamentous fungi in the subphylum Entomophthoramycotina, which are principally encountered in the tropics.

EPIDEMIOLOGY

- Mucormycosis is acquired primarily via inhalation of environmental sporangiospores in immunocompromised hosts. The infection may break through antifungal prophylaxis regimens used to reduce the risk of aspergillosis.
- Entomophthoramycosis typically causes indolent subcutaneous infections localized to the sinuses, head and face (conidiobolomycosis), or trunk and arms (basidiobolomycosis) from inhalation or minor trauma. Gastrointestinal basidiobolomycosis has occurred in Arizona and the Near East and is perhaps acquired by ingestion.

MICROBIOLOGY

- Most common culture-confirmed cases in the literature are *Rhizopus* species (47%), *Mucor* species (18%), *Cunninghamella bertholletiae* (7%), *Apophysomyces elegans* (5%), *Lictheimia (Absidia)* species (5%), *Saksenaea* species (5%), and *Rhizomucor pusillus* (4%), with other species (8%) accounting for the remaining cases.
- *Conidiobolus coronatus* and *Conidiobolus incongruus* cause conidiobolomycosis. *Basidiobolus ranarum* causes basidiobolomycosis.

DIAGNOSIS

- A high index of suspicion in immunocompromised patients is essential because most signs, symptoms, and radiographic signs are nonspecific. Cultures have a poor sensitivity. Diagnosis is typically established by histopathologic documentation of "ribbon-like" angioinvasive hyphae in tissue, though this is prone to error.

TREATMENT

- Lipid formulations of amphotericin B are the drug of choice. Some patients can then be transitioned to oral posaconazole if absorption is adequate.

PREVENTION

- Given the rarity of mucormycosis and entomophthoramycosis, primary prophylaxis is not recommended. Secondary or potentially indefinite prophylaxis should be considered for immunocompromised patients with previous episodes of mucormycosis, depending on the status of underlying immunosuppression.

188 *Sporothrix schenckii*

John H. Rex and Pablo C. Okhuysen

MICROBIOLOGY AND EPIDEMIOLOGY

- A dimorphic fungus, with budding yeast in tissue and a mold in culture
- Worldwide distribution, especially in tropical and subtropical regions
- Acquisition is associated with exposure to soil, plants, plant products (hay, straw, sphagnum moss), and a variety of animals (especially cats)
- Grows slowly on fungal culture from involved tissues

DIAGNOSIS

- Lymphocutaneous diseases: presentation with an indolent papulonodular lesion, sometimes ulcerating, should suggest the diagnosis. Secondary lesions along lymphangitic channels are characteristic. Biopsy will show pyogranulomas without visible organisms; culture will be positive.
- The most common extracutaneous form is osteoarticular. Pulmonary disease (usually cavitary) and meningeal disease are also well described. All are diagnosed by culture with organisms not commonly seen on examination of tissues and fluids except in cavitary pulmonary disease.
- Multifocal dissemination may also occur, in immunocompromised subjects: cultures of skin lesions and joints are usually positive, whereas blood and bone marrow cultures are only occasionally positive.
- Serodiagnostic methods remain experimental.

THERAPY

- Itraconazole at 200 mg/day orally is the treatment of choice for lymphocutaneous disease, with 3 to 6 months of therapy typically needed for complete resolution.
- Therapy with a saturated solution of potassium iodide is also effective for lymphocutaneous disease, although associated with many side effects.
- Itraconazole is also active in extracutaneous disease, but extended therapy may be required. In difficult settings, amphotericin B is also employed. Improvement of immune status (e.g., introduction of antiretroviral therapy in subjects with human immunodeficiency virus coinfection, reduction of immunosuppressive agents) is useful.

189 Agents of Chromoblastomycosis
Duane R. Hospenthal

DEFINITION
- Chronic fungal infection limited to the skin and subcutaneous tissue
- Scaly nodular, tumorous, verrucous, plaque, or cicatricial lesions, typically affecting the lower extremities
- Defined by the microscopic presence of muriform cells

EPIDEMIOLOGY
- Worldwide distribution, with most cases occurring in tropical and subtropical regions
- Largest numbers of cases reported from Madagascar, Brazil, Mexico, Venezuela, and Costa Rica
- Male predominance, ages 40 to 69; commonly associated with outdoor activities such as farming or woodcutting and with absence of footwear

MICROBIOLOGY
- Most commonly caused by *Fonsecaea pedrosoi*
- Less commonly caused by *Cladophialophora carrionii, Fonsecaea monophora, Fonsecaea nubica, Phialophora verrucosa,* or *Rhinocladiella aquaspersa*
- Other dark-walled fungi rarely reported as causative agents

DIAGNOSIS
- Presence of muriform cells (also called sclerotic, copper penny, or Medlar bodies) pathognomonic
- Muriform cells observed microscopically in skin scrapings prepared with potassium hydroxide or in routinely stained skin biopsy specimens
- Culture on standard mycologic media possible but not always necessary

THERAPY
- No proven treatment identified
- Small lesions treated successfully with surgical excision, liquid nitrogen or topical heat application, or photocoagulation; use of curettage and electrocautery discouraged because of reports of disease spread after their use
- Oral itraconazole or terbinafine in combination with local liquid nitrogen therapy most effective therapy
- Posaconazole used successfully in small number of patients refractory to itraconazole or terbinafine

PREVENTION
- No vaccine available
- Need for footwear and proper protective clothing

190 Agents of Mycetoma

Duane R. Hospenthal

DEFINITION

- Mycetoma is an infection of the skin and subcutaneous tissue characterized by a triad of localized swelling, draining sinuses, and grains (aggregates of infecting organisms).
- It most commonly affects a single site, typically involving the lower extremity, and especially the foot.
- Eumycetoma (eumycotic mycetoma) is mycetoma caused by fungi, most commonly *Madurella mycetomatis.*
- Actinomycetoma (actinomycotic mycetoma) is mycetoma caused by bacteria, most commonly *Nocardia brasiliensis.*

EPIDEMIOLOGY

- Distribution is worldwide with most cases occurring in tropical and subtropical regions.
- Largest numbers of cases are reported from Africa, Latin America, and the Indian subcontinent.
- Mycetoma occurs predominantly in men, ages 20 to 40, typically with occupations that expose them to the environment.

MICROBIOLOGY

- *M. mycetomatis, Madurella grisea,* and *Pseudallescheria boydii* are the most common causes of eumycetoma, although many other genera and species of fungi have been reported as etiologic agents.
- *N. brasiliensis, Actinomadura madurae, Streptomyces somaliensis,* and *Actinomadura pelletieri* are the most common causes of actinomycetoma, although disease secondary to other species of *Actinomadura, Nocardia,* and *Streptomyces* has been described.

DIAGNOSIS

- Clinical presentation of the classic triad of chronic, painless, soft tissue swelling with draining sinuses that discharge grains is pathognomonic.
- Microscopic examination of the grains can differentiate between eumycetoma and actinomycetoma.
- Culture of causative agent from grains can better direct selection of antimicrobial therapy.
- Radiographic techniques (plain radiographs, ultrasound, computed tomography, and magnetic resonance imaging) can be used adjunctively in making (or excluding) the diagnosis and determining its extent.

THERAPY

- Small lesions may be treated successfully with surgical excision alone.
- Actinomycetoma is typically treated with medical therapy alone.
- Eumycetoma commonly requires combined medical and surgical therapy.
- No single therapy has proved most effective for either form of mycetoma.
- Most actinomycetoma regimens include parenteral aminoglycosides and oral sulfa drugs.

- Less severe actinomycetoma may be treated with 6 to 24 months of trimethoprim-sulfamethoxazole.
- Eumycetoma is typically treated with a regimen of an oral azole antifungal drug for 6 to 24 months combined with debulking surgery.

PREVENTION

- No vaccine is available.
- Use of footwear and proper protective clothing should protect against this infection.

191 Cryptococcosis (*Cryptococcus neoformans* and *Cryptococcus gattii*)

John R. Perfect

HISTORY

- The life cycle represents both asexual (clinical) and sexual (recombination) cycles with the impact of sexual cycle on pathogenesis.

TAXONOMY

- There are 19 cryptococcal species with two major pathogenic species, *C. neoformans* and *C. gattii.*
- At present, the following taxonomic divisions have been proposed: *Cryptococcus neoformans* var. *grubii* (serotype A), with three genotypes (VNI, VNII, VNB); *Cryptococcus neoformans* var. *neoformans* (serotype D or VNIV); and five other cryptic species: *Cryptococcus gattii, Cryptococcus bacillisporus, Cryptococcus deuterogattii, Cryptococcus tetragattii,* and *Cryptococcus decagattii* (serotypes B/C or VGl-lV).

IDENTIFICATION

- Biochemical tests, including urease, melanin production, and appearance of capsule
- Cultures or DNA-based tests

ECOLOGY

- *C. neoformans* (serotypes A and D) found in pigeon guano to rotting trees
- *C. gattii* found in eucalyptus to coniferous trees (landscape of niche may be changing)

EPIDEMIOLOGY

- Not routine constituent of human biota but can colonize humans without disease
- Widespread asymptomatic infections in the exposed populations
- Risk factors for disease (acquired immunodeficiency syndrome [AIDS], corticosteroid treatment, transplantation, cancer, monoclonal antibodies, sarcoidosis, autoantibodies to granulocyte-macrophage colony-stimulating factor, idiopathic CD4 lymphocytopenia); primarily cell-mediated immunity defect (see Table 191-1)
- Antiretroviral therapy (ART) impact on clinical cryptococcosis is impressive in patients with AIDS.
- A million new cases of cryptococcosis per year, with more than 600,000 deaths worldwide at the peak of the human immunodeficiency virus (HIV) epidemic and probably reduced with ART availability

PATHOGENICITY

- Virulence factors (capsule, melanin, high temperature growth, urease, phospholipase)
- Understanding at the genetic and molecular level

HOST RESPONSES

- Efficient protection requires intact cell-mediated, innate, and humoral immunity.

TABLE 191-1 Conditions Known or Possibly Associated with Predisposition to *Cryptococcus neoformans* Infections

HIV infection
Lymphoproliferative disorders
Sarcoidosis
Corticosteroid therapy
Hyper-IgM syndrome
Hyper-IgE syndrome
   Autoantibodies to GM-CSF
Monoclonal antibodies (e.g., infliximab intercept, adalimumab, alemtuzumab)
Systemic lupus erythematosus*
HIV-negative CD4+ T-cell lymphocytopenia
Diabetes mellitus†
Organ transplantation*
Peritoneal dialysis
Cirrhosis

GM-CSF, granulocyte-macrophage colony-stimulating factor; HIV, human immunodeficiency virus.
*Immunosuppressive therapy may account for the predisposition.
†Diabetes mellitus has historically been considered a risk factor for cryptococcal infection. However, diabetes is a common disease, and it is unclear whether this condition is truly a specific risk factor for cryptococcosis.
Modified from Casadevall A, Perfect JR. *Cryptococcus neoformans*. Washington, DC: ASM Press; 1998:410.

PATHOGENESIS

- Three factors: (1) host defenses, (2) virulence of strain, and (3) size of inocula
- Cryptococcosis considered primarily a reactivation disease

CLINICAL MANIFESTATIONS (SEE TABLE 191-2)

- Major sites are the central nervous system and lung.
- Other sites with unique considerations are the skin, prostate, peritoneum, and eye.
- Cryptococci can infect any organ of the human body.
- Disease primarily depends on host immunity (either from too little or too much [immune reconstitution inflammatory syndrome, IRIS]).

LABORATORY DIAGNOSIS

- Microscopy (India ink and histopathologic stains including mucicarmine)
- Culture of cerebrospinal fluid (CSF), blood, bronchoalveolar lavage
- Cryptococcal antigen on CSF and serum is sensitive and specific as detected by latex agglutination, enzyme-linked immunosorbent assay, and lateral flow

MANAGEMENT

- The Infectious Diseases Society of American Guidelines in 2010 established road maps for therapies and strategies (www.idsociety.org/Organism/#Fungi).
- Direct antifungal drug resistance uncommonly arises during therapy.
- Treatment is best studied for cryptococcal meningitis in HIV-infected patients (2013 guidelines at http://aidsinfo.nih.gov/guidelines/html/4/adult-and-adolescent-oi-prevention-and-treatment-guidelines/333/cryptococcosis). Treatment is initiated with amphotericin B, preferably with the liposomal formulation at 3 to 4 mg/kg daily, the alternatives being the lipid complex at 5 mg/kg or conventional amphotericin B at 0.7 mg/kg/day. Any one of these can be used plus flucytosine 25 mg/kg every 6 hours (100 mg/kg per day) for at least 2 weeks and until clinically improved. In severely ill patients or those with high intracranial pressure, delaying ART during these 2 weeks may prevent IRIS from complicating management. Patients who respond to amphotericin B may be switched to fluconazole, 400 to 800 mg/day, for 8 to 10 weeks as a consolidation phase. Finally, a suppressive phase is begun with fluconazole 200 mg once daily. Antifungal therapy can be stopped after 1 to 2 years in patients who respond to ART with a CD4 count above 100/µL for at least 3 months, a nondetectable viral load, and a negative or low serum cryptococcal antigen.

TABLE 191-2   Clinical Manifestations of Cryptococcosis

Central Nervous System	Genitourinary Tract
Acute, subacute, chronic meningitis	Prostatitis
Cryptococcomas of brain (abscesses)	Renal cortical abscess
Spinal cord granuloma	Positive urine culture from occult source
Chronic dementia (from hydrocephalus)	Genital lesions
Lung	**Bone and Joints**
Nodules (single or multiple)	Osteolytic lesion (single or multiple sites)
Lobar infiltrates	Arthritis (acute/chronic)
Interstitial infiltrates	**Muscle**
Cavities	Myositis
Endobronchial masses	**Heart, Blood Vessels**
Endobronchial colonization	Cryptococcemia
Acute respiratory distress syndrome	Endocarditis (native and prosthetic)
Mediastinal adenopathy	Mycotic aneurysm
Hilar adenopathy	Myocarditis
Pneumothorax	Pericarditis
Pleural effusions/empyema	Infected vascular graft
Miliary pattern	**Gastrointestinal Tract**
Skin	Esophageal nodule
Papules and maculopapules	Nodular or ulcerated lesions in stomach or intestines (may resemble Crohn's disease)
Subcutaneous abscess	
Vesicles	Hepatitis
Plaques	Peritonitis
Cellulitis	Pancreatic mass
Purpura	**Breast**
Acne	Breast abscess
Draining sinuses	Lymph nodes
Ulcers	Lymphadenopathy
Bullae	**Thyroid**
Herpetiformis-like	Thyroiditis
Molluscum contagiosum–like	Thyroid mass
Eye	**Adrenal Gland**
Papilledema	Adrenal insufficiency
Extraocular muscle paresis	Adrenal mass
Keratitis	**Head and Neck**
Chorioretinitis	Gingivitis
Endophthalmitis	Sinusitis
Optic nerve atrophy	Salivary gland enlargement

Modified from Casadevall A, Perfect JR. *Cryptococcus neoformans*. Washington, DC: ASM Press; 1998:409.

- Complications of cryptococcal meningitis requiring special attention are (1) increased intracranial pressure, which can lead to blindness, permanent dementia, and death; (2) hydrocephalus, which may require placement of a ventriculoperitoneal shunt; and (3) immune reconstitution syndrome, which may be mistaken for therapeutic failure.

192 | *Histoplasma capsulatum* (Histoplasmosis)

George S. Deepe, Jr.

DEFINITION

- Histoplasmosis is the most frequent cause of fungal respiratory infection and has a broad spectrum of clinical manifestations ranging from a self-limited, acute, influenza-like illness to a progressive disseminated infection that is life threatening.

EPIDEMIOLOGY

- The fungus is typically found in the midwestern and southeastern United States and in Central and South America.
- Indigenous cases have been reported worldwide.
- The fungus thrives in decaying bird guano (starlings and blackbirds) and bat guano.
- Patients with acquired immunodeficiency syndrome (AIDS) or receiving immunosuppressive drugs, including tumor necrosis factor-α inhibitors, are predisposed to disseminated infection.

MICROBIOLOGY

- The fungus exists in the mycelial form in nature.
- The mycelia produce two sizes of conidia—micro and macro. The former are thought to induce disease because they are small enough to reach the bronchioles and alveoli.
- Conversion to the yeast phase is driven by temperature.

DIAGNOSIS

- Serology is useful for all but AIDS patients. Complement-fixation titers of 1 : 32 or greater are indicative of active disease. The presence of the H immunodiffusion band signifies active disease. An M band does not discriminate between current or remote infection.
- The *Histoplasma* antigen test either from urine or serum is particularly useful in diagnosis of extrapulmonary disease. It is also useful for following response to therapy.
- Tissue and buffy coat examination is useful for detecting the organism.
- See Table 192-1 for diagnostic tests.

THERAPY

- Pulmonary histoplasmosis: mild to moderate—no treatment or itraconazole 200 mg 3 times daily, followed by 200 mg twice a day for 6 to 12 weeks; moderate to severe—lipid-formulated amphotericin B, 3 to 5 mg/kg or deoxycholate amphotericin B, 0.7 to 1 mg/kg, for 1 to 2 weeks, followed by itraconazole for total of 10 to 11 weeks; cavitary—itraconazole as described above.
- Disseminated disease: moderate to severe—same as moderate-to-severe pulmonary disease; in children can use deoxycholate amphotericin B, 1 mg/kg for 4 to 6 weeks.
- Rheumatologic manifestations—nonsteroidals
- Mediastinal lymphadenitis—no treatment or, if symptomatic, itraconazole as described above
- See Table 192-2 for treatment options.

PREVENTION

- Prophylaxis for immunosuppressed patients—itraconazole 200 mg daily
- Avoid construction sites, spelunking, and remodeling of unoccupied homes or farm habitats.

TABLE 192-1	Diagnostics for Histoplasmosis	
INFECTION SITE	**DISEASE SEVERITY**	**DIAGNOSTIC**
Lung		
Acute	Mild-moderate	H and M bands and complement fixation.
	Moderate to severe	As above. Serum or urine antigen, or both, also may be positive in up to 70%. Bronchoalveolar fluid antigen may be useful. Culture of bronchoalveolar lavage fluid and silver stain of concentrated lavage fluid. Sputum culture.
Chronic cavitary		H and M bands and complement fixation. Culture of bronchoalveolar lavage fluid and silver stain of concentrated lavage fluid. Sputum cultures.
Disseminated		
	Acute	Serum or urine antigen, or both. H and M bands and complement fixation. These are not useful in AIDS patients. Examination of the buffy coat for yeast cells in phagocytes. Biopsy of bone marrow or liver with silver stain and culture. Blood culture.
	Chronic	Serum or urine antigen, or both. H and M bands and complement fixation. Biopsy of tissue with silver stain and culture.
Central nervous system		Serum or urine antigen, or both. CSF antigen. Culture of CSF. H and M bands and complement fixation are not as useful.
Mediastinal		
	Lymphadenitis	H and M bands and complement fixation.
	Granuloma	H and M bands and complement fixation.
	Fibrosis	H and M bands and complement fixation.
Rheumatologic	Arthralgias	H and M bands and complement fixation.
Pericarditis		H and M bands and complement fixation.
Endocarditis/Endovascular		H and M bands and complement fixation. Serum or urine antigen, or both. Culture and silver stain of valve.

AIDS, acquired immunodeficiency syndrome; CSF, cerebrospinal fluid.

TABLE 192-2   Treatment of Histoplasmosis

INFECTION SITE	DISEASE SEVERITY	TREATMENT
Lung		
Acute	Mild-Moderate	None or itraconazole 200 mg 3 times daily for 3 days followed by 200 mg twice a day for 6-12 wk.
	Moderate-Severe	Lipid-formulated amphotericin B, 3-5 mg/kg, or deoxycholate amphotericin B, 0.7-1 mg/kg, daily for 1-2 wk followed by itraconazole 200 mg 3 times a day for 3 days followed by 200 mg twice a day for a total duration of 12 wk. For children, itraconazole 5-10 mg/kg or deoxycholate amphotericin B, 1 mg/kg daily.
Chronic cavitary		Itraconazole 200 mg 3 times a day for 3 days followed by twice daily for at least 1 yr and as long as 2 yr.
Disseminated		
	Acute	Lipid-formulated amphotericin B, 3-5 mg/kg, or deoxycholate amphotericin B, 0.7-1 mg/kg, daily for 1-2 wk followed by itraconazole 200 mg 3 times a day for 3 days followed by 200 mg twice a day for at least 12 mo. For children, deoxycholate amphotericin B (1 mg/kg) daily for 4-6 wk or 2-4 wk followed by itraconazole 5-10 mg/kg daily. Total duration = 3 mo.
	Chronic	Itraconazole 200 mg 3 times a day for 3 days followed by 200 mg twice a day for at least 1 yr. Serum levels should be monitored to ensure adequate concentrations.
Central nervous system		Liposomal amphotericin B, 5 mg/kg daily for 4-6 wk followed by itraconazole administered as above for at least 1 yr and resolution of symptoms and negative cerebrospinal fluid antigen.
Mediastinal		
	Lymphadenitis	No treatment. If symptomatic (e.g., dysphagia), itraconazole 200 mg twice daily for 12 wk. Corticosteroids (60 mg with a rapid taper) may be used to diminish lymph node size.
	Granuloma	Same as lymphadenitis. Corticosteroids are not necessary.
	Fibrosis	Surgical intervention with stents. Antifungals are not useful.
Rheumatologic	Arthralgias, etc.	Nonsteroidals
Pericarditis		Nonsteroidals or corticosteroids. If the latter, treat with itraconazole (200 mg × 3 for 3 days and then once a day) until corticosteroids have been discontinued.
Endocarditis/ Endovascular		Surgical removal of the valve combined with lipid-formulated amphotericin B, 5 mg/kg daily for 6 wk. Lifelong suppression may be considered in some who are not surgical candidates with itraconazole 200 mg once or twice a day.

Data from Wheat LJ, Freifeld AG, Kleiman MB, et al. Clinical practice guidelines for the management of patients with histoplasmosis: 2007 update by the Infectious Diseases Society of America. *Clin Infect Dis.* 2007;45: 807-825.

193 Blastomycosis

Robert W. Bradsher, Jr.

DEFINITION

- Infection by Blastomyces dermatitidis

MICROBIOLOGY AND EPIDEMIOLOGY

- Broad-based single budding yeast
- *Blastomyces dermatitidis:* dimorphic; grows 25° to 28°C as a mold and at 37°C as yeast
- Visible in wet preparations of potassium hydroxide or calcofluor white by fluorescent microscopy
- Primarily in North America—Mississippi, Ohio, and St. Lawrence River Valleys and Great Lakes regions
- Point source outbreaks, often around lakes or rivers with recreational or occupational exposures
- Endemic or sporadic cases most commonly in normal hosts, although immune-suppressed hosts can be infected and could reactivate infection from prior subclinical infection
- Cellular immunity is the primary host defense to control the infection

CLINICAL MANIFESTATIONS

- Pulmonary portal of infection with pneumonia the most common finding
- Extrapulmonary infection to skin and subcutaneous tissue most common but also bone, prostate, central nervous system (CNS), or essentially any organ

DIAGNOSIS

- Diagnosis by visualization of organism with fungal stains or by culture of specimens. No colonization or contamination with this fungus
- Antibody tests lack of sensitivity
- Antigen testing of urine may be useful for diagnosis, but cross-reactions occur with other dimorphic fungal infections

TREATMENT (SEE TABLE 193-1)

- Itraconazole is the drug of choice for mild-to-moderate pulmonary or non-CNS extrapulmonary infection
- Amphotericin B (usually lipid) is the treatment for severe infection until improvement and then itraconazole
- CNS infection with lipid amphotericin B, followed by voriconazole or fluconazole

TABLE 193-1 Treatment of Blastomycosis*

INDICATION	THERAPY
Moderately severe or severe pulmonary blastomycosis or immunosuppressed patients	Liposomal amphotericin B 3-5 mg/kg or conventional amphotericin B 0.7-1 mg/kg once daily for 6-8 wk. After improvement, consider switching to itraconazole 200 mg PO once or twice daily.[†]
Pregnant	Liposomal amphotericin B 3-5 mg/kg or conventional amphotericin B 0.7-1 mg/kg once daily for 6-8 wk.
Brain abscess or meningitis	Amphotericin B as above until improved. For step-down treatment, consider itraconazole 200 mg PO 2-3 times daily, fluconazole 800 mg daily, or voriconazole 6 mg/kg for 2 doses, then 4 mg/kg q12h, IV or PO.
Mild-to-moderate pulmonary blastomycosis	Itraconazole 200 mg PO once or twice daily.[†]

IV, intravenous; PO, by mouth.

*Total duration of therapy at least 6 months. Disseminated, central nervous system, osteoarticular, or cavitary pulmonary manifestations may require longer treatment.

[†]Consider monitoring trough levels of native drug in patients not responding to itraconazole. Levels above 1 μg/mL by high-performance liquid chromatography are considered desirable, although data are scant.

194 Coccidioidomycosis (*Coccidioides* Species)

John N. Galgiani

DEFINITION

- The dimorphic fungi, *Coccidioides immitis* and *Coccidioides posadasii,* cause a systemic fungal infection, coccidioidomycosis, also known as *San Joaquin Valley fever.*

EPIDEMIOLOGY

- Coccidioidomycosis is endemic to arid regions of the Western Hemisphere.
- Approximately 150,000 new U.S. infections occur annually with 60% originating in Arizona and 30% in California. Of these, 50,000 produce significant illness.
- Infections most frequently occur during dry seasons, and the incubation period until first symptoms ranges from 1 to 3 weeks.
- The most common illness is a community-acquired pneumonia, lasting weeks to months whether treated or not with antifungal agents. Progressive pneumonia or hematogenous dissemination to other organs is a serious complication that requires treatment.
- Patients with diabetes are more likely to suffer pulmonary complications.
- Dissemination is frequent in patients with impaired cellular immunity.

MICROBIOLOGY

- *Coccidioides* has been found in desert soil and associated with animal burrows but is sparsely distributed, even within the most highly endemic regions.
- Throughout the 20th century, coccidioidomycosis was recognized as caused by a single fungal species, *C. immitis.* This population contains two genetically and geographically distinct clades, now recognized as separate species: *C. immitis* predominantly found in California and *C. posadasii* in all other endemic regions.
- On most laboratory media, growth by apical mycelial elongation is visible within a week.
- Alternate hyphal cells autolyze, leaving behind single 3- to 5-μm cells (arthroconidia) that can become airborne and capable of being inhaled deep into airways.
- In mammalian tissue, an arthroconidium remodels into a spherical cell that enlarges isotropically to form large mature spherules with scores of endospores developing within.
- Endospores, when released during spherule rupture, can develop into a new spherule within host tissue or revert to mycelial growth if removed from the infection.
- A sexual phase has not been observed, but population genetics suggest that one exists. Sequence analysis indicates that *Coccidioides* is an ascomycete.

DIAGNOSIS

- Isolation of *Coccidioides* in culture from a clinical specimen is diagnostic of infection.
- Recognizing endospore-containing spherules in wet mounts or histologic sections is also definitive.
- Diagnosis in most patients is made presumptively by detecting anticoccidioidal antibodies in serum or cerebrospinal fluid.

- Complement-fixing anticoccidioidal antibodies are quantitated by serial dilution titration. More extensive infections are frequently associated with higher titers, and clinical improvement is associated with decreasing titers.
- Immunodiffusion techniques are routinely used to provide a qualitative mimic of the complement-fixing antibody test and also to detect other *Coccidioides*-specific antibodies, often IgM, which occur earlier.
- Proprietary enzyme immunoassay kits that measure anticoccidioidal IgM and IgG antibodies are in wide use. They are more sensitive in detecting early coccidioidal infections but may not be as specific.
- A test for coccidioidal antigens is commercially available and is most frequently positive in patients with extensive infection.

THERAPY

- Healthy patients with uncomplicated coccidioidal pneumonia usually improve with general supportive management whether or not antifungal drugs are used. If antifungal treatment is initiated for such patients, it usually consists of fluconazole given orally at a dose of 400 mg per day for periods ranging from 3 months to 1 year.
- Patients with severe early pneumonia sufficient to require intensive care hospitalization are often treated with intravenous amphotericin B initially until the respiratory status stabilizes or improves.
- When infection results in chronic fibrocavitary pneumonia or extrapulmonary dissemination, antifungal therapy involves oral fluconazole (400 mg daily or higher) or itraconazole (200 mg twice or three times daily). Treatment would normally be continued for at least 1 year. In such patients, it is not infrequent for treatment to continue for several years because relapse off treatment is common.
- In some patients, surgery is essential in addition to antifungal drugs to control infection.
- Treatment of coccidioidal meningitis is most frequently managed with oral fluconazole in doses of 400 to 800 mg daily. This treatment is lifelong for all patients. Patients who develop hydrocephalus usually require the placement of an internal ventricular shunt.

PREVENTION

- A preventive vaccine for coccidioidomycosis is not available.

195 Dermatophytosis (Ringworm) and Other Superficial Mycoses

Roderick J. Hay

DEFINITION

- Dermatophyte infections are superficial infections of the stratum corneum of the skin or of keratinized appendages, such as hair or nails, arising from it. Other superficial infections are caused by *Candida* and *Malassezia* spp. or less common organisms (e.g., *Piedraia*).

EPIDEMIOLOGY

- Globally, the superficial fungal infections of the skin affect more than 900,000 million individuals. Most have no underlying abnormality, although individual conditions such as seborrheic dermatitis and oropharyngeal candidiasis may be early signs of human immunodeficiency virus infection.

MICROBIOLOGY

- The main fungi involved are dermatophyte species of the genera *Trichophyton*, *Microsporum*, and *Epidermophyton* and yeasts such as *Candida* or *Malassezia* spp. Less commonly, other mold fungi (e.g., *Scytalidium*) are implicated.

DIAGNOSIS

- Direct microscopy of the skin and culture is diagnostic. Molecular diagnostic techniques are in development.

THERAPY

- Topical treatments include azole antifungal agents and terbinafine. Selenium sulfide and zinc pyrithione have specific activity against *Malassezia*. Oral therapies are itraconazole and fluconazole; oral terbinafine is used mainly for dermatophyte infections (see Table 195-1).

PREVENTION

- There are no major preventive programs, although early identification of infection limits spread in communities, such as schools.

TABLE 195-1 Treatment of Dermatophytosis

DERMATOPHYTOSIS, CLINICAL DISEASE PATTERN	TREATMENT
Tinea pedis	
Interdigital	*Topical cream/ointment:* terbinafine, imidazoles (miconazole, econazole, clotrimazole, etc.), undecenoic acid, tolnaftate
"Dry type"	*Oral:* terbinafine, 250 mg/day for 2-4 wk; itraconazole, 400 mg/day for 1 wk per month (repeated if necessary); fluconazole 200 mg weekly for 4-8 wk
Tinea corporis	
Small, well-defined lesions	*Topical cream/ointment:* terbinafine, imidazoles (e.g., miconazole, econazole, clotrimazole)
Larger lesions	*Oral:* terbinafine, 250 mg/day for 2 weeks; itraconazole, 200 mg/day for 1 wk; fluconazole, 250 mg weekly for 2-4 wk
Tinea capitis	Griseofulvin, 10-20 mg/kg/day for minimum 6 wk
	Terbinafine
	<20 kg: 62.5 mg/day
	20-40 kg: 125 mg/day
	>40 kg: 250 mg/day
	Itraconazole, 4-6 mg/kg pulsed dose weekly
Onychomycosis	Fluconazole, 3-8 mg/kg pulsed dose weekly
Fingernails	Terbinafine, 250 mg daily for 6 wk
	Itraconazole, 400 mg/day for 1 wk each month, repeated for 2-3 mo
	Fluconazole, 200 mg weekly for 8-16 wk
Toenails	Terbinafine, 250 mg daily for 12 wk
	Itraconazole, 400 mg/day for 1 wk each month, repeated for 2-4 mo
	Fluconazole, 200 mg weekly for 12-24 wk

Chapter 195 Dermatophytosis (Ringworm) and Other Superficial Mycoses

196 Paracoccidioidomycosis

Angela Restrepo, Angela María Tobón, and Luz Elena Cano

MICROBIOLOGY AND EPIDEMIOLOGY

- Paracoccidioidomycosis is caused by *Paracoccidioides brasiliensis,* which contains four different phylogenetic lineages (S1, PS2, PS3, and PS4). A new species, *Paracoccidioides lutzii,* has been recognized within *P. brasiliensis* and also causes paracoccidioidomycosis.
- *Paracoccidioides* spp. are thermally dimorphic fungi, identified by multiple-budding yeast cells (pilot's wheel).
- These fungi exhibit slow mycelial growth for more than 20 days at 22° to 24° C. The yeast form appears ±10 days at 36° to 37° C.
- Direct microscopy and histopathology allow prompt diagnosis.
- These fungi are restricted to Latin American countries in unknown habitats.
- The largest endemic areas are found in Brazil.
- Most patients are males and work (or have worked) in agriculture within the endemic areas.
- Two progressive disease forms exist: (1) acute/subacute in children, adolescents, and immunocompromised individuals and (2) chronic in adults at least 30 years of age.

CLINICAL MANIFESTATIONS

- In the acute/subacute form, a severe disease, there is fever, weight loss, lymphadenopathy and hepatosplenomegaly. Multiple skin and mucosal lesions occur in half of the cases.
- In the chronic form, there are pulmonary infiltrates on chest radiographs (>90% of the cases) and lesions in mucous membranes and skin. Adrenal lesions with adrenal insufficiency are common.
- Specific diagnosis is usually late due to confusion with other more prevalent diseases (e.g., tuberculosis). Lack of physicians' awareness is a problem.
- Lung imaging studies are essential in adult patients. Healing by fibrosis creates serious complications.
- In tissues, granuloma formation is an important clue to diagnosis. Budding yeast cells are found in lesions.
- Serology shows that anti–*P. brasiliensis* antibodies are detectable in most patients. Quantitative tests allow treatment follow-up. Antigen determination also is useful in certain patients.
- Human immunodeficiency virus comorbidity is uncommon.

TREATMENT (SEE TABLE 196-1)

- Itraconazole is the treatment of choice for most patients, at 200 to 400 mg/day for 9 to 12 months.
- Amphotericin B deoxycholate is reserved for severe cases, at 1 mg/kg/day until achieving a 2-g total dose. This should be followed by oral medications.
- Trimethoprim-sulfamethoxazole (TMP-SMX) is given as TMP, 160 to 240 mg, and SMX, 800 to 1200 mg per day for 12 to 24 months, depending on disease severity.
- Regular follow-up observations (clinical, laboratory oriented) are mandatory.

TABLE 196-1 Antifungal Therapy for Paracoccidioidomycosis

ANTIFUNGAL PRESCRIBED (ADMINISTRATION ROUTE)	MINIMAL TREATMENT DURATION BASED ON ORGAN INVOLVEMENT*	DOSE	ADVERSE EFFECTS	RESPONSE (%)	RELAPSES (%)
TMP-SMX (PO/IV)	Minor: 12 mo Moderate: 18-24 mo	*Adults* TMP: 160-240 mg/day SMX: 800-1200 mg/day Divided into two doses per day *Children* TMP: 8-10 mg/kg SMX: 40-50 mg/kg Divided into two doses per day	Leukopenia Hypersensitivity-reactions, such as rash	80	20
Amphotericin B deoxycholate (IV)	Until patient improves and can be treated by the oral route Achieve a total dose of 2 g†	1 mg/kg/day	Nephrotoxicity Hypokalemia Nausea/vomiting Fever Anemia	70	25
Ketoconazole (PO)	9-12 mo	200-400 mg/day	Hormonal alterations Increase in hepatic enzymes Nausea/vomiting	90	11
Itraconazole (PO)	6-9 mo	*Adults* 600 mg/day for 3 days; continue 200 mg/day *Children (<30/kg and >5 yr)* 5-10 mg/kg/day	Nausea/vomiting ↑ Hepatic enzymes Drug interactions	94-98	3-5
Voriconazole (PO/IV)	6 mo	Initial dose: 400 mg each 12 hr for one day, then 200 mg each 12 hr Diminish the dose to 50% if weight is <40 kg	Visual alterations ↑ Hepatic enzymes Skin rash Photosensitivity Hallucinations Periostitis	88	No data

IV, intravenous; PO, orally; TMP-SMX, trimethoprim-sulfamethoxazole.
*Shown only with the aim of guiding therapy. Total duration must be defined in accordance with clinical and immune-based tests, as well with the mycosis clinical form.
†Should always be continued with TMP-SMX or itraconazole oral therapy, once clinical improvement has been obtained.

Uncommon Fungi and Related Species

Duane R. Hospenthal

PSEUDALLESCHERIA BOYDII

Definition
- Infection of the lungs, bones and joints, or central nervous system (CNS); may be disseminated
- Also causes mycetoma

Epidemiology
- Typically occurs in the immunocompromised or following trauma
- CNS infection in immunocompetent persons after near-drowning
- Organism can be found in soil and fresh water, especially stagnant or polluted

Microbiology
- *P. boydii (Scedosporium apiospermum)* is a group of at least five species.
- Identification is typically made by identification of microscopic structures from culture.

Diagnosis
- Diagnosis is made by culture recovery from infected site.
- Because *P. boydii* may colonize airways, sputum cultures may not reflect infection.

Therapy
- Voriconazole is likely the most effective agent.

SCEDOSPORIUM PROLIFICANS

Definition
- Disseminated infection and bone and joint infections are most common.
- *S. prolificans* may cause onychomycosis and infections of the eye and wounds.

Epidemiology
- Disseminated infection commonly occurs in the severely immunocompromised.
- Localized infection occurs in immunocompetent individuals after trauma.
- The organism can be found in soil and colonizing the respiratory tract.

Microbiology
- Identification is made by culture.

Diagnosis
- Diagnosis is made by culture recovery from the infected site.
- Because *S. prolificans* may colonize airways, sputum cultures may not reflect infection.

Therapy
- No effective therapy. Consider voriconazole with amphotericin B.

DARK-WALLED FUNGI (*BIPOLARIS, EXOPHIALA, EXSEROHILUM, PHIALOPHORA, CURVULARIA*, OTHERS)

Definition
- This infection involves fungi that have melanin in their cell wall and may appear dark walled in tissue.
- Infection is often termed *phaeohyphomycosis* and typically presents as localized skin and soft tissue infections, CNS infections, or allergic sinusitis.
- Dark-walled fungi that cause chromoblastomycosis and mycetoma are not included in the agents of phaeohyphomycosis.

Epidemiology
- Infection is commonly acquired from minor trauma or inhalation.
- Fungi are found in soil, organic material, plants, and air.
- They may be spread through contaminated products (e.g., injectable steroids).

Microbiology
- The most common agents of phaeohyphomycosis are *Alternaria, Bipolaris, Cladophialophora, Curvularia, Exophiala, Exserohilum,* and *Wangiella*

Diagnosis
- Diagnosis is made by recovery of these organisms in culture from the site of infection.
- Cell walls may appear dark brown or golden on histopathology (hematoxylin and eosin). Use of a Fontana-Masson stain may allow easier identification of these fungi.

Therapy
- Surgical débridement of lesions or colonizing fungi in the case of allergic fungal sinusitis
- Amphotericin B in life-threatening infections
- Voriconazole and itraconazole are typically effective but prolonged therapy needed

FUSARIUM SPP.

Definition
- Can cause disseminated infection in immunocompromised patients
- Common cause of keratitis and other eye infections in contact lens wearers and following trauma
- Skin and soft tissue infection after trauma, onychomycosis; can cause mycetoma

Epidemiology
- Common plant pathogens; found in soil and organic debris
- Has been recovered in hospital water supplies

Microbiology
- *F. solani* is the most common pathogen, although other species may also cause infection.
- *Fusarium* produces banana- (or crescent)-shaped multicellular macroconidia in culture.

Diagnosis
- Recovery of the fungus from culture of an otherwise sterile site
- One of the few molds that are commonly recovered from blood culture

Therapy
- Optimum therapy is not known.
- Recovery from neutropenia is essential in response to therapy of disseminated infection.
- Amphotericin B or voriconazole is suggested.

TRICHOSPORON SPP.

Definition
- Most commonly presents as disseminated infection

Epidemiology

- Typically an infection of the immunocompromised; may be associated with central venous catheter
- Fungi found colonizing the skin, gastrointestinal, respiratory, or genital tract
- Found in soil and water
- Breakthrough infections in patients receiving echinocandins

Microbiology

- Most common pathogen is *T. asahii*.
- *Trichosporon* are identified by their unique ability to produce septate hyphae, arthroconidia, and budding yeast.
- Appears yeastlike on initial culture

Diagnosis

- By recovery of the organism from the blood or lesion biopsy

Therapy

- Azole antifungal (voriconazole, itraconazole, isavuconazole, posaconazole, or fluconazole)

MALASSEZIA FURFUR
Definition

- Catheter-related bloodstream infection
- Also causes pityriasis versicolor

Epidemiology

- Typically associated with parenteral lipid infusion
- Commonly reported in neonates

Microbiology

- May be difficult to grow from positive blood cultures without lipid supplementation

Diagnosis

- Recovery of fungus from blood culture

Therapy

- Catheter removal and discontinuation of parenteral lipids
- Susceptible to most antifungals (voriconazole, fluconazole, or amphotericin B)

Prevention

- Limiting use of parenteral lipids

OTHER UNCOMMON YEASTS
Definition

- Other less common yeasts may also cause catheter-related bloodstream infection.

Epidemiology

- Typically associated with use of central venous catheters and immunocompromise

Microbiology

- Include *Saprochaete capitata (Blastoschizomyces capitatus), Pichia anomala, Rhodotorula species,* and *Saccharomyces cerevisiae*

Diagnosis

- Made by recovery of the yeast in blood culture

Therapy
- Removal of central venous catheter
- Antifungals based on recovered yeast

PENICILLIUM MARNEFFEI
Definition
- Acute disseminated infection of persons infected with human immunodeficiency virus (HIV) in Southeast Asia
- Infection similar to acute disseminated histoplasmosis in patients with acquired immunodeficiency syndrome
- Rarely, localized infection in apparently immunocompetent persons

Epidemiology
- Limited to Southeast Asia. More common in rainy season, in young adult males with HIV infection, typically with low CD4 cell counts

Microbiology
- Typical *Penicillium*-like structures on microscopic examination of culture
- Cultures produce red pigment that diffuses into the agar.

Diagnosis
- Typically made from recovery of the organism in blood
- May also be recovered in culture of skin lesions, lymph nodes, or bone marrow aspirates
- Serologic testing may be available in endemic regions.

Therapy
- Amphotericin B in life-threatening presentations
- Itraconazole or voriconazole in initial therapy (not life-threatening)
- Itraconazole secondary prophylaxis in HIV-infected patients

LACAZIA LOBOI
Definition
- Chronic nodular or keloidal skin infection, commonly of the ears or face

Epidemiology
- Limited to Central and South America
- Infection also found in dolphins

Microbiology
- Has not been recovered in culture
- Identified as closely related to *Paracoccidioides brasiliensis* by molecular techniques

Diagnosis
- Based on clinical presentation and finding typical structures on histopathology
- Globose (yeast) cells end-to-end in short "strings"

Therapy
- Surgical removal

AGENTS OF ADIASPIROMYCOSIS (*EMMONSIA* SPP.)
Definition
- Disease secondary to host immune response to nonreplicating fungal conidia, termed *adiaspores*
- Chiefly a pulmonary disease; may range from asymptomatic to rapidly leading to respiratory failure and occasionally death
- May also present as ocular nodules

Epidemiology

- Seen with occupational inhalation to dusts in men, average age 40
- Outbreak in Brazilian children in association with diving and freshwater sponges

Microbiology

- Secondary to *Emmonsia* species, usually *E. crescens*
- Dimorphic fungi closely related to *Blastomyces dermatitidis*

Diagnosis

- Identification is limited to observation of typical structures on histopathology showing adiaspores, up to 500 μm in diameter, nondividing, and surrounded by granulomata composed of epithelioid and giant cells.

Therapy

- Corticosteroids appear to be useful.

EMMONSIA PASTEURIANA
Definition

- Disseminated infection most commonly afflicting HIV-infected persons

Epidemiology

- Severely immunocompromised persons
- Largest report from South Africa

Microbiology

- *Emmonsia pasteuriana* or closely related fungus
- Thermally dimorphic fungus

Diagnosis

- Recovery of the dimorphic fungus from skin biopsy or blood culture

Therapy

- Responses to amphotericin B and triazole antifungals have been reported

PROTOTHECA SPP.
Definition

- Localized skin or subcutaneous infection caused by algal pathogen
- Rare reports of disseminated or deep infection

Epidemiology

- Likely cause infection after traumatic inoculation
- Organisms colonize skin, gastrointestinal and respiratory tract

Microbiology

- Disease is typically due to *P. wickerhamii* or *P. zopfii*.
- Unicellular algae lack chlorophyll.
- *Prototheca* spp. grow on fungal culture media with yeastlike colonial morphology.
- Microscopic appearance in tissue is diagnostic.

Diagnosis

- Recovery of algae in culture is diagnostic.
- Yeast biochemical panels commonly identify *Prototheca*.

Therapy

- Surgical excision with amphotericin B or itraconazole

PYTHIUM SPP.

Definition
- Vascular infections in persons with iron overload such as thalassemia or ocular infections following trauma
- Skin and subcutaneous and disseminated infection possible

Epidemiology
- Worldwide distribution, but most commonly reported from Thailand
- Risk factors: thalassemia-hemoglobinopathy syndrome and trauma
- Presumed association with work in swampy (e.g., rice paddy) environment
- High morbidity (eye or limb loss) and mortality

Microbiology
- Fungus-like protist, *Pythium*, grows rapidly as mold on fungal culture.

Diagnosis
- Recovery of the organism from culture is diagnostic.
- Local serologic testing may be available.

Therapy
- Can perform surgical resection or amputation.
- No satisfactory medical therapy is known.
- Doxycycline, minocycline, tigecycline, linezolid, and macrolides have activity in vitro.

RHINOSPORIDIUM SEEBERI

Definition
- Localized polypoidal infection, chiefly of the nose, upper airway, and conjunctiva

Epidemiology
- Worldwide distribution, but most commonly reported from southern India and Sri Lanka

Microbiology
- Has not been grown in culture
- Identified as a protist by molecular methods

Diagnosis
- Made by microscopic observation of typical structures—thick-walled cysts (100 to 350 μm) filled with numerous spores

Therapy
- Surgical excision with electrocautery of lesion base

198 *Pneumocystis* Species

Peter D. Walzer, A. George Smulian, and Robert F. Miller*

DEFINITION

- *Pneumocystis* spp. are genetically distinct, host-specific opportunistic fungal pathogens widely found in nature.
- *Pneumocystis jirovecii,* found in humans, causes pneumonia ("*Pneumocystis* pneumonia" or "PCP") in immunocompromised patients.

EPIDEMIOLOGY

- Infection is acquired by inhalation of the cyst form of the organism.
- Primary infection occurs in the first 2 years of life in most people.
- Person-to-person transmission and outbreaks of PCP in immunosuppressed patients have been reported.
- Environmental factors influence PCP hospitalizations.
- Colonization is common, associated with obstructive airway disease.

DIAGNOSIS

- PCP in patients with human immunodeficiency virus (HIV): slow development, milder disease, 10% to 12% mortality
- PCP in non-HIV patients: rapid development, severe disease, 30% to 50% mortality
- Gold standard: microscopic demonstration of organism in respiratory tract specimens by immunofluorescence or special stains
- Other methods (polymerase chain reaction, β-D-glucan levels) are promising but are considered investigational

TREATMENT

- Trimethoprim-sulfamethoxazole (TMP-SMX) 15 to 20 mg/kg/day (TMP) and 75 to 100 mg/kg/day (SMX) IV or PO in divided doses every 6 to 8 hours for 14 to 21 days is the treatment of choice for mild, moderate, or severe PCP.
- *Mild-to-moderate PCP:* Oral dose can be given as TMP-SMX double strength 2 tablets orally three times a day.
- Several alternative regimens are available depending on the severity of PCP.
- Prednisone 40 mg PO twice daily on days 1 to 5, 40 mg PO every day on days 6 to 10, and 20 mg PO every day on days 11 to 21 are given as adjunctive therapy for moderate-to-severe PCP (PaO_2 ≤70 mm Hg, or alveolar-arterial O_2 gradient >35 mm Hg).
- Start prednisone as soon as possible or within the first 3 days after beginning antimicrobial therapy.
- Prednisone is mainly indicated for HIV-positive patients.

---

*All material in this chapter is in the public domain, with the exception of any borrowed figures or tables.

PREVENTION

- TMP-SMX 1 DS tablet orally every day or 1 SS tablet orally every day is the drug of choice for primary and secondary prophylaxis.
- Alternative regimens are available.
- Strong evidence supports isolation of PCP patients from contact with other immunocompromised hosts.

199 Microsporidiosis

Louis M. Weiss

DEFINITION

- Microsporidia are obligate eukaryotic intracellular pathogens related to fungi.
- Taxonomy of the phylum is based on ultrastructural descriptions of the spores and life cycle.
- Molecular phylogeny, based on rRNA sequences, is also utilized for classification.

EPIDEMIOLOGY

- The phylum Microsporidia contains at least 1200 species distributed into more than 190 genera.
- Several different genera and species of microsporidia cause disease in humans, including *Nosema, Vittaforma, Pleistophora, Encephalitozoon, Enterocytozoon, Trachipleistophora, Anncaliia, Tubulinosema, Endoreticulatus,* and *Microsporidium.*
- Microsporidiosis occurs in both immunocompromised and immune-competent hosts.
- These pathogens can be transmitted by food or water and are likely zoonotic.
- Diarrhea or keratoconjunctivitis are the most common presenting manifestations of infection, but infection can occur in any organ system.

DIAGNOSIS

- Diagnosis can be made by finding characteristic spores in body fluids (e.g., stool, urine, conjunctival scraping, etc., using stains, such as chromotrope 2R or Uvitex 2B).
- Definitive identification of the microsporidia causing an infection can be done using ultrastructural examination or molecular techniques.
- Patients with diarrhea or keratoconjunctivitis should have urine examined to look for disseminated infection.
- Species-specific diagnosis is useful for guiding treatment.

THERAPY

- Systemic albendazole and fumagillin are active therapeutic agents for the treatment of microsporidiosis.
- Topical fumagillin is useful for microsporidian keratoconjunctivitis.
- Immune restoration such as combination antiretroviral treatment in patients with acquired immunodeficiency syndrome often results in resolution of infection.

PREVENTION

- There are limited data on effective preventive strategies for microsporidiosis, but the most effective prophylaxis is restoration of immune function in immunocompromised hosts.
- The usual sanitary measures that prevent contamination of food and water will decrease the chance of infection.
- Hand washing and general hygienic habits reduce the chance of contamination of the conjunctiva and cornea with microsporidian spores.

200 *Entamoeba* Species, Including Amebic Colitis and Liver Abscess

William A. Petri, Jr., and Rashidul Haque

DEFINITION
- Amebiasis is defined as human infection by *Entamoeba* species, including *E. histolytica*, which is the cause of amebic colitis, liver abscess, and, rarely, brain abscess; *E. moshkovskii*, which causes diarrhea; and *E. dispar*, which is nonpathogenic.

EPIDEMIOLOGY
- Amebiasis is spread by fecal-oral transmission, and in addition to person to person can be waterborne and foodborne.
- Most infections are in impoverished communities in the developing world.
- Amebic colonization, diarrhea, and colitis are most common in infants through the preschool years.
- Amebic liver and brain abscess occur 90% of the time in young men.
- *E. histolytica* is a common cause of diarrhea in returning international travelers.
- Men who have sex with men (MSM) are at risk of both human immunodeficiency virus (HIV) and amebiasis, and one should consider the possibility of HIV in the setting of amebiasis in MSM.

MICROBIOLOGY
- Cyst form is infectious, environmentally stable, and resistant to chlorination.
- Trophozoite is the tissue-invasive stage.

DIAGNOSIS
- Stool ova and parasite exam should not be used because they are insensitive and nonspecific. Instead, diagnosis is best accomplished in the laboratory through a combination of fecal antigen detection or quantitative polymerase chain reaction for fecal parasite DNA, in combination with serologic tests for antiamebic antibodies (which can be negative early in illness).
- Colonoscopy and abdominal imaging techniques (ultrasound, computed tomography, and magnetic resonance imaging) are useful adjuncts for diagnosis of intestinal and extraintestinal disease, respectively.

THERAPY (SEE TABLE 200-1)
- Noninvasive infection is treated with paromomycin: 30 mg/kg/day orally in three divided doses per day × 5 to 10 days.
- Invasive infection is treated with tinidazole 2 g once daily for 5 days, followed by paromomycin (to prevent relapse from gut lumen parasites).
- Consider percutaneous drainage for liver abscesses of 5 cm or greater in diameter or if they are in the left lobe.

PREVENTION
- Prevention is accomplished by sanitation and clean water.
- Vaccine is under development.

TABLE 200-1 Drug Therapy for Treatment of Amebiasis

DRUG	ADULT DOSAGE	SIDE EFFECTS
Amebic Liver Abscess*		
Metronidazole[†]	750 mg PO tid × 10 days	Primarily GI side effects: anorexia, nausea, vomiting, diarrhea, abdominal discomfort, or unpleasant metallic taste; disulfiram-like intolerance reaction to alcoholic beverages; neurotoxicity, including seizures, peripheral neuropathy, dizziness, confusion, irritability
or		
Tinidazole	2 g PO once daily × 5 days	Primarily GI side effects and disulfiram-like intolerance reaction to alcoholic beverages for 5 days
Followed by a luminal agent		
Paromomycin	30 mg/kg/day PO in three divided doses per day × 5-10 days	Primarily GI side effects: diarrhea, GI upset
or		
Diloxanide furoate	500 mg PO tid × 10 days	Primarily GI side effects: flatulence, nausea, vomiting Pruritus, urticaria
Amebic Colitis[‡]		
Tinidazole	2 g PO once daily × 5 days	Same as for amebic liver abscess
Plus a luminal agent (same as for amebic liver abscess)		
Asymptomatic Intestinal Colonization		
Treatment with luminal agent as for amebic liver abscess		

GI, gastrointestinal; PO, by mouth.

*Amebic liver abscess may necessitate antiparasitic treatment plus percutaneous or surgical drainage. Nitazoxanide may be effective therapy as well, but clinical experience is limited.

[†]Drug of choice for treatment of amebic liver abscess.

[‡]Amebic colitis may necessitate antiparasitic treatment plus surgical treatment.

Modified from Haque R, Huston CD, Hughes M, et al. Current concepts: amebiasis. *N Engl J Med.* 2003;348: 1565-1573.

201 Free-Living Amebae

Anita A. Koshy, Brian G. Blackburn, and Upinder Singh

MICROBIOLOGY AND EPIDEMIOLOGY

- Free-living amebae are protists that are common in the environment worldwide but rarely cause recognized human infections. The trophozoite stages of these organisms feed on bacteria and debris in the environment.
  - *Naegleria fowleri* is widely distributed globally and has been isolated from fresh water, most commonly in warm environments.
  - *Acanthamoeba* spp. are ubiquitous members of the environment and are found worldwide in soil and fresh water.
  - *Balamuthia mandrillaris* is also likely widely distributed and has been isolated from soil.

CLINICAL MANIFESTATIONS AND DIAGNOSIS

- *N. fowleri* typically causes a fulminant meningoencephalitis in healthy, immunocompetent young patients, in association with swimming in warm fresh water. The disease is nearly always fatal.
  - The cerebrospinal fluid (CSF) profile of patients with *N. fowleri* primary amebic meningoencephalitis (PAM) is similar to that seen in bacterial meningitis (high white blood cell count, low glucose, high protein), but with a negative Gram stain and culture. Motile trophozoites can sometimes be seen on wet mount of the CSF.
  - Neuroimaging studies in patients with PAM are usually nonspecific.
- *Acanthamoeba* spp. and *B. mandrillaris* cause the subacute onset of focal neurologic deficits and mental status changes (granulomatous amebic encephalitis [GAE]) related to central nervous system mass lesions. *Acanthamoeba* is mostly seen in immunocompromised and debilitated individuals, whereas *Balamuthia* occurs in both immunocompromised and immunocompetent patients. The case-fatality rate for these infections is also high.
  - In the United States, *Balamuthia* GAE may be more common in male Hispanic patients than in other groups.
  - CSF studies of patients with GAE are usually nonspecific, and it is rare to isolate organisms from the CSF.
  - Neuroimaging studies generally reveal multiple space-occupying lesions in the brain, with or without contrast enhancement.
  - Biopsy of involved tissues (skin, brain, etc.) can be diagnostic, usually via histopathologic examination/immunohistochemical staining or polymerase chain reaction (PCR).
- *Acanthamoeba* spp. and *B. mandrillaris* can involve other sites (lungs, sinuses, adrenals, and skin).
- *Acanthamoeba* spp. also cause sight-threatening keratitis in otherwise healthy individuals in association with contact lens use. Diagnosis depends on a high clinical suspicion, in conjunction with in vivo confocal microscopy or demonstration of *Acanthamoeba* in corneal scrapings or biopsy specimens by histopathologic examination, culture, or PCR.

THERAPY

- Therapeutic regimens for free-living amebic infections of humans are not well defined.
- Treatment for *N. fowleri* PAM should include high-dose intravenous amphotericin products; intrathecal amphotericin may also provide some benefit, and the addition of azoles, rifampin, miltefosine, or other antimicrobials should be considered.
- *Acanthamoeba* keratitis should be treated with topical chlorhexidine or polyhexamethylene biguanide; adjunctive surgical therapy may also be necessary.
- *Acanthamoeba* GAE should be treated with combination antimicrobial regimens, possibly including pentamidine, an azole, a sulfonamide, miltefosine, and flucytosine. However, the most efficacious regimen is not currently known.
- *B. mandrillaris* GAE should be treated with combination antimicrobial regimens, possibly including pentamidine, flucytosine, a sulfonamide, albendazole, an azole, a macrolide, amphotericin, and/or miltefosine. However, the most efficacious regimen is not currently known.
- Surgical débridement may play an adjunctive role in the management of both forms of GAE.

202 Malaria (*Plasmodium* Species)

Rick M. Fairhurst* and Thomas E. Wellems

DEFINITION

- The history of travel and exposure in a malaria-endemic area is typical.
- Uncomplicated malaria is often confused with the "flu": fever, accompanied by headaches, body aches, and malaise.
- Severe malaria can present with any one of the following: diminished consciousness, convulsions, respiratory distress, prostration, hyperparasitemia, severe anemia, hypoglycemia, jaundice, renal insufficiency, hemoglobinuria, shock, cessation of eating and drinking, repetitive vomiting, or hyperpyrexia.

EPIDEMIOLOGY

- Malaria is endemic in tropical and subtropical areas of Africa, South America, Asia, and Oceania.
- Malaria is transmitted by the bite of a female *Anopheles* mosquito.
- Transmission can also occur by blood transfusion, imported mosquitoes, or autochthonous mosquitoes infected by immigrants.

MICROBIOLOGY

- Plasmodia are parasitic protozoa of the Apicomplexa phylum.
- *Plasmodium falciparum*, *Plasmodium vivax*, *Plasmodium ovale*, *Plasmodium malariae*, and *Plasmodium knowlesi* are the major human malaria parasites.

LABORATORY DIAGNOSIS

- Identification of parasites is through Giemsa-stained thick and thin blood smears.
- Rapid diagnostic tests are available (e.g., BinaxNOW in the United States).

THERAPY

- Treatment depends primarily on disease severity, drug-resistance epidemiology, patient age, and pregnancy status.
- Uncomplicated malaria due to:
  - Chloroquine-sensitive *P. falciparum* (Mexico, Central America west of the Panama Canal, Haiti, the Dominican Republic, and most areas of the Middle East), *P. vivax*, *P. ovale*, *P. malariae*, and *P. knowlesi*, as well as uncomplicated malaria, due to:
    - Oral treatment with chloroquine phosphate
  - Chloroquine-resistant *P. falciparum* (most areas of the world) or chloroquine-resistant *P. vivax* (Papua New Guinea and Indonesia)
    - Oral treatment with atovaquone-proguanil, artemether-lumefantrine, quinine plus doxycycline, or mefloquine (dihydroartemisinin-piperaquine is registered and available in some countries outside the United States)

---

*All material in this chapter is in the public domain, with the exception of any borrowed figures or tables.

- Prevent relapsing *P. vivax* and *P. ovale* malaria with primaquine phosphate (contraindicated in pregnant/breast-feeding women and glucose-6-phosphate dehydrogenase [G6PD]-deficient persons)
- Severe malaria
  - Intravenous treatment with quinidine gluconate (only drug commercially available in the United States), artesunate (available only from the Centers for Disease Control and Prevention in the United States), or quinine dihydrochloride (not available in the United States)

PREVENTION
- Chemoprophylaxis decisions should be based on drug-resistance epidemiology, patient age, and pregnancy status.
  - Areas with chloroquine-sensitive malaria: chloroquine phosphate
  - Areas with mefloquine-sensitive malaria: mefloquine
  - All areas: atovaquone-proguanil or doxycycline
  - Areas with mostly *P. vivax:* primaquine (contraindicated in pregnant women and G6PD-deficient persons)
- Mosquito repellents and avoidance measures

203 Leishmania Species: Visceral (Kala-Azar), Cutaneous, and Mucosal Leishmaniasis

Alan J. Magill

DEFINITION

- Leishmaniasis is infection with *Leishmania* species of protozoa acquired by the bite of a *Phlebotomus* or *Lutzomyia* sand fly.

CLINICAL MANIFESTATIONS

- The syndrome classifications of leishmaniasis are cutaneous, mucosal (mucocutaneous), and visceral (kala-azar). Uncommon skin manifestations are diffuse cutaneous leishmaniasis, post–kala-azar dermal leishmaniasis, leishmaniasis recidivans, and disseminated leishmaniasis.

DIAGNOSIS

- Giemsa stain, culture, and polymerase chain reaction assay are performed.

TREATMENT

- Treatment of skin lesions includes topical, oral, and systemic regimens. Visceral leishmaniasis and New World mucosal leishmaniasis are treated parenterally by an amphotericin B formulation, pentavalent antimony, and miltefosine.

204 Trypanosoma Species (American Trypanosomiasis, Chagas' Disease): Biology of Trypanosomes

Louis V. Kirchhoff*

DEFINITION

- Chagas' disease, or American trypanosomiasis, is an infection caused by the single-cell protozoan parasite *Trypanosoma cruzi*.

MICROBIOLOGY

- *T. cruzi* is spread among its various mammalian hosts, including domestic and wild animals as well as humans, by bloodsucking triatomine insects, also called cone-nosed or kissing bugs.
- The parasites multiply in the gut of these insects, and their feces contain forms that can infect mammals. When contaminated feces touch vulnerable mammalian tissues such as the conjunctivae, oral and nasal mucosal surfaces, or skin abrasions, transmission can take place.
- Once the parasites gain a foothold in a mammalian host, they alternate between multiplying intracellular forms and free-swimming forms in the bloodstream that spread the infection internally or get swept up by feeding vectors, thus completing the cycle.
- *T. cruzi* can also be transmitted from mother to fetus, through blood products and organs obtained from infected donors, and in laboratory accidents.
- Infection with *T. cruzi* in humans is lifelong.

EPIDEMIOLOGY

- Chagas' disease is endemic in all South and Central American countries and also in Mexico.
- The infection is not endemic in any of the Caribbean islands.
- About 8 million persons are chronically infected with *T. cruzi,* roughly 56,000 new infections occur each year, and about 12,000 persons die of the illness annually. An estimated 300,000 immigrants with Chagas' disease currently live in the United States.
- During recent decades, large numbers of people in the endemic countries have been migrating from rural areas to the cities, and at the same time many millions of people have emigrated from the endemic countries to industrialized regions, particularly the European Union and the United States, thus urbanizing and globalizing the disease.

CLINICAL MANIFESTATIONS

- Between 10% and 30% of persons who are chronically infected with *T. cruzi* ultimately develop cardiac or gastrointestinal symptoms that are caused by pathologic processes related to the persistent presence of the parasite.
- Chronic cardiac Chagas' disease typically involves rhythm disturbances and cardiomyopathy.
- Gastrointestinal problems can include megaesophagus and megacolon.
- Immunosuppression of persons who harbor *T. cruzi* chronically can result in life-threatening reactivation of the infection.

---

*All material in this chapter is in the public domain, with the exception of borrowed figures.

DIAGNOSIS

- The diagnosis of acute or congenital Chagas' disease is made by parasitologic methods, typically direct microscopic examination of blood, hemoculture, or polymerase chain reaction–based assays.
- Chronic *T. cruzi* infection is diagnosed serologically, and many enzyme-linked immunosorbent assays, immunofluorescence assays, and chemiluminescence tests are available commercially for this purpose.

THERAPY

- Nifurtimox and benznidazole are the only two drugs available for treating *T. cruzi* infections (available from the Centers for Disease Control and Prevention Drug Service).
- Parasitologic cure rates for these drugs are high for acute and congenital infections but unfortunately very low in persons with long-standing infections.
- There are no convincing data from randomized controlled trials indicating that treatment of chronically infected persons with either drug significantly delays pathogenesis or affects long-term outcomes.

PREVENTION

- No vaccine or prophylactic drugs are available for reducing transmission of *T. cruzi*.
- In the endemic countries, reducing transmission depends primarily on educating at-risk populations, housing improvement, and spraying insecticides to eliminate vectors in dwellings.
- Serologic screening of blood and organ donors is also a key element in the control of Chagas' disease.
- In many of the endemic countries, enormous progress has been made in both vector control and blood screening and in the United States, Canada, and the European Union with the latter.

205 Agents of African Trypanosomiasis (Sleeping Sickness)

Louis V. Kirchhoff*

DEFINITION

- Human African trypanosomiasis (HAT), also known as sleeping sickness, is caused by two protozoan parasite subspecies: *Trypanosoma brucei gambiense* (West African trypanosomiasis) and *Trypanosoma brucei rhodesiense* (East African trypanosomiasis).

MICROBIOLOGY

- The trypanosomes that cause HAT are transmitted among their mammalian hosts by tsetse flies. The flies become infected when they take a blood meal from an infected mammal. There is a developmental cycle in the flies, after which infective parasites migrate to the salivary glands and are injected into a new host when the flies take subsequent blood meals. In their mammalian hosts African trypanosomes are found primarily in the bloodstream and, to a lesser extent, in perivascular areas of the brain and other tissues. In contrast to *Trypanosoma cruzi*, the parasite that causes Chagas' disease, African trypanosomes do not have an intracellular phase. They avoid immune destruction by antibodies by periodically changing their glycoprotein coats through a molecular process called *antigenic variation*.

EPIDEMIOLOGY

- HAT occurs only in sub-Saharan Africa, where endemic foci are found in about 20 countries.
- HAT is much less of a problem today than in the past. Fewer than 10,000 new cases are reported annually to the World Health Organization. Although this number reflects substantial underreporting, there is no doubt that control efforts implemented in many endemic countries during the past 15 years have achieved considerable success. Each year in industrialized countries HAT is diagnosed in a sprinkling of persons who have traveled to endemic areas, but given the large numbers of persons who make such trips, the incidence of such cases is extremely low.

CLINICAL MANIFESTATIONS

- Two clinical stages exist. Stage 1 (hemolymphatic disease) is characterized by fever, adenopathy, and headache. Stage 2 (central nervous system or encephalitic disease) involves mainly neuropsychiatric signs and symptoms.
- The primary difference between the clinical patterns of *gambiense* and *rhodesiense* HAT is that the latter follows a much more rapid course and can lead to death in a matter of months, whereas *gambiense* HAT typically develops a chronic pattern that can last for years.
- Untreated HAT almost inevitably ends in death.
- It is important for caregivers attending to travelers with fever and other nonspecific symptoms who have been in endemic areas to include HAT in the differential diagnosis.

---

*All material in this chapter is in the public domain, with the exception of borrowed figures.

DIAGNOSIS

- Given the life-threatening nature of untreated HAT, a high index of suspicion should be maintained with persons who have been in areas endemic for HAT.
- Numerous other illnesses common in the tropics cause symptoms similar to those seen in both the early and late stages of sleeping sickness.
- A definitive diagnosis of African trypanosomiasis requires demonstration of the parasite. Examination of blood smears and cerebrospinal fluid for parasites is the cornerstone of HAT diagnosis.
- There is a growing role for polymerase chain reaction and related molecular methods in the diagnosis of HAT.
- Diagnostic approaches and treatment should be discussed in detail with appropriate staff at the Centers for Disease Control and Prevention.

THERAPY

- Treatment is complicated because it varies according to the clinical stage of the disease and the trypanosome subspecies causing the infection.
- Toxicity of the drugs used to treat HAT is a major problem.

PREVENTION

- Individuals can reduce their risk of acquiring infections with African trypanosomes by avoiding areas known to harbor infected insects, wearing clothing that reduces the biting of the flies, and using insect repellent.
- Chemoprophylaxis is not recommended because of the high toxicity of the drugs that are active against African trypanosomes, and no vaccine is available to prevent transmission of the parasites.

206 *Toxoplasma gondii*

José G. Montoya, John C. Boothroyd,
and Joseph A. Kovacs

DEFINITION

- *Toxoplasma gondii* is a ubiquitous coccidian protozoan that usually causes asymptomatic infection in humans but can cause significant disease in congenitally infected infants and immunodeficient patients and occasionally in immunocompetent individuals.

EPIDEMIOLOGY

- Toxoplasmosis is a worldwide zoonosis that can infect a wide range of animals and birds.
- Transmission to humans is mainly by ingestion of viable tissue cysts in meat or of food or water contaminated with oocysts. Less commonly, there is congenital transmission or transplantation of an infected organ.
- Positive immunoglobulin G (IgG) representing prior infection increases with age; seroprevalence is ≈11% in the United States and up to ≈78% in other parts of the world.
- Congenital transmission occurs almost exclusively when the mother becomes infected during pregnancy. Retinochoroiditis can occur after congenital infection or recently acquired infection. Infection in human immunodeficiency virus (HIV)/acquired immunodeficiency syndrome patients almost always results from reactivation of latent infection. Among organ transplant patients, disease can result from either newly acquired infection from the transplanted organ or from reactivation of latent infection.

MICROBIOLOGY

- *Toxoplasma* organisms are exclusively intracellular. The sexual phase occurs in felines. Excreted oocysts require 1 to 5 days to become infectious. Tachyzoites actively replicate in essentially all cell types. Tissue cysts with intracystic bradyzoites maintain organism viability during latent infection.
- Tachyzoites replicate well in tissue culture and are responsible for clinical manifestations during primary infection or reactivation of latent infection.
- Multiple strains are identified by genotyping. Strains differ in virulence, with the most virulent strains so far reported being found in South America.

DIAGNOSIS

- Direct detection of the organism is by polymerase chain reaction (PCR) assay, histopathology with immunoperoxidase staining, or, less commonly, by tissue culture or mouse inoculation.
- Serologic assays can help distinguish acute from chronic infection and can identify patients at risk for reactivation. Immunoglobulin M (IgM)-positive test results should be confirmed at a reference laboratory (e.g., the Palo Alto Medical Foundation–*Toxoplasma* Serology Laboratory [PAMF-TSL]; www.pamf.org/serology/).
- Maternal infection is often asymptomatic; serology shows acute infection, and IgM-positive test results must be confirmed at a reference laboratory. Congenital infection may be asymptomatic or appear with neurologic or ocular manifestations; this form is diagnosed in utero by PCR of amniotic fluid or after birth by serology or PCR.

- Chorioretinitis may be asymptomatic or show visual loss; ophthalmologic examination and PCR of vitreous or aqueous fluid are performed. The Goldmann-Witmer coefficient (anti-*Toxoplasma* IgG/total IgG in aqueous fluid divided by anti-*Toxoplasma* IgG/total IgG in serum) can be helpful.
- HIV-infected patients usually present with focal neurologic symptoms. Patients are usually IgG positive and IgM negative, computed tomography or magnetic resonance imaging may show one or more contrast-enhancing lesions, cerebrospinal fluid PCR is specific but not sensitive, brain biopsy sensitivity is improved by immunoperoxidase staining, and diagnosis is often presumptive and extends to a response to empirical therapy.
- Immunodeficient patients present with encephalopathy, seizures, pneumonia, and fever. Diagnosis is based on positive PCR or histopathology. Hematopoietic stem cell transplantation (HSCT) requires pretransplant serology; solid-organ transplantation requires pretransplant serology in the donor and recipient.

THERAPY

- Immunocompetent patients: These patients usually require no therapy if asymptomatic; they may benefit from treatment if symptoms are severe or persist.
- Immunocompromised patients: The therapy dosage is pyrimethamine (200-mg load, then 50 to 75 mg/day) plus sulfadiazine (1000 to 1500 mg every 6 hours) plus leucovorin (10 to 20 mg/day). The dosage is then decreased to maintenance dosing of pyrimethamine (25 to 50 mg/day) plus sulfadiazine (500 to 1000 mg every 6 hours) plus leucovorin (10 to 20 mg/day) after 3 to 6 weeks if a clinical response occurs. Alternatives include pyrimethamine, as above, plus leucovorin plus either clindamycin (intravenous [IV] or oral [PO]; 600 mg every 6 hours) or atovaquone (1500 mg every 12 hours). Another alternative is trimethoprim-sulfamethoxazole (TMP-SMX) (IV or PO; 5 mg/kg of TMP every 12 hours). Corticosteroids are given only for clinically significant edema or mass effect, and anticonvulsants are given only after a seizure.
- HIV patients: Start antiretroviral therapy (ART) after 2 to 3 weeks; stop anti-*Toxoplasma* medications if the CD4 count is greater than 200 cells/mm^3 for more than 6 months. High relapse rate occurs without ART and maintenance therapy.
- Acute infection in pregnant women less than or equal to 18 weeks of gestation: Give spiramycin (1 g every 8 hours; available at no cost through the PAMF-TSL and the U.S. Food and Drug Administration) until delivery. If infection in the fetus is documented or suspected, or if at greater than 18 weeks of gestation, give pyrimethamine (50 mg every 12 hours for 2 days, then 50 mg/day) plus sulfadiazine (initial dose 75 mg/kg, followed by 50 mg/kg every 12 hours; maximum, 4 g/day), plus folinic acid (10 to 20 mg/day). Before 14 to 18 weeks of gestation, give no pyrimethamine or leucovorin.
- Congenitally infected infant: Give pyrimethamine (1 mg/kg every 12 hours for 2 days, then 1 mg/kg/day for 2 or 6 months); then this dose is given every Monday, Wednesday, and Friday; plus sulfadiazine (50 mg/kg every 12 hours) plus folinic acid (10 mg three times weekly) for at least 12 months.
- Chorioretinitis patients: If therapy is clinically indicated, give pyrimethamine (100-mg loading dose over 24 hours, then 25 to 50 mg/day) plus sulfadiazine (1 g every 6 hours) plus leucovorin (10 to 20 mg/day) for 4 to 6 weeks. TMP-SMX, one double-strength tablet every 3 days, can prevent relapse.

PREVENTION AND PROPHYLAXIS

- Avoid undercooked meat and potentially contaminated food or water; clean cat litter daily.
- Immunocompromised patients: Give TMP-SMX, one double-strength or single-strength tablet daily. An alternative is dapsone (50 mg/day) plus pyrimethamine (50 mg/wk) plus leucovorin (25 mg/wk). If the patient has HIV, start if the CD4 count is less than 100 to 200 cells/mm^3; discontinue if the patient is on ART and the CD4 count is greater than 200 cells/mm^3 for at least 3 months (primary prophylaxis) or 6 months (secondary prophylaxis). For HSCT recipients, start TMP-SMX after engraftment. If the patient is a solid-organ transplant recipient, start at transplantation if classified as D$^+$ or R$^+$.

207 Giardia lamblia

David R. Hill and Theodore E. Nash

DEFINITION

- Giardiasis, caused by the protozoan *Giardia lamblia*, is a common cause of sporadic, endemic, and epidemic diarrhea throughout the world.
- Infected persons can have acute diarrhea with malaise, cramping and bloating, chronic diarrhea with malabsorption, or asymptomatic infection. Asymptomatic infection is most common in children, particularly in low-income settings, and may contribute to poor nutrition.

EPIDEMIOLOGY

- *Giardia* is one of the most widely distributed enteric parasites.
- In the United States, there are approximately 20,000 documented infections annually, with estimated infections of more than 100,000; it is most frequently reported in children aged 1 to 9 years and adults aged 35 to 45 years.
- In low-income countries, *Giardia* infects nearly all children by the age of 10 years.
- Transmission of this fecal-oral parasite is most common through person to person transmission and through untreated or inadequately treated surface water.
- Although specific human genotypes (assemblages A and B) are found in some animals, epidemics of giardiasis caused by animals have not been reliably observed. Animals typically harbor other assemblages.

DIAGNOSIS

- A clinical syndrome of diarrhea lasting 7 to 10 days, and often associated with weight loss, is helpful in distinguishing giardiasis from other enteric infections.
- Useful epidemiologic risk factors are a history of travel, drinking untreated surface water, having young children in daycare, or engaging in sexual practices with the potential for fecal-oral transmission.
- Stool examination for ova and parasites is the traditional method of diagnosis.
- Antigen detection is widely available and is more sensitive and specific than stool examination for ova and parasites. Polymerase chain reaction assay is becoming more widely used and can identify the assemblage.

THERAPY

- Tinidazole is the drug of choice, taken in a single dose (see Table 207-1).
- Alternatives are metronidazole, nitazoxanide, and albendazole.
- Potential adverse events associated with treatment should be discussed with the patient.
- Treatment during pregnancy requires special considerations.
- Post-*Giardia* lactose intolerance should be considered if treatment appears to fail. If parasites are present, then re-treatment with a drug of a different class is usually successful.

TABLE 207-1 Treatment of Giardiasis

Drug (FDA Pregnancy Category)*	DOSAGE	
	Adult	Pediatric
Tinidazole (C)	2 g, single dose	50 mg/kg, single dose (maximum, 2 g)
Metronidazole[†] (B)	250 mg tid × 5-7 days	5 mg/kg tid × 7 days
Nitazoxanide (B)	500 mg bid × 3 days	Age 12-47 mo: 100 mg bid × 3 days
		Age 4-11 yr: 200 mg bid × 3 days
Albendazole[†] (C)	400 mg qd × 5 days	15 mg/kg/day × 5-7 days (maximum, 400 mg)
Paromomycin[†] (NC)	500 mg tid × 5-10 days	30 mg/kg/day in 3 doses × 5-10 days
Quinacrine[‡] (C)	100 mg tid × 5-7 days	2 mg/kg tid × 7 days
Furazolidone[‡] (C)	100 mg qid × 7-10 days	2 mg/kg qid × 10 days

FDA, U.S. Food and Drug Administration; NC, not categorized.

*FDA pregnancy categories: B, Animal reproduction studies have failed to demonstrate a risk to the fetus, and there are no adequate and well-controlled studies in pregnant women. C, Animal reproduction studies have shown an adverse effect on the fetus, and there are no adequate and well-controlled studies in humans, but potential benefits may warrant use of the drug in pregnant women despite potential risks.

[†]Not an FDA-approved indication.

[‡]No longer produced in the United States; may be obtained from some compounding pharmacies.

PREVENTION

- Prevention of giardiasis requires the proper handling and treatment of drinking and recreational water supplies, good personal hygiene, and protection of food supplies from contamination.
- Bringing water to a boil, filtration, and careful halogenation can be effective measures to treat small volumes of water.

208 *Trichomonas vaginalis*

Jane R. Schwebke

MICROBIOLOGY AND EPIDEMIOLOGY

- *Trichomonas vaginalis* is a flagellated parasite.
- Infection is through sexual transmission.
- Susceptibility to human immunodeficiency virus (HIV) infection may be increased.

DIAGNOSIS

- Infection causes vaginitis in women and may cause urethritis in men; it is often asymptomatic.
- In women, most cases are diagnosed using wet prep microscopy of vaginal fluid as the point of care test, but this lacks sensitivity.
- Gold standard for diagnosis is nucleic acid amplification testing.

THERAPY

- Metronidazole is the usual therapy.
- Resistance to metronidazole may occur.
- Tinidazole may be more effective.

PREVENTION

- Sexual partners should be treated.
- Condoms prevent infection.

209 *Babesia* Species

Jeffrey A. Gelfand and Edouard G. Vannier

DEFINITION

- Babesiosis is an emerging infectious disease caused by hemoprotozoan parasites of the genus *Babesia*.

EPIDEMIOLOGY AND MICROBIOLOGY

- The main etiologic agent of babesiosis in the United States is *Babesia microti*, a parasite typically found in white-footed mice and primarily transmitted to humans during the blood meal of an infected *Ixodes scapularis* nymphal tick.
- *B. microti* can also be transmitted via transfusion of blood products, primarily packed red blood cells. Transplacental transmission is rare.
- Babesiosis is a nationally notifiable disease in seven highly endemic states (Connecticut, Massachusetts, Minnesota, New Jersey, New York, Rhode Island, and Wisconsin) and 12 other jurisdictions.
- Risk factors for severe babesiosis include age older than 50 years, splenectomy, human immunodeficiency virus infection, malignancy, and immunosuppression therapies for transplantation or cancer.

DIAGNOSIS

- Fever is the salient symptom. Chills and sweats are common. Less frequent symptoms include headache, myalgia, anorexia, arthralgia, and nausea.
- Diagnosis is made on Giemsa-stained thin blood smears. Trophozoites often appear as rings. Tetrads of merozoites are pathognomonic. Other features that distinguish babesiosis from malaria include the lack of brownish deposit in rings, the absence of gametocytes, and the presence of extracellular merozoites.
- If parasites are not visualized on a smear and babesiosis is suspected, polymerase chain reaction assay–based amplification of parasite DNA should be performed. Serology confirms the diagnosis.
- Laboratory findings are consistent with hemolytic anemia and include low hematocrit, low hemoglobin, elevated lactate dehydrogenase level, and elevated reticulocyte count. Thrombocytopenia and elevated liver enzyme values are common.

THERAPY (SEE TABLE 209-1)

- Mild *B. microti* illness should be treated with a single 7- to 10-day course of oral atovaquone (750 mg orally every 12 hours) *plus* oral azithromycin (500 mg orally once, then 250 mg daily). Symptoms should be expected to abate within 48 hours and to resolve within 3 months.
- Severe *B. microti* illness requires hospitalization. Initial therapy should consist of a 7-to 10-day course of clindamycin (300 to 600 mg intravenously every 6 hours or 600 mg orally every 8 hours) *plus* oral quinine (650 mg orally every 8 hours). Despite therapy, half of hospitalized patients develop complications and about 10% die.

TABLE 209-1	Treatment of Human Babesiosis		
ORGANISM	SEVERITY	ADULTS	CHILDREN
Babesia microti*	Mild†	Atovaquone 750 mg q12h PO plus azithromycin 500 mg PO on day 1 and 250 mg/day PO from day 2 on	Atovaquone 20 mg/kg q12h PO (maximum 750 mg/dose) plus azithromycin 10 mg/kg PO on day 1 (maximum 500 mg/dose) and 5 mg/kg/day PO from day 2 on (maximum 250 mg/dose)
	Severe‡§	Clindamycin 300-600 mg q6h IV or 600 mg q8h PO plus quinine 650 mg q8h PO	Clindamycin 7-10 mg/kg q6-8h IV or 7-10 mg/kg q6-8h PO (maximum 600 mg/dose) plus quinine 8 mg/kg q8h PO (maximum 650 mg/dose)
Babesia divergens*		Immediate complete RBC exchange transfusion plus clindamycin 600 mg q6-8h IV plus quinine 650 mg q8h PO	Immediate complete RBC exchange transfusion plus clindamycin 7-10 mg/kg q6-8h IV (maximum 600 mg/dose) plus quinine 8 mg/kg q8h PO (maximum 650 mg/dose)

Note: Monitor patients on quinine with electrocardiography; monitor quinine serum levels in the setting of hepatic or renal disease.

IV, intravenously; PO, orally; RBC, red blood cell.

*Treatment for 7 to 10 days, but duration may vary.

†Atovaquone (750 mg twice daily) combined with higher doses of azithromycin (600 to 1000 mg/day) has been used in immunocompromised patients. With this regimen, symptoms and parasitemia resolve faster.

‡Consider partial or complete RBC exchange transfusion in cases of high-grade parasitemia (≥10%), severe anemia (<10 g/dL), or pulmonary, renal, or hepatic compromise. Even when parasitemia is less than 10%, consider exchange transfusion if acute respiratory distress syndrome or syndrome resembling a systemic inflammatory response syndrome is present.

§In asplenic individuals and in immunocompromised patients, persistent or relapsing babesiosis should be treated for at least 6 weeks, including 2 weeks during which parasites are no longer detected.

- If symptoms persist or relapse, antimicrobial therapy should last 6 weeks, including 2 weeks during which parasites are no longer seen on blood smear.
- Partial or complete red blood cell exchange transfusion is recommended when high-grade parasitemia (≥10%) or severe anemia (≤10 g/dL) occurs, or when pulmonary, renal, or hepatic systems are compromised.

PREVENTION

- No vaccine is available. Individuals at risk should avoid highly endemic areas.

210 Cryptosporidiosis (*Cryptosporidium* Species)

A. Clinton White, Jr.

DEFINITION

- Cryptosporidiosis is caused by infection with oocysts of *Cryptosporidium* species.

EPIDEMIOLOGY

- Cryptosporidiosis has a global distribution with a higher prevalence in resource-poor countries.
- Cryptosporidiosis is a major cause of prolonged diarrhea and malnutrition in children in resource-poor countries.
- Cryptosporidiosis is a major cause of diarrhea in adults infected by human immunodeficiency virus (HIV).
- Cryptosporidiosis is associated with person-to-person and waterborne transmission in wealthy countries.
- The major species, *Cryptosporidium hominis*, primarily infects humans.
- Zoonotic species, including *Cryptosporidium parvum*, are also common in humans.

MICROBIOLOGY

- *Cryptosporidium* species are apicocomplexan protozoan parasites.

CLINICAL MANIFESTATIONS

- Most patients present with diarrhea that is frequently prolonged.

DIAGNOSIS

- Diagnosis depends on demonstration of the organism in stool by antigen detection, nucleic acid amplification, or microscopy with acid-fast or fluorescent stains.

MANAGEMENT

- For immunocompromised hosts, there is no effective therapy, but reversal of immune defects is critical (e.g., treating underlying HIV with antiretroviral therapy).
- Nitazoxanide alone is effective in immunocompetent hosts but not in severely immunocompromised patients.

PREVENTION

- Water treatment and hand hygiene are key measures to prevent infection.

211 Cyclospora cayetanensis, Cystoisospora (Isospora) belli, Sarcocystis Species, Balantidium coli, and Blastocystis Species

Kathryn N. Suh, Phyllis Kozarsky, and Jay S. Keystone

CYCLOSPORA AND *CYSTOISOSPORA (ISOSPORA)*
Epidemiology

- Both are opportunistic pathogens in immunocompromised hosts but also infect noncompromised patients.
- *Cyclospora:* distribution is worldwide and is endemic in developing areas, with outbreaks in developed areas.
- *Cystoisospora:* occurrence is primarily in tropical and subtropical climes, especially South America, Africa, and Southeast Asia.
- Contaminated food and water are primary sources.
- Oocysts can survive in environment for months but must sporulate to become infective.

Diagnosis

- Acute or chronic diarrhea occurs with other constitutional and gastrointestinal symptoms.
- Oocysts in stool may be visualized using modified acid-fast stain.
- Multiple stool examinations may be required.

Therapy

- Trimethoprim-sulfamethoxazole, 1 double-strength tablet twice daily for 7 to 10 days, or ciprofloxacin, 500 mg orally twice daily for 7 days, is effective (see Tables 211-1 and 211-2).

SARCOCYSTIS SPECIES
Epidemiology

- Distribution is mainly tropical and subtropical, especially in Southeast Asia and Malaysia.
- Infection is widely distributed in various animals; human disease is very rare after consumption of infected raw or undercooked animal flesh.
- *Sarcocystis suihominis* and *Sarcocystis hominis* are the main causes of human disease.

Diagnosis

- Infection is generally asymptomatic.
- Rarely, self-limited gastrointestinal illness or myositis (fever, myalgias) occurs after exposure in endemic areas.
- Sporocysts or oocysts may be visible in stool; muscle biopsy may be required.

Therapy

- None; albendazole has been used.

BALANTIDIUM COLI
Epidemiology

- Distribution is worldwide, with infections in Latin America, Southeast Asia, Papua New Guinea, and the Middle East most common.

TABLE 211-1   Therapy (Adult) for Cyclosporiasis

DRUG*	THERAPEUTIC DOSAGE	PROPHYLACTIC DOSAGE
Trimethoprim-sulfamethoxazole	One DS tablet[†] PO bid for 7-10 days	One DS tablet PO three times weekly
Ciprofloxacin	500 mg PO bid for 7 days	500 mg PO three times weekly
Nitazoxanide	500 mg PO bid for 7 days	

DS, double strength; PO, orally.
*Drugs are listed in order of preference.
[†]One DS tablet contains 160 mg trimethoprim/800 mg sulfamethoxazole.

TABLE 211-2   Therapy (Adult) for Cystoisosporiasis

DRUG*	THERAPEUTIC DOSAGE	PROPHYLACTIC DOSAGE
Trimethoprim-sulfamethoxazole	One DS tablet[†] PO bid for 10 days	One DS tablet PO daily or three times weekly
Ciprofloxacin	500 mg PO bid for 7 days	500 mg PO daily or three times weekly

DS, double strength; PO, orally.
*Drugs are listed in order of preference.
[†]One DS tablet contains 160 mg trimethoprim/800 mg sulfamethoxazole.

TABLE 211-3   Therapy (Adult) for Balantidiasis

DRUG*	DOSAGE
Tetracycline	500 mg PO qid for 10 days
Metronidazole	750 mg PO tid for 5 days
Iodoquinol	650 mg PO tid for 20 days

PO, orally.
*Drugs are listed in order of preference.

- Pigs are primary reservoirs and shed cysts in stool.
- Cysts in contaminated food or water are infective.

Diagnosis
- The infection is generally asymptomatic; occasionally a diarrheal illness is reported.
- Trophozoites are visible in stool.

Therapy
- Tetracycline, metronidazole, or iodoquinol is used (see Table 211-3).

BLASTOCYSTIS SPECIES
Epidemiology
- Distribution is worldwide, primarily in developing countries, but prevalence varies markedly.

Diagnosis
- Role in human disease is unclear; diarrhea, flatulence, and abdominal discomfort are most commonly reported symptoms.
- Microscopic diagnosis is challenging; trichrome stain is the most sensitive.
- Polymerase chain reaction assay is more sensitive and specific but not widely available.

Therapy
- Therapy is often unsatisfactory.
- Trimethoprim-sulfamethoxazole, metronidazole, or iodoquinol is used (see Table 211-4).

TABLE 211-4 Therapy (Adult) for Blastocystosis	
DRUG*	DOSAGE
Metronidazole	750 mg PO tid or 1.5 g daily, for 10 days
Trimethoprim-sulfamethoxazole	One DS tablet[†] bid or two DS tablets daily for 7 days
Iodoquinol	650 mg PO tid for 20 days
Nitazoxanide	500 mg bid for 3 days
Paromomycin	25-35 mg/kg divided tid for 7 days

DS, double strength; PO, orally.
*Drugs are listed in order of preference.
†One DS tablet contains 160 mg trimethoprim/800 mg sulfamethoxazole.

212 Human Illness Associated with Harmful Algal Blooms

J. Glenn Morris, Jr.

DEFINITION

- Illnesses of primary concern caused by preformed toxins produced by algal species include ciguatera fish poisoning, paralytic shellfish poisoning, and amnesic shellfish poisoning.

EPIDEMIOLOGY AND MICROBIOLOGY

- Depending on the agent, illness is caused by ingestion of toxins in seafood or by inhalation or skin contact.
- Occurrence of illness is usually linked with blooms of specific toxic algal species (see Table 212-1). Harmful algal bloom–related illnesses in the United States have been reported from Atlantic, Pacific, and Gulf Coasts, Hawaii and Alaska, and the Caribbean (see Fig. 212-1).

DIAGNOSIS

- Diagnosis is based on clinical presentation (see Table 212-1).

THERAPY

- Therapy is supportive. The syndrome of hypotension/bradycardia seen in severe cases of ciguatera fish poisoning may require atropine; respiratory support may be necessary in severe cases of paralytic shellfish poisoning.

PREVENTION

- Prevention is based on avoidance of fish or shellfish that contain toxins. Environmental monitoring of shellfish for toxins responsible for paralytic, amnesic, and neurotoxic shellfish poisoning is conducted by state and local health departments.

TABLE 212-1 Human Illness Associated with Harmful Algal Blooms

SYNDROME	CAUSATIVE ORGANISMS	TOXIN PRODUCED	CLINICAL MANIFESTATIONS
Ciguatera fish poisoning	*Gambierdiscus* spp. and others	Ciguatoxin	Acute gastroenteritis, followed by paresthesias and other neurologic symptoms
Paralytic shellfish poisoning	*Alexandrium* spp. and others	Saxitoxins	Acute paresthesias and other neurologic manifestations; may progress rapidly to respiratory paralysis
Neurotoxic shellfish poisoning	*Karenia brevis*	Brevetoxins	Gastrointestinal and neurologic symptoms; formation of toxic aerosols by wave action can produce respiratory irritation and asthma-like symptoms
Diarrhetic shellfish poisoning	*Dinophysis* spp.	Okadaic acid and others	Acute gastroenteritis, abdominal pain
Amnesic shellfish poisoning	*Pseudonitzschia* spp.	Domoic acid	Gastroenteritis, followed by memory loss, neurologic manifestations; may progress to amnesia, coma, and death
Azaspiracid shellfish poisoning	*Azadinium* spp. and others	Azaspiracid	Acute gastroenteritis, abdominal pain
Lyngbya or *Cyanobacteria* exposure syndromes	*Lyngbya* spp.	Lyngbyatoxin A, debromaplysiatoxin	"Swimmers' itch," particularly in inguinal area; sore eyes, ears; headache; possibly gastrointestinal symptoms
	Microcystis spp.	Microcystins	(??)
Pfiesteria-associated syndrome	*Pfiesteria* spp. (?)	Unidentified to date	Deficiencies in learning and memory; acute respiratory and eye irritation; acute confusional syndrome

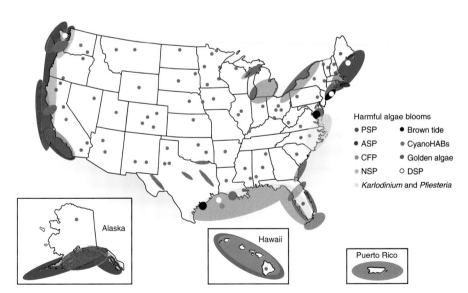

Harmful algae blooms
- PSP
- ASP
- CFP
- NSP
- Brown tide
- CyanoHABs
- Golden algae
- DSP
- *Karlodinium* and *Pfiesteria*

FIGURE 212-1 Sites and types of harmful algal blooms along the U.S. coast. ASP, amnesic shellfish poisoning; CFP, ciguatera fish poisoning; CyanoHABs, cyanobacterial harmful algal bloom; DSP, diarrhetic shellfish poisoning; NSP, neurotoxic shellfish poisoning; PSP, paralytic shellfish poisoning. (From U.S. National Office for Harmful Algal Blooms/Woods Hole Oceanographic Institution.)

213 Intestinal Nematodes (Roundworms)

James H. Maguire

DEFINITION

- Intestinal nematodes or roundworms are helminthic parasites of the human gastrointestinal tract (see Table 213-1).
- *Ascaris* and *Trichuris* (whipworm) are acquired by ingestion of contaminated soil.
- *Strongyloides* and hookworms *(Ancylostoma, Necator)* are acquired by exposure to larvae in soil.
- Only *Enterobius* (pinworm) is transmitted from person to person by ingestion of eggs or by contact with fomites.

EPIDEMIOLOGY

- Soil-transmitted helminths called *Strongyloides* are prevalent in tropics and subtropics. They infect more than 1 billion persons, primarily those with limited access to clean water and sanitation.
- In temperate areas and industrialized countries, *Strongyloides* are found primarily among immigrants and travelers returning from the tropics and subtropics.

MICROBIOLOGY

- *Ascaris* nematodes, hookworms, and *Trichuris* whipworms cannot replicate in a human host; hence, there is no person-to-person transmission. The duration of infection is the lifespan of adult worms, usually less than a few years.
- *Strongyloides* can replicate in human hosts; hence, infection is acquired via person-to-person contact and contact with larvae on soil. Infection persists for decades, and numbers of worms can increase without exogenous reinfection, especially in persons receiving corticosteroids or with human T-cell lymphotropic virus-1 infection.
- Pinworms are common in all parts of the world, particularly in children.
- Pinworms spread readily by person-to-person contact and ingestion of eggs shed in the environment, and infected persons frequently reinfect themselves and others in family.
- Hookworms, *Ascaris,* and *Strongyloides* migrate through the lung, but whipworms and pinworms do not.

DIAGNOSIS

- Intestinal parasite infections: usually cause light, few, or no symptoms but often elicit peripheral blood eosinophilia
- Soil-transmitted helminths: in children with moderate infections and those at risk of malnutrition
- Suggestive clinical syndromes: *Ascaris*: intestinal or biliary obstruction; hookworm: iron-deficiency anemia; *Trichuris*: intestinal prolapse, dysentery; *Strongyloides*: abdominal pain, diarrhea, larva currens, disseminated infection (immune compromised); pinworm: anal itching
- *Ascaris* nematodes, hookworms, and *Trichuris* whipworms: readily diagnosed by microscopic examination of the stool for characteristic eggs

TABLE 213-1 Features of Major Intestinal Nematodes

NEMATODE	TRANSMISSION	DIRECT PERSON-TO-PERSON TRANSMISSION	GEOGRAPHIC DISTRIBUTION	DURATION OF INFECTION	LOCATION OF ADULT WORM(S)	TREATMENT*
Ascaris lumbricoides	Ingestion of infective eggs	No	Warm, humid areas; temperate zones in warmer months	1-2 yr	Free in lumen of small bowel, primarily jejunum	Albendazole Mebendazole Pyrantel Ivermectin Levamisole Piperazine
Trichuris trichiura (whipworm)	Ingestion of infective eggs	No	Warm, humid areas; temperate zones in warmer months	1-3 yr	Anchored in superficial mucosa of cecum and colon	Albendazole Mebendazole
Necator americanus, Ancylostoma duodenale (hookworm)	Penetration of skin by filariform larvae	No	Warm, humid areas; temperate zones in warmer months	3-5 yr (Necator); 1 yr (Ancylostoma)	Attached to mucosa of mid to upper portion of small bowel	Albendazole Mebendazole Levamisole Pyrantel
Strongyloides stercoralis	Penetration of skin or bowel mucosa by filariform larvae	Yes	Primarily warm, humid areas, but can be worldwide	Lifetime of host	Embedded in mucosa of duodenum, jejunum	Ivermectin[†] Albendazole Thiabendazole
Enterobius vermicularis (pinworm)	Ingestion of infective eggs	Yes	Worldwide	1 mo	Free in lumen of cecum, appendix, adjacent colon	Albendazole Mebendazole Pyrantel Ivermectin Levamisole Piperazine

*Nitazoxanide has been shown to be effective in the treatment of ascariasis, trichuriasis, and enterobiasis in several trials in Mexico. Tribendimidine, which is licensed in China, was shown to be efficacious against Ascaris and had moderate efficacy against Strongyloides in a randomized trial.
†Drug of choice.

- Strongyloides: serology more sensitive than stool examination
- Pinworm: cellophane tape method

THERAPY

- Soil-transmitted helminths and pinworms; albendazole, mebendazole, or pyrantel
- Single dose effective for Ascaris, hookworm; multiple doses for Trichuris; repeat single dose after 2 weeks for pinworm
- Strongyloides: two daily doses of ivermectin; prolonged therapy for hyperinfection or disseminated infection

PREVENTION

- Sanitation, provision of clean water, wearing shoes, hand washing
- Periodic mass drug administration for soil-transmitted helminths
- Strongyloides: suspect, diagnose, and treat before immunosuppressive therapy

214 Tissue Nematodes (Trichinellosis, Dracunculiasis, Filariasis, Loiasis, and Onchocerciasis)

James W. Kazura

DEFINITION
- Tissue nematode infections cause a spectrum of disease manifestations ranging from asymptomatic cases to chronic pathologic processes and, occasionally, severe illness and death.

EPIDEMIOLOGY
- Infections with tissue nematodes occur throughout the world and have the highest prevalence in tropical regions where obligatory insect vectors are present.
- Trichinellosis
- Dracunculiais
- Filariases

MICROBIOLOGY
- The life cycles of these parasites are complex with five distinct stages that involve their human host and, where applicable, insect vectors.
- Trichinellosis
- Dracunculiais
- Filariases

DIAGNOSIS
- Parasites are identified microscopically in body fluids, or diagnostic assays are used to detect parasite antigens.

THERAPY
- Anthelmintic drugs are available for many infections.
- For trichinellosis, no drugs are available for treatment of newborn larvae or maturing first-stage larvae. Corticosteroids and mebendazole are sometimes utilized in severe disease. During the enteral stage of infection (1 to 2 weeks after eating contaminated meat), mebendazole or albendazole can be used to eliminate adult worms from the small intestine.
- For lymphatic filariasis, diethylcarbamazine is more active against *Wuchereria bancrofti* than *Brugia malayi*.
- Diethylcarbamazine is also used to treat tropical pulmonary eosinophilia and loiasis.
- Ivermectin is used to treat onchocerciasis.

PREVENTION
- Controlling insect vectors and mass administration of anthelmintic drugs to endemic populations reduces and may potentially eliminate transmission of medically significant tissue nematode infections.

Trematodes (Schistosomes and Liver, Intestinal, and Lung Flukes)

James H. Maguire*

DEFINITION
- Trematodes or flukes are flatworms that live in blood vessels, biliary tract, intestines, and lungs of humans and lower animals.
- Included are the schistosomes and the foodborne trematodes—liver flukes *(Fasciola, Clonorchis, Opisthorchis),* intestinal flukes (various species), and lung fluke *(Paragonimus).*

EPIDEMIOLOGY
- Schistosomes are prevalent in tropical and subtropical Africa, the Middle East, Southeast Asia, East Asia, the Philippines, and limited areas in the Caribbean and South America in areas with inadequate sanitation or access to clean water.
- Foodborne trematodes are most prevalent in Southeast and East Asia but also in other parts of the world where persons ingest raw or undercooked fish, crayfish, or plants produced in fresh water contaminated with human or animal feces or (for *Paragonimus*) sputum.

MICROBIOLOGY
- Persons become infected with schistosomes when the larval parasites (cercariae) shed by freshwater snails (intermediate hosts) penetrate bare skin.
- Persons become infected with foodborne trematodes by ingesting the larval parasites (metacercariae) encysted in fish, aquatic vegetation, or crustaceans (second intermediate host) that were infected with cercariae shed from snails (first intermediate host).

DIAGNOSIS
- Trematode infections are frequently light and may cause few or no symptoms but often elicit peripheral blood eosinophilia.
- Suggestive clinical syndromes during the first weeks after initial infection include acute illness with fever, urticaria, eosinophilia, and other symptoms when larval flukes are migrating through the body and maturing; ectopic migration can lead to disease of the central nervous system, the skin, and other parts of the body.
- Suggestive clinical syndromes during chronic infections include intestinal schistosomes (diarrhea, intestinal polyps, portal hypertension), urinary schistosomes (hematuria, bladder cancer), liver flukes (biliary obstruction), intestinal flukes (diarrhea, abdominal discomfort), and lung flukes (cough, hemoptysis, cavitary lung lesions).
- Diagnosis is made by microscopic identification of characteristic eggs in stool, urine, or sputum or by identification of larval or adult worms in tissue.
- Serology, available for some trematode infections, may be more sensitive than microscopic examination, especially during acute infections.

---

*All material in this chapter is in the public domain, with the exception of any borrowed figures or tables.

THERAPY

- Praziquantel is the drug of choice for all trematode infections except fascioliasis, for which triclabendazole is preferred (see Table 215-1).

PREVENTION

- For schistosomiasis, preventive methods include sanitation, provision of clean water, snail control, and avoidance of contact with contaminated fresh water.
- For foodborne trematodes, prevention of infection includes maintaining freshwater bodies free of contamination by humans and lower animals, snail control, and proper cooking of aquatic fish, plants, and crustaceans.
- Periodic screening and treatment or mass drug administration for populations at risk for infection are essential.

TABLE 215-1   Features of Schistosomes and Other Important Trematodes

PARASITE	SNAIL INTERMEDIATE HOST (GENUS)	SECOND INTERMEDIATE HOST	GEOGRAPHIC DISTRIBUTION	LOCATION OF ADULT WORMS	TREATMENT
Schistosomes*					
Schistosoma mansoni	Biomphalaria	None	South America, Africa, Caribbean, Arabian peninsula	Mesenteric venules	Praziquantel, 40 mg/kg/day in 1 or 2 doses × 1 day Oxamniquine[†]
Schistosoma japonicum	Onchomelania	None	China, Philippines, Indonesia, Thailand	Mesenteric venules	Praziquantel, 60 mg/kg/day in 3 doses × 1 day
Schistosoma mekongi	Neotricula	None	Cambodia, Laos	Mesenteric venules	Praziquantel, 60 mg/kg/day in 3 doses × 1 day
Schistosoma intercalatum, Schistosoma guineensis	Bulinus	None	Central and West Africa	Mesenteric venules	Praziquantel, 40 mg/kg/day in 1 or 2 doses × 1 day
Schistosoma haematobium	Bulinus	None	Africa, Middle East	Venules of lower urinary tract	Praziquantel, 40 mg/kg/day in 1 or 2 doses × 1 day Metriphonate[†]
Liver Flukes					
Clonorchis sinensis	Bithynia, Parafossarulus	Freshwater fish	China, Taiwan, Korea, Japan, Vietnam	Bile, pancreatic ducts	Praziquantel, 75 mg/kg/day in 3 doses × 1-2 days Albendazole,[‡] 10 mg/kg/day × 10 days
Opisthorchis viverrini	Bithynia	Freshwater fish	Thailand, Laos, Cambodia	Bile, pancreatic ducts	Praziquantel, 75 mg/kg/day in 3 doses × 1-2 days Albendazole,[‡] 10 mg/kg/day × 10 days
Opisthorchis felineus	Bithynia	Freshwater fish	Eastern Europe, former Soviet Union	Bile, pancreatic ducts	Praziquantel, 75 mg/kg/day in 3 doses × 1-2 days Albendazole,[‡] 10 mg/kg/day × 10 days
Fasciola hepatica	Lymnaea	Watercress, other aquatic plants	Americas, Europe, Asia, western Pacific, North Africa	Bile ducts	Triclabendazole,[§] × 10 mg/kg × 1 day Nitazoxanide[¶]

Continued

TABLE 215-1 Features of Schistosomes and Other Important Trematodes—cont'd

PARASITE	SNAIL INTERMEDIATE HOST (GENUS)	SECOND INTERMEDIATE HOST	GEOGRAPHIC DISTRIBUTION	LOCATION OF ADULT WORMS	TREATMENT
Intestinal Flukes					
Fasciolopsis buski	*Segmentina*	Aquatic plants	Far East, India	Small intestine	Praziquantel, 25 mg/kg/day × 1 day Niclosamide,[‡] 1 g × 1 day Triclabendazole[¶]
Heterophyes heterophyes	*Pirenella, Cerithidea*	Freshwater fish	Far East, Egypt, Middle East, southern Europe	Small intestine	Praziquantel, 25 mg/kg/day × 1 day Triclabendazole[¶]
Metagonimus yokogawai	*Semisulcospira*	Freshwater fish	Far East, Russia, southern Europe	Small intestine	Praziquantel, 25 mg/kg/day × 1 day Triclabendazole[¶]
Lung Flukes					
Paragonimus westermani; other species	*Semisulcospira, Onchomelania, Thiara*	Freshwater crabs, crayfish	Far East, South Asia, Philippines, West Africa, South and Central America	Lungs	Praziquantel, 75 mg/kg/day in 3 doses × 2 days Triclabendazole,[‡] 10 mg/kg day × 3 days

*Some experts recommend higher doses (e.g., praziquantel 60 mg/kg/day in divided doses for all species), multiple doses (e.g., for 2 or 3 days), or a repeated dose at 4 to 6 weeks to achieve higher rates of cure in persons not exposed to reinfection.
[†]Not available or limited availability.
[‡]Alternative drug.
[§]In the United States it is available (from the manufacturer, Novartis, from Victoria Pharmacy in Zurich, Switzerland) for compassionate use after approval of patient Investigational New Drug (IND) by the U.S. Food and Drug Administration.
[¶]Limited data.

216 | Tapeworms (Cestodes)

Charles H. King and Jessica K. Fairley

DEFINITION
- Cestodes are flatworms (platyhelminths) that cause human parasitic infection in the form of intestinal tapeworms or invasive larval cysts (i.e., neurocysticercosis or echinococcosis) (see Table 216-1).

EPIDEMIOLOGY
- *Diphyllobothrium latum,* fish tapeworm, is associated with eating undercooked fresh-water fish and endemic worldwide.
- *Hymenolepis nana* is the most common tapeworm worldwide and transmitted person to person.
- *Taenia saginata* (beef tapeworm) occurs in cattle-breeding areas of the world.
- *Taenia solium* (pork tapeworm), and consequently neurocysticercosis, is endemic to resource-limited areas, including Mexico, Central and South America, Asia, and Africa.
- *Echinococcus granulosus* infection occurs worldwide in livestock-raising areas and primarily is associated with domestic dogs.
- *Echinococcus multilocularis* has a life cycle that involves wild canines and is endemic only in the Northern Hemisphere.

MICROBIOLOGY
- Mature tapeworms reside in intestines of carnivorous animals.
- Eggs are shed and then pass to an intermediate host, causing cystic infection via dissemination of oncospheres into host tissues.
- Definitive carnivore host ingests cyst-infected tissue, and tapeworm then develops in intestines.

DIAGNOSIS
- Diagnosis of intestinal tapeworms relies on examination of stool for evidence of eggs or tapeworm segments (proglottids).
- Neurocysticercosis is diagnosed by typical appearance on imaging scans and supported by clinical symptoms and serologic testing.
- Echinococcosis is diagnosed by typical scan imagery and supported by serology.

THERAPY
- Mainstay of therapy for intestinal tapeworms is praziquantel or niclosamide.
- Neurocysticercosis therapy depends on the location and stage of the cyst.
- Parenchymal neurocysticercosis is generally treated with a combination of anthelmintic agents and corticosteroids (albendazole or praziquantel).
- Echinococcosis, depending on the stage and species, often requires surgery in combination with anthelmintic agents.

TABLE 216-1 Common Cestode Parasites of Humans, Their Typical Vectors, and Their Usual Symptoms

PARASITE SPECIES	DEVELOPMENTAL STAGE FOUND IN HUMANS	COMMON NAME	TRANSMISSION SOURCE	SYMPTOMS ASSOCIATED WITH INFECTION
Diphyllobothrium latum	Tapeworm	Fish tapeworm	Plerocercoid cysts in freshwater fish	Usually minimal; with prolonged or heavy infection, vitamin B_{12} deficiency
Hymenolepis nana	Tapeworm, cysticercoids	Dwarf tapeworm	Infected humans	Mild abdominal discomfort
Taenia saginata	Tapeworm	Beef tapeworm	Cysts in beef	Abdominal discomfort, proglottid migration
Taenia solium	Tapeworm	Pork tapeworm	Cysticerci in pork	Minimal
Taenia solium (Cysticercus cellulosae)	Cysticerci	Cysticercosis	Eggs from infected humans	Local inflammation, mass effect; if in central nervous system, seizures, hydrocephalus, arachnoiditis
Echinococcus granulosus	Larval cysts	Hydatid cyst disease	Eggs from infected dogs	Mass effect leading to pain, obstruction of adjacent organs; less commonly, secondary bacterial infection, distal spread of daughter cysts
Echinococcus multilocularis	Larval cysts	Alveolar cyst disease	Eggs from infected canines	Local invasion and mass effect leading to organ dysfunction; distal metastasis possible
Taenia multiceps	Larval cysts	Coenurosis, bladder worm	Eggs from infected dogs	Local inflammation and mass effect
Spirometra mansonoides	Larval cysts	Sparganosis	Cysts from infected copepods, frogs, snakes	Local inflammation and mass effect

PREVENTION

- Improved sanitation is essential.
- Education programs on symptoms of infection and keeping livestock in corrals away from humans should be implemented.
- Livestock at market or slaughterhouse should be screened for cysts.
- Dogs should be screened and treated to eliminate *Echinococcus granulosus*.
- Prolonged freezing or thorough cooking will kill cysts in tissue.

217 | Visceral Larva Migrans and Other Uncommon Helminth Infections

*Theodore E. Nash**

VISCERAL LARVA MIGRANS
Definition

- Visceral larva migrans (toxocariasis) is caused by *Toxocara canis* and less frequently by *Toxocara cati* and other helminths. It commonly occurs in children and may be manifested by fever, wheezing, hepatomegaly, and other generalized symptoms.

Diagnosis

- Diagnosis is based on the finding of larvae in affected tissues and the presence of eosinophilia.

Treatment

- Most patients recover without therapy.
- Anti-inflammatory drugs may be considered, and albendazole, mebendazole, and diethyl-carbamazine have been tried but are of uncertain efficacy.

OCULAR LARVA MIGRANS
Definition

- Ocular larva migrans is caused by *Toxocara canis* larvae in the eye and results in a chorio-retinal granuloma or occasionally in panuveitis. Retinal detachment may also occur. There is no specific therapy.

OTHER UNCOMMON HELMINTHS

- Other helminthic infections discussed in the chapter are anisakiasis, cutaneous larva migrans, eosinophilic meningitis, gnathostomiasis, angiostrongyliasis, eosinophilic gastroenteritis, dirofilariasis, capillariasis, nanophyetiasis, and swimmer's itch.

---

*All material in this chapter is in the public domain, with the exception of any borrowed figures or tables.

218 Lice (Pediculosis)

James H. Diaz

DEFINITION

- Pediculosis is a complex of three different human infestations (head lice, body lice, and pubic lice) with two species of bloodsucking lice: *Pediculus humanus* var. *capitis* or *corporis* and *Phthirus pubis.*

EPIDEMIOLOGY

- Head lice, or pediculosis capitis, are transmitted primarily by head-to-head contact rather than by fomites.
- Head lice afflict millions of people annually, mostly school-aged children.
- Body lice, or pediculosis corporis, are transmitted primarily by bodily contact rather than by fomites.
- Body lice are associated with poor hygiene and primarily infest the indigent, institutionalized, homeless, refugees, and immunocompromised.
- Pubic lice infestations (phthiriasis) are transmitted primarily during sexual contacts and often coexist with other sexually transmitted diseases.

MICROBIOLOGY

- Body lice can transmit several bacterial diseases, including (1) relapsing fever caused by *Borrelia recurrentis,* (2) trench fever caused by *Bartonella quintana,* and (3) epidemic typhus caused by *Rickettsia prowazekii. B. quintana* has been isolated in head lice from homeless persons in the United States, establishing the potential for transmission of trench fever by head lice in addition to body lice.

DIAGNOSIS

- Lice infestations are diagnosed by clinical inspection demonstrating live adult lice, nymphs, and viable eggs, or nits, in their precise human anatomic niches.
- Recently, dermoscopy has been used to immediately distinguish viable nits from hatched, empty nits.
- Dermoscopy may provide a more sensitive screening tool for head lice infestations than inspection alone.

THERAPY

- A combination of pharmacologic therapy with topical or oral (ivermectin) pediculicides and physical removal of viable nits by wet combing is required.
- Pharmacotherapy should begin with the least toxic pediculicides, such as pyrethrins.
- Topical or oral ivermectin preparations should be reserved for pyrethrin-resistant cases.

PREVENTION

- Combinations of sanitizing the environment and eliminating all human reservoirs of head lice in households, apartments, housing complexes, homeless shelters, classrooms, and schools are recommended.
- Prevention strategies for pubic lice are similar to the prevention strategies for body lice and should include hot cycle washing and drying of all clothing and bedding; institution of basic personal hygiene and sanitation measures; and treatment of sexual contacts with active body or pubic lice infestations.

219 Scabies

James H. Diaz

DEFINITION
- Scabies is an infestation by the itch or scabies mite *Sarcoptes scabiei* var. *hominis* and has become a significant reemerging ectoparasitosis in its most severe form as crusted or Norwegian scabies among the homeless, institutionalized older adults, the mentally retarded, and the immunocompromised.

EPIDEMIOLOGY
- The worldwide annual prevalence of scabies has been estimated to be about 300 million cases.
- Scabies occurs worldwide in both genders, at all ages, and among all ethnic and socioeconomic groups. Scabies is hyperendemic throughout the developing world, especially in sub-Saharan Africa, India, the Aboriginal regions of northern Australia, and the South Pacific Islands, especially the Solomon Islands.
- Crusted or Norwegian scabies is highly transmissible in the hospital environment.

MICROBIOLOGY
- The human scabies mite is an obligate parasite and completes its entire life cycle on its human hosts as females burrow intradermally to lay eggs and larvae emerge and mature to reinfest the same or new hosts. The entire incubation period from eggs to full-grown mites lasts 14 to 15 days.
- The human incubation period from initial infestation to symptom development is 3 to 6 weeks in initial infestations and as short as 1 to 3 days in reinfestations as a result of prior sensitization to mite antigens.

DIAGNOSIS
- The diagnosis of scabies is made by epidemiologic considerations and clinical observations.
- A clinical diagnosis may be confirmed by low-power microscopic examination of a burrow skin scraping that excavates the female mite.
- Skin biopsy may help confirm the diagnosis in atypical cases.
- Newer diagnostic methods for scabies include enhanced microscopic techniques (dermoscopy), immunologic detection of specific scabies antibodies, and molecular identification of scabies DNA.

THERAPY
- Both topical 5% permethrin and oral ivermectin appear most effective for individual classic scabies.
- The management of crusted (Norwegian) scabies may require combined, intense scabicidal therapies with both topical 5% permethrin and oral ivermectin, especially in high-risk community and institutional outbreaks.

PREVENTION

- Aggressive treatment of infested patients and all close household, institutional, and sexual contacts, especially in cases of highly infectious crusted (Norwegian) scabies, is required.
- Disposal or hot wash-dry sterilization (by machine washing and drying at 60°C [140°F] or higher) of all contaminated clothing and bedding of index cases is essential.
- Provision of improved access for personal hygiene and health care for all displaced, homeless, or institutionalized persons should be implemented.

220 Myiasis and Tungiasis

James H. Diaz

MYIASIS
Definition
- Myiasis is an ectoparasitic infestation of viable or necrotic tissues by the dipterous larvae of higher flies. Furuncular myiasis is the most common clinical manifestation of myiasis and occurs when one or more fly larvae penetrate the skin, causing pustular lesions that resemble boils or furuncles.

Epidemiology
- Myiasis is an opportunistic infestation that occurs in travelers returning from tropical jungles and in vulnerable populations living in endemic areas of the tropics.

Microbiology
- In human botfly furuncular myiasis, botfly larvae rapidly burrow into the skin with sharp mandibles to begin their developmental instar stages, which can last 6 to 12 weeks and cause draining, boil-like lesions, or furuncles.

Diagnosis
- The diagnosis of myiasis is usually by clinical inspection and examination, often with microscopy. Some immunodiagnostic tests have been developed to detect the antibodies to the antigens of specific fly species causing myiasis.

Therapy
- Furuncular myiasis may be treated conservatively by coaxing embedded larvae from furuncles by smothering their respiratory spiracles with occlusive coatings of petrolatum (Vaseline), clear fingernail polish, tobacco tar, pork fat, raw beefsteak, or bacon strips. However, unsuccessful occlusive therapy may asphyxiate larvae and necessitate their surgical or vacuum extraction. Along with larval removal, myiasis wounds should be cleansed and conservatively débrided, tetanus prophylaxis administered, and bacterial secondary infections treated with antibiotics.

Prevention
- Methods include control of domestic and livestock animal larval infestations; sanitary disposal of animal carcasses and offal to deny flies their preferred breeding grounds; proper management of any open human wounds or cutaneous infections; cementing floors to deny floor maggot flies their preferred egg-laying surfaces; sleeping on raised beds or cots in screened huts or tents; wearing long-sleeved shirts and pants, which can be pyrethrin- or pyrethroid-impregnated; spraying exposed skin with diethyl toluamide (*N,N*-diethyl-meta-toluamide [DEET])–containing repellents; and ironing both sides of all clothes and diapers left outside to dry in tumbu fly habitats.

TUNGIASIS
Definition
- Tungiasis is a painful, cutaneous infestation with the gravid female jigger flea that usually occurs on the feet but may occur anywhere where bare skin touches soil containing gravid female fleas.

Epidemiology
- In travelers returning to accessible health care infrastructures in developed nations, tungiasis is an exotic infestation, with a minimal parasite burden and a simple surgical cure, but in the impoverished and underserved communities of developing tropical nations, tungiasis is a recurrent infestation of the feet with a high parasite burden causing significant morbidity, including autoamputation.

Microbiology
- In tungiasis, the gravid female jigger (chigoe) flea penetrates bare skin usually on the feet (or heels), under or near the toenails or in the interdigital web spaces, to feed on blood and tissue juices and to incubate hundreds of developing eggs within days; it swells to 2000 times its size and then expels eggs over a period of 3 weeks or less before dying and leaving its shriveled carcass in a contaminated wound tract.

Diagnosis
- The diagnosis of tungiasis is usually by clinical inspection and examination, often with microscopy.

Therapy
- Tungiasis is treated by extracting all embedded fleas immediately with sterile needles or curets, administering tetanus prophylaxis, and treating secondary wound infections with appropriate topical or oral antibiotics.

Prevention
- Methods include wearing shoes, which can be sprayed with pyrethroid or diethyl toluamide–containing solutions; not sitting naked on bare ground; insecticide treatment of flea-infested domestic and stray animals and pets with 10% pyrethrin or pyrethroid sprays, or 1% to 4% malathion powder; bathing the feet of domestic and stray dogs and pigs with insecticide solutions, such as 2% trichlorfon (Neguvon); and spraying or dusting households, especially those with dirt floors, with 1% to 4% malathion.

221 Mites, Including Chiggers

James H. Diaz

DEFINITION
- Mites are among the smallest arthropods, with more than 3000 species, only about 25 of which, mostly chigger, animal, plant, and scabies mites, are of any medical importance.

EPIDEMIOLOGY
- Most mites are simply biting nuisances that can cause highly symptomatic maculopapular eruptions and do not transmit infectious diseases.

MICROBIOLOGY
- Only biting larvae of Asian scrub typhus chiggers (*Leptotrombidium* spp.) can transmit scrub typhus caused by *Orientia tsutsugamushi* (formerly *Rickettsia tsutsugamushi*), and only biting house mouse mites *(Liponyssoides sanguineus)* can transmit rickettsialpox caused by *Rickettsia akari.*

DIAGNOSIS
- Clinical diagnoses are highly sensitive and specific in the presence of a mite-bite outbreak.
- Mite-transmitted scrub typhus and rickettsialpox present clinically in a similar fashion with fever, bite eschar, regional lymphadenopathy, conjunctival injection, central nervous system symptoms in severe scrub typhus (e.g., confusion, delirium, coma, or transient hearing loss), and centrifugal rash in scrub typhus.

THERAPY
- Treatment of chigger bites is supportive with soap and water cleansing, warm water soaks, and topical and local anesthetics and antihistamines. Impetigo and secondary infections are potential complications that would necessitate antibiotic treatment.
- Both scrub typhus and rickettsialpox respond to treatment with oral doxycycline.

PREVENTION
- Chigger bites can be prevented with campsite spraying of pyrethrin or pyrethroid-containing insecticides; by spraying or impregnating pyrethrin and pyrethroid-containing repellents on clothing and sleeping bags; and by applying diethyl toluamide–containing insect repellents (*N,N*-diethyl-meta-toluamide [DEET]) to exposed skin.
- Rickettsialpox can be prevented by improving rodent reservoir control in campgrounds, homes, apartments, barns, sheds, and, especially, crowded public housing.
- There are no vaccines for scrub typhus or rickettsialpox.
- Weekly doses of 200 mg of doxycycline can prevent *O. tsutsugamushi* infections in endemic regions.

222 Ticks, Including Tick Paralysis

James H. Diaz

DEFINITION
- Ticks can transmit the broadest range of infectious microbes among all arthropods, including bacteria, viruses, and parasites.
- Gravid ticks may also transmit paralytic salivary toxins during blood-feeding.

EPIDEMIOLOGY
- Ticks are among the most competent and versatile of all arthropod vectors of infectious diseases.
- Tick-transmitted Lyme borreliosis or Lyme disease is now the most common arthropod-borne infectious disease in the United States and Europe.
- Most tick-borne infectious diseases can also be transmitted to humans by blood transfusions and organ transplants, and babesiosis can be transmitted congenitally.

MICROBIOLOGY
- Ticks of all ages and both genders may remain infectious for generations without having to reacquire infections from host reservoirs.
- New tick-transmitted pathogenic species are constantly being described in the United States.

DIAGNOSIS
- Ticks can transmit several pathogens during one blood-feeding, resulting in coinfections that can complicate differential diagnosis and treatment.
- The diagnosis of tick-transmitted infectious diseases is based on combinations of tick-bite history and characteristic lesions, such as erythema migrans and eschars, microscopic identification of pathogens in blood and tissue biopsy specimens, serologic and immunocytologic tests, and nucleic acid serotyping.

THERAPY
- Most tick-transmitted bacterial diseases remain sensitive to doxycycline, amoxicillin, and chloramphenicol.
- The tick-transmitted viral diseases can be managed only supportively.
- Babesiosis is caused by a malaria-like parasite and must be treated with combinations of antimalarial agents and azithromycin or clindamycin.

PREVENTION
- Combinations of immunization, prophylactic antibiotics, personal protective measures, landscape management, and wildlife management are all effective strategies for the prevention and control of tick-borne infectious diseases.
- A single 200-mg dose of doxycycline administered within 72 hours of a tick bite is more than 80% effective in preventing Lyme disease.

223 Kawasaki Disease

Jane C. Burns

DEFINITION

- Kawasaki disease (KD) is an acute, self-limited pediatric vasculitis that is the most common cause of acquired heart disease in children. Coronary artery aneurysms develop in 25% of untreated patients.

EPIDEMIOLOGY

- KD affects children of all ethnicities worldwide. Children of Asian and African-American descent are disproportionately affected. There is no evidence for person-to-person transmission. Temporospatial clustering of cases has been observed.

ETIOLOGY

- The cause of KD is unknown. According to the current paradigm, KD is triggered in genetically susceptible children after exposure to a widely dispersed agent.

DIAGNOSIS

- The diagnosis is established by fulfillment of four of five clinical criteria in a child with fever and no other apparent cause. Clinical criteria include bilateral conjunctival injection; a polymorphous rash; oropharyngeal changes including erythematous, fissured lips, erythematous oropharynx without discrete lesions, and strawberry tongue; extremity changes including edema of the dorsa of the hands and feet, palm and sole erythema, and periungual desquamation during the convalescent phase; and a cervical lymph node mass measuring at least 1.5 cm. Coronary artery abnormalities are detected by transthoracic echocardiography.

THERAPY

- High-dose intravenous immune globulin (IVIG, 2 g/kg) plus aspirin is the standard therapy for KD. If administered within the first 10 days after fever onset, the incidence of coronary artery aneurysms is reduced from 25% to 5%. A subset of patients (10% to 20%) may be relatively resistant to IVIG and require additional anti-inflammatory therapy.

PREVENTION

- There is no known intervention that can prevent KD.

Special Problems

224 Infections Caused by Percutaneous Intravascular Devices

Susan E. Beekmann and David K. Henderson*

DEFINITION

- Infections caused by peripheral and central intravenous catheters, including nontunneled central catheters and tunneled (Hickman or Broviac) catheters with or without the Groshong tip, peripherally inserted central venous catheters (PICCs), totally implanted intravascular access devices (ports), pulmonary artery catheters, and arterial lines

EPIDEMIOLOGY

- Rates of central line–associated bloodstream infections (CLABSIs) in 2009 ranged from 1.05 (pooled mean hemodialysis rate) to 1.14 (pooled mean inpatient ward rate) to 1.65 (pooled mean intensive care unit rate) bacteremias per 1000 central venous catheter (CVC) days.
- These rates reflect a 58% reduction in total estimated CLABSIs from 2001 to 2009; the reduction in incidence of *Staphylococcus aureus* CLABSIs was greater than for any other pathogen.
- The majority of CLABSIs now occur in inpatient wards and outpatient hemodialysis centers.

MICROBIOLOGY

- Staphylococci predominate as the most frequently encountered pathogens in device-related infections; coagulase-negative staphylococci are the single most common cause of these infections, whereas *S. aureus* bacteremias have decreased.
- CLABSIs increasingly are caused by multiresistant gram-negative rods.

DIAGNOSIS

- Clinical markers show a poor correlation with intravenous device–related bacteremia.
- Blood culture results positive for coagulase-negative staphylococci, *S. aureus*, or *Candida* spp., in the absence of any other identifiable source of infection, increase the possibility of intravenous device–related bacteremia.
- Quantitative or semiquantitative culture of the catheter combined with two blood cultures (one peripheral and one through the catheter) is most accurate for short-term central catheters.
- Paired quantitative blood culture was determined to be the most accurate diagnostic method for long-term devices, including tunneled and totally implanted catheters.
- Differential time to positivity (between cultures drawn through the catheter and peripherally) compares favorably with quantitative blood cultures for the diagnosis of CLABSIs.

PREVENTION

- Many CLABSIs can be prevented using simultaneous implementation of an array of practice improvements (i.e., "bundles").

---

*All material in this chapter is in the public domain, with the exception of any borrowed figures or tables.

- All health care personnel involved in catheter insertion and maintenance should complete an educational program regarding catheter-associated infections.
- Chlorhexidine solutions should be used for skin preparation before catheter insertion.
- Maximal sterile barriers should be used during insertion of CVCs.
- Do not routinely replace CVCs, PICCs, hemodialysis catheters, peripheral arterial catheters, or pulmonary artery catheters to prevent infection.
- Antimicrobial-impregnated catheters, if used, should only be used as part of a comprehensive nosocomial bacteremia prevention strategy.

225 Nosocomial Pneumonia

Michael Klompas

DIAGNOSIS

- Classic clinical signs for ventilator-assisted pneumonia (VAP) include fever, leukocytosis, purulent secretions, worsening oxygenation, infiltrates, and pathogenic cultures. These signs are neither sensitive nor specific. Paucity of neutrophils or lack of organisms on Gram stain make VAP unlikely, but their presence is not specific. Stable oxygenation/ventilator settings argue against clinically significant disease.
- Quantitative bronchoalveolar lavage (BAL) cultures are 51% sensitive, are 77% specific, and have a positive predictive value of 67% for histologically confirmed VAP.
- Randomized controlled trials of quantitative BAL cultures versus endotracheal aspirates for diagnosis have found no difference in duration of mechanical ventilation, length of stay, mortality, superinfection, or acquired resistance rates. Endotracheal aspirates are therefore preferred.
- Obtain diagnostic studies to guide therapy: blood and endotracheal aspirate cultures, urine pneumococcal and legionella antigens, ± viral studies.

MICROBIOLOGY

- Most common pathogens: *Staphylococcus aureus, Pseudomonas aeruginosa, Klebsiella* sp., and *Acinetobacter* sp. Drug resistance is common: 50% of *S. aureus* isolates are methicillin-resistant, 25% to 30% of *Pseudomonas* and *Klebsiella* isolates are ceftazidime and cefepime resistant, and 60% of *Acinetobacter* isolates are carbapenem resistant.
- Risk factors for methicillin-resistant *S. aureus* (MRSA) and multidrug-resistant gram-negative pathogens include recent broad-spectrum antibiotics, prolonged hospitalization, poor functional status, hemodialysis, and severe illness.

TREATMENT

- Initiate broad-spectrum antibiotics as soon as pneumonia is suspected. Use vancomycin or linezolid plus two antipseudomonal agents for empiric therapy. Consider a loading dose of vancomycin 25 to 30 mg/kg for seriously ill patients. Include anaerobic coverage if there is frank aspiration.
- Reassess the likelihood of pneumonia daily; if the diagnosis no longer seems likely, then stop antibiotics.
- Narrow treatment as soon as susceptibilities are available. Avoid double coverage. If cultures are negative and the patient is improving, trim or stop antibiotics.
- Vancomycin and linezolid are similarly effective for MRSA. Dose vancomycin 15 to 20 mg/kg every 8 to 12 hours. The goal trough is 15 to 20 mg/L. There is an increased risk of clinical failure if the vancomycin minimal inhibitory concentration is greater than 1 mg/L.
- Treat 7 to 8 days, but shorter for patients with rapid clinical improvement and longer for patients who are slow to improve or who have complications such as bacteremia, abscess, or empyema. Daily procalcitonin monitoring can safely shorten the duration of antibiotics.
- Adjunctive aerosolized antibiotics in addition to intravenous therapy enhance clearance of pulmonary cultures but have no impact on clinical cure rates or patient outcomes. Vibrating

mesh plate is preferred for delivery. Aerosolization may be as effective as intravenous drug delivery, but nephrotoxicity is equally likely. Data are sparse.

PREVENTION

- VAP rates are subjective and nonspecific. Therefore, preferentially select interventions proven to improve concrete outcomes.
- Noninvasive positive pressure ventilation, continuous aspiration of subglottic secretions, and ventilator-weaning protocols (especially paired daily spontaneous awakening and breathing trials) shorten the average duration of mechanical ventilation.
- Digestive decontamination decreases mortality, but there are ongoing concerns about the potential impact on antibiotic resistance rates, especially in units with high baseline resistance rates.

226 Nosocomial Urinary Tract Infections

Thomas M. Hooton

DEFINITION

- Nosocomial urinary tract infection (UTI) refers to UTI acquired in any institutional setting providing health care.
- Catheter-associated (CA)-bacteriuria is composed mostly of CA-asymptomatic bacteriuria (CA-ASB).
- CA-ASB should be distinguished from CA-UTI because treatment is usually indicated only for the latter.
- Significant bacteriuria: $\geq 10^3$ CFU/mL in a symptomatic person is an indicator of CA-UTI, whereas $\geq 10^5$ CFU/mL in an asymptomatic person is an indicator of CA-ASB.

EPIDEMIOLOGY

- Nosocomial UTIs, 97% of which are catheter associated, account for up to 40% of nosocomial infections in U.S. hospitals each year.
- Approximately 15% to 25% of patients in general hospitals have a catheter inserted at some time during their stay.
- About 5% to 10% of long-term care facility residents are managed with urethral catheterization.
- The incidence of bacteriuria associated with indwelling urethral catheterization with a closed drainage system is approximately 3% to 8% per day.
- The duration of catheterization is the most important risk factor for CA-bacteriuria.
- CA-bacteriuria comprises a large reservoir of antibiotic-resistant organisms and is a frequent target for inappropriate antimicrobial therapy.

MICROBIOLOGY

- A broad range of bacteria can cause nosocomial UTI, and many are resistant to multiple antimicrobial agents.
- CA-bacteriuria is caused by a broad range of bacteria, including *Escherichia coli,* other Enterobacteriaceae, nonfermenters such as *Pseudomonas aeruginosa,* and gram-positive cocci, including coagulase-negative staphylococci and *Enterococcus* spp.
- Funguria, mostly candiduria, is reported in 3% to 32% of catheterized patients.

DIAGNOSIS

- The majority of patients with CA-bacteriuria are asymptomatic, and signs and symptoms commonly associated with UTI, such as fever, dysuria, urgency, flank pain, or leukocytosis, are nonspecific.
- In the catheterized patient, pyuria does not differentiate CA-ASB from CA-UTI, but its absence suggests that CA-UTI is not the cause of symptoms.

THERAPY (SEE TABLE 226-1)

- Screening and treatment of ASB are not recommended except in pregnant women and some patients who undergo genitourinary surgery.

TABLE 226-1 Empirical Management of Catheter-associated Urinary Tract Infection

Antimicrobial Agent* and Dosing

Mild to Moderate, Afebrile (Dosage Duration: 5-7 Days)

Ciprofloxacin 500 mg PO twice daily or 1 g (extended release) PO once daily[†]
Levofloxacin 750 mg PO once daily[†]

Severe Illness or Febrile, or Both (Dosage Duration: 5-14 Days)

Ciprofloxacin 400 mg IV twice daily[†]
Levofloxacin 500-750 mg IV once daily[†]
Ceftriaxone 1-2 g IV once daily[‡]
Cefepime 1 g IV twice daily[‡]
Piperacillin-tazobactam 3.375 g IV q6h[‡]
Meropenem 500 mg–1 g IV q8h[‡]
Imipenem-cilastatin 500 mg IV q6-8h[†]
Doripenem 500 mg IV q8h[‡]
Ertapenem 1 g IV once daily[‡]
Gentamicin 5-7 mg/kg IV once daily[†] ± ampicillin 1-2 g IV q6h[§]

In Choosing an Empirical Agent, Consider the Following

Severity of illness and comorbidities
Antimicrobial susceptibility of prior urinary tract infection strains
Local resistance data
Exposure to same class in past 3-6 mo—choose alternative agent
Consider adding vancomycin if Gram stain shows gram-positive cocci
Use a carbapenem (meropenem, imipenem, doripenem, or ertapenem) if an extended-spectrum β-lactamase strain is known or suspected
Tailor regimen based on susceptibility data, and transition to oral medications (usually a fluoroquinolone), as soon as condition allows

*If resistance to the antimicrobial agent is a concern because of the prevalence of resistance in the community, especially in a severely ill patient, an initial intravenous dose of a broader-spectrum agent, such as meropenem, should be given.
[†]Pregnancy category C—animal studies have shown an adverse effect on the fetus; use only if potential benefit justifies the potential risk to the fetus.
[‡]Pregnancy category B—no clear risk to fetus based on animal or human studies, or both.
[§]Pregnancy category D—associated with human fetal risk; use only if the potential benefit justifies the potential risk to the fetus.
Modified from Hooton TM. Clinical practice. Uncomplicated urinary tract infection. *N Engl J Med.* 2012;366: 1028-1037.

- Urine cultures should be obtained before treatment of nosocomial UTI.
- Recommended treatment duration for CA-UTI ranges from 7 to 21 days, depending on the severity.
- Asymptomatic nosocomial candiduria rarely requires treatment.

PREVENTION

- Reducing exposure to urinary catheterization is the most effective way to prevent CA-bacteriuria.
- Indwelling urethral catheterization places the patient at greater risk for CA-bacteriuria than condom or intermittent catheterization.
- A closed catheter drainage system is indicated in all catheterized patients.
- Routine use of antimicrobial-coated urinary catheters is not supported by available data.
- Routine use of systemic antimicrobial agents to prevent CA-bacteriuria should be discouraged.
- Use of multiple infection control techniques and strategies simultaneously *(bundling)* is recommended to prevent CA-bacteriuria.

227 Health Care–Acquired Hepatitis

Kent A. Sepkowitz

DEFINITION

- Viral hepatitis can be acquired by patients or health care workers (HCWs) during the process of health care delivery.

EPIDEMIOLOGY

- Transmission between patients and HCWs is rare, but the risk remains.
- Dialysis patients and workers are at particular risk for hepatitis C virus (HCV) and, if unvaccinated, for hepatitis B virus (HBV).
- Increasingly, transmissions to patients are seen in long-term care and can be traced to unsafe injection practices.

DIAGNOSIS

- Identification of an outbreak is difficult unless a cluster of cases occurs.
- Most investigations are identified in conjunction with public health authorities.
- Use of a genotype to determine homology is useful in investigation.

POSTEXPOSURE TREATMENT

- Hepatitis A: Both immune globulin and hepatitis A vaccine have been used effectively.
- Hepatitis B: Treat all exposed nonimmune persons. If exposed but without HBV antibody, administer hepatitis B immune globulin with or without initiation of vaccine series. The role of antivirals has not been determined. Use a similar approach for exposed patients.
- Hepatitis C: Treat only if the exposed person has evidence of acute infection. Use of currently approved therapies has not been studied in this context but is likely effective.

VACCINATION

- Hepatitis A vaccine is not routinely recommended for HCWs.
- Hepatitis B vaccine or formal declination is mandated for HCWs.
- No vaccine is available for HCV.

228 Transfusion- and Transplantation-Transmitted Infections

Matthew J. Kuehnert and Sridhar V. Basavaraju*

DEFINITION

- Transfusion- and transplant-transmitted infections occur when a pathogen is spread from the donor to recipients through blood, organs, or other tissue.

EPIDEMIOLOGY

- Transfusion- and transplant-transmitted infections are unusual but occur when a donor has an infection but screening is not effective or when a pathogen is not screened. The risk of infection transmitted through organ transplantation is likely greater than through blood or tissue, due to the lack of inclusion criteria for organ donors.

MICROBIOLOGY

- Transfusion of blood product has transmitted infections by bacteria, viruses, parasites, and prions.
- Solid organ transplantation has transmitted infections caused by viruses, bacteria, fungi, mycobacteria, and parasites.
- Encephalitis following solid organ transplantation has resulted from transmission of West Nile Virus, lymphocytic choriomeningitis virus, rabies, and *Balamuthia mandrillaris*.

DIAGNOSIS

- Diagnosis is dependent on clinical recognition that a recipient has an infection that could have been from a transfusion or transplant.

THERAPY AND PREVENTION

- Better donor screening, or prompt recognition when transfusion- or transplant-transmitted infection occurs, can improve recipient outcomes.

---

*The findings and conclusions in this chapter are those of the authors and do not necessarily represent the official position of the Centers for Disease Control and Prevention.

229 Prophylaxis and Empirical Therapy of Infection in Cancer Patients

Elio Castagnola, Małgorzata Mikulska, and Claudio Viscoli

RISK FACTORS FOR INFECTIONS IN CANCER PATIENTS
- Neutropenia is the most important, particularly if severe (<100 polymorphonuclear neutrophils) and prolonged (7 to 10 days).
- Other risk factors include mucositis; underlying disease and its status; intensity of chemotherapy; the use of biologic response modifiers, especially monoclonal antibodies, such as alemtuzumab or rituximab; presence of central venous catheter; and genetic factors.

EPIDEMIOLOGY AND ETIOLOGY
- Epidemiology of bloodstream infections in neutropenia is constantly changing, and after years of the predominance of gram-positive cocci, gram-negative rods have been emerging in many centers as the most frequent pathogens.
- This shift has been accompanied by an increasing rate of resistant pathogens, such as extended-spectrum β-lactamase–producing Enterobacteriaceae, carbapenem-resistant gram-negative pathogens, methicillin-resistant *Staphylococcus aureus*, methicillin-resistant *Staphylococcus epidermidis*, or vancomycin-resistant enterococci.
- The main challenge is the management of multidrug-resistant (MDR) gram-negative bacteria for which few therapeutic options exist.
- Invasive fungal diseases (IFDs) in hematology patients are caused mainly by *Aspergillus*, in turn caused by a widespread use of *Candida*-active fluconazole prophylaxis (the emergence of fluconazole-resistant strains is the natural consequence), whereas in solid-organ tumors, candidemia remains the most frequent IFD.

PROPHYLAXIS (SEE TABLE 229-1)
- In general, antibacterial, antifungal, and antiviral prophylaxis is indicated in patients receiving induction chemotherapy for acute myelogenous leukemia (AML).
- Influenza and varicella vaccination of household contact and health care workers is recommended.
- Influenza and pneumococcal vaccination of patients, especially during less aggressive treatment phases, is recommended.
- Fluoroquinolones are recommended only for patients with prolonged (7 to 10 days) neutropenia in centers where resistance to fluoroquinolones is less than 20%.
- Primary antifungal prophylaxis in cancer patients is usually recommended if the incidence of IFD is higher than 15%.
  - Fluconazole is recommended as yeast-active prophylaxis in AML patients receiving anthracycline regimens.
  - Posaconazole as mold-active prophylaxis is recommended for patients receiving chemotherapy for AML or myelodysplastic syndrome.
- Secondary antifungal prophylaxis should be administered to patients with previous IFD who receive high-intensity chemotherapy or a transplant.
- Prophylaxis against *Pneumocystis jirovecii* (usually with trimethoprim-sulfamethoxazole three times per week) is beneficial in patients with deficits of T-cellular immunity,

TABLE 229-1 Suggested Prophylaxis for Infections in Cancer Patients

	DRUG	SCHEDULE	COMMENTS
Antibacterial	Ciprofloxacin	500 mg bid	Adults receiving chemotherapy for acute leukemia or autologous HSCT; starting with chemotherapy and continuing until resolution of neutropenia or initiation of empirical antibacterial therapy for febrile neutropenia
	Levofloxacin	500 mg once daily	
	Amoxicillin-clavulanate	25 mg/kg (max., 1000 mg) bid	Children receiving chemotherapy for acute leukemia
Antifungal	Posaconazole	Oral solution 200 mg tid orally with a (fatty) meal	Patients receiving chemotherapy for acute myelogenous leukemia or myelodysplastic syndrome
	Fluconazole	400 mg once daily	Patients receiving chemotherapy for acute myelogenous leukemia with cytarabine plus anthracycline regimens (administered for 7 and 3 days, respectively) and high-dose cytarabine-containing regimens
	Other		Secondary prophylaxis according to isolated pathogen and/or clinical presentation
Pneumocystis jirovecii	Trimethoprim-sulfamethoxazole	One-double strength tablet (160/800 mg) three times weekly, *or* 25 mg/kg of TMP-SMX (5 mg/kg of TMP), max., 1920 mg (two double-strength capsules) in 2 divided doses for 3 consecutive days/wk	All patients receiving chemotherapy with steroids, including those with solid tumors (e.g., brain cancer)
	Dapsone	2 mg/kg/day (max., 100 mg), on alternate days three times/wk	In patients who cannot tolerate TMP-SMX
	Aerosolized pentamidine	300 mg once a month with nebulizer	In patients who cannot tolerate TMP-SMX; effective, but it is more difficult to administer
	Atovaquone	750 mg twice daily or 1500 mg once daily	In patients who cannot tolerate TMP-SMX
Antiviral	Acyclovir *or*	2000 mg (40 mg/kg in children) in 4-5 divided doses or in adult >40 kg: 800 mg twice daily	Patients with positive anti-HSV antibodies and severe mucositis or receiving treatment for acute leukemia
	Valacyclovir	500 mg twice daily for HSV prophylaxis For VZV exposure 1 g three times daily	VZV-susceptible patients exposed to chickenpox who did not receive prompt administration of specific immunoglobulins
	Lamivudine	100 mg once daily	Patients with chronic inactive HBV infection (HBsAg-positive, HBV DNA low level or negative) Patients with resolved HBV infection (HBsAg-negative and HBcAb-positive) if receiving rituximab or allogeneic HSCT
Tuberculosis	Isoniazid	300 mg once daily	Patients with latent tuberculosis Efficacy not specifically evaluated in cancer patients
Central venous catheter	None	Good skin preparation and the use of sterile technique at time of device insertion Good maintenance procedures	All patients with indwelling central venous catheter

Continued

TABLE 229-1 Suggested Prophylaxis for Infections in Cancer Patients—cont'd

	DRUG	SCHEDULE	COMMENTS
Others	Growth factors	Filgrastim 300 µg/day (in children: 5 µg/kg/day) either subcutaneously or as an intravenous infusion over at least 1 hr, or pegylated filgrastim, 6 mg every 14 days	For the prevention of febrile neutropenia in patients who have a high risk of this complication based on age, medical history, disease characteristics, and myelotoxicity of the chemotherapy regimen Secondary prophylaxis with G-CSFs is recommended for patients who experienced a neutropenic complication from a prior cycle of chemotherapy (for which primary prophylaxis was not received), in which a reduced dose of chemotherapy may compromise disease-free or overall survival or treatment outcome Efficacy not fully demonstrated for pegylated filgrastim
	Immunoglobulins	Polyclonal immunoglobulins: 400 mg/kg every 21-28 days	Patients with chronic lymphocytic leukemia after the second episode of severe bacterial infection Patients with leukemia or lymphoma with hypogammaglobulinemia (<400 mg/dL) and severe bacterial infections (reasonable, but not proved)
		Specific anti-VZV (VariZIG) 125 IU for every 10 kg of body weight (max., 625 IU)	In high-risk contact with a negative history of varicella within 96 hours after exposure to chickenpox
	Vaccines	Influenza Varicella	Influenza and varicella (negative contacts) vaccination of household contact and health care workers Influenza vaccination of patients, especially during less aggressive treatment phases
		Pneumococcus	Conjugated-polysaccharide 13-valent antipneumococcal vaccine
	Isolation procedures	Perform hand hygiene with an alcohol-based hand rub or by washing hands with soap and water if soiled, before and after all patient contacts or contact with the patients' potentially contaminated equipment or environment Use contact precautions (gowns and gloves) Ensure adherence to standard environmental cleaning with an effective disinfectant	Patients colonized or infected with multidrug-resistant pathogens (such as VRE, KPC, etc.) or infected with other pathogens for which contact isolation precautions are advisable (*Clostridium difficile*, norovirus, etc.); of note, alcohol-based hand rubs are not sporicidal

G-CSFs, granulocyte colony-stimulating factors; HBcAb, hepatitis B core antibody; HBsAg, hepatitis B surface antigen; HBV, hepatitis B virus; HSCT, hematopoietic stem cell transplantation; HSV, herpes simplex virus; IU, international unit; KPC, *Klebsiella pneumoniae* carbapenemase; max., maximum; TMP-SMX, trimethoprim-sulfamethoxazole; VRE, vancomycin-resistant enterococci; VZV, varicella-zoster virus.

particularly with chronic lymphocytic leukemia, or in those receiving high-dose corticosteroids or alemtuzumab.
- Antiherpes prophylaxis with acyclovir or valacyclovir should be offered to patients with acute leukemia or receiving alemtuzumab.
- Varicella postexposure prophylaxis with specific immunoglobulins or acyclovir is recommended for high-risk varicella-zoster virus–susceptible patients.
- Lamivudine is recommended for cancer patients with chronic inactive hepatitis B receiving high-dose chemotherapy, particularly if containing rituximab, and for selected patients with a resolved hepatitis B virus infection.

MANAGEMENT OF FEBRILE NEUTROPENIA (SEE FIGS. 229-1 AND 229-2)
- Blood cultures
- Assessment of the risk of severe infection (e.g., Multinational Association for Supportive Care in Cancer score; see Table 229-2)
- Assessment of the risk of infection caused by resistant pathogens; risk is high in case of
  - Colonization or previous infection caused by resistant bacteria
  - Local epidemiology with high incidence of infections caused by resistant pathogens
- Choice of the appropriate therapy
  - Oral versus intravenous
  - Inpatient versus outpatient setting

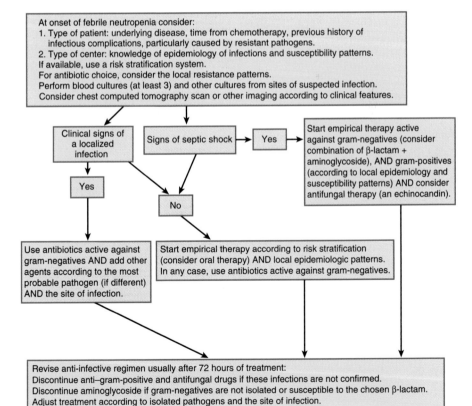

FIGURE 229-1 Possible initial approach to a patient with febrile neutropenia.

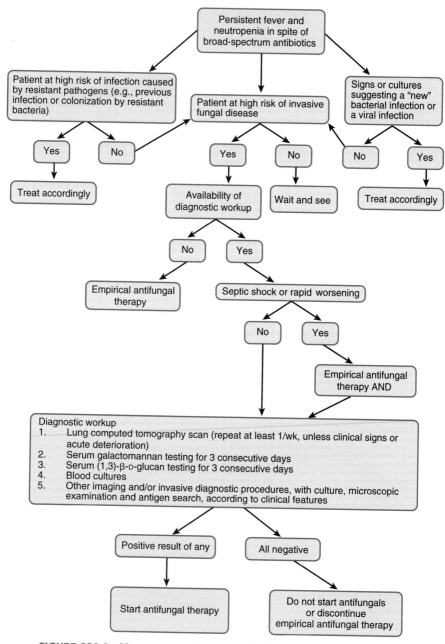

FIGURE 229-2 Management of persistently febrile neutropenic patient.

TABLE 229-2 Factors Associated with Low Risk of Severe Infection or Associated with an Uncomplicated Clinical Course in Febrile Neutropenic Cancer Patients

	MASCC SCORE	
	Clinical Parameters	Score
Clinical data available at onset of febrile neutropenia or soon after admission	1. Burden of illness: no or mild symptoms	5
	2. No hypotension	5
	3. No chronic obstructive pulmonary disease	4
	4. Solid tumor or no previous fungal infection	4
	5. No dehydration	3
	6. Outpatient status	3
	7. Burden of illness: moderate symptoms	3
	8. Patient's age <60 yr	2

MASCC, Multinational Association for Supportive Care in Cancer.
Points attributed to the variable "burden of illness" are not cumulative. The maximal theoretical score is therefore 26.
Low-risk patient: score ≥21.

- Escalation versus deescalation strategy
  - Escalation strategy usually starts with anti-*Pseudomonas* β-lactam monotherapy.
  - Deescalation strategy starts with a combination of anti-*Pseudomonas* β-lactam plus other agents covering the most probable resistant pathogens; these other agents should be discontinued if no resistant pathogen is isolated.
- Empirical antifungal therapy (adding antifungal agent in patients persistently febrile despite broad-spectrum antibiotics) could be replaced by diagnostic-driven strategy based on the use of diagnostic tools, such as a chest computed tomography scan and fungal serum markers (galactomannan and β-D-glucan).
- In the era of increasing antibiotic resistance and few agents active against MDR pathogens, antimicrobial stewardship in cancer centers is mandatory and should include
  - Infection-control practices
  - Local surveillance of antibiotic resistance, antibiotic consumption, and patient outcomes
  - Promoting appropriate antibiotic use (timely deescalation, appropriate dosing)
  - Establishing antibiotic regiments for empirical therapy appropriate for local epidemiology

230 Infections in Recipients of Hematopoietic Stem Cell Transplants

Jo-Anne H. Young and Daniel J. Weisdorf

TYPES OF DONORS OF STEM CELLS FOR HEMATOPOIETIC STEM CELL TRANSPLANTATION (HSCT)

- Syngeneic: donor is an identical twin sibling
- Autologous: the recipient donates to self
- Allogeneic: the donated material comes from a different individual than the recipient

SPECIFIC TYPES OF ALLOGENEIC DONORS

- Matched related or partially matched related donor, such as a sibling with the same or similar human leukocyte antigen (HLA) type
- Unrelated donor or matched unrelated donor
- Haploidentical: parent, cousin, sibling, or child is the donor; one HLA haplotype matched. Although haploidentical or other HLA mismatched transplants may lead to a high incidence of graft-versus-host disease (GVHD), administration of cyclophosphamide early post-transplant and T-cell depletion of the grafts may limit risks of GVHD.
- Cord: umbilical cord blood usually partially HLA matched, not matched for blood type; sometimes two cords used to provide blood with sufficient cells
- Haplo-cord: haploidentical peripheral blood stem cells plus cord blood cells; haplo-cord engrafts rapidly but may not be sustained yet provides neutrophil production until the cord engrafts

TYPES OF CELLS USED IN HSCT

- Peripheral blood stem cells, usually filgrastim (granulocyte colony-stimulating factor) mobilized; may be CD34 selected for T-cell depletion
- Umbilical cord blood: usually associated with delayed engraftment but less GVHD
- Bone marrow: collected by aspiration harvest from matched related or matched unrelated donor; associated with less chronic GVHD
- Donor lymphocyte infusion: donor cells sorted for lymphocytes; given after engraftment or after relapse for antitumor or antiviral effect but can stimulate GVHD

PREPARATION OF PATIENT FOR CELL INFUSION ("CONDITIONING REGIMEN")

- Myeloablative: total-body irradiation plus cyclophosphamide or busulfan; can be without irradiation
- Nonmyeloablative (reduced intensity): using lower-dose total-body irradiation or with anti-thymocyte globulin, most often with fludarabine

OUTCOMES

- Engraftment: absolute neutrophil count rises to more than 500 cells/μL by day 42
- Primary graft failure: no engraftment by day 42
- Mixed chimerism: persistence of host and donor hematopoiesis
- Relapse: return of the underlying malignant condition

COMPLICATIONS

- Mucositis: mucosal inflammation that serves as a portal of entry for oral or intestinal infections; common with methotrexate-containing regimens. Palifermin may reduce mucositis.
- Hemorrhagic cystitis: often occurs in conjunction with cyclophosphamide early after transplant, despite the use of mesna and forced diuresis; viral causes more common later after transplant, including adenovirus or BK virus
- Engraftment syndrome (immune reconstitution syndrome): fever with or without rash and/or pulmonary infiltrates at engraftment
- Veno-occlusive disease, also called sinusoidal obstruction syndrome: triad of jaundice, weight gain, and ascites leading to multiorgan failure, usually occurring in the first 3 to 4 weeks after transplantation
- Diffuse alveolar hemorrhage: bleeding into alveoli, usually during the second or third week after transplant; diagnosed by progressive bloody returns on lung lavage and treated with corticosteroids
- Graft-versus-host disease: inflammation and cell death (apoptosis) in skin, liver, gut, or lung. Acute form usually occurs until day 100. Chronic form generally occurs later and has features resembling but distinct from scleroderma. The risk is higher in the elderly and with grafts from partially matched donors. Calcineurin inhibitors (cyclosporine, tacrolimus), less often sirolimus, and mycophenolate mofetil are started soon after transplant to decrease the incidence and severity of GVHD. High-dose corticosteroids (and other agents) are used to treat GVHD.
- Posterior reversible encephalopathy syndrome: neurotoxicity from hypertension, calcineurin inhibitors, or fludarabine
- Bronchiolitis obliterans organizing pneumonia and obliterative bronchiolitis: pneumonitis associated with small airway injury, sometimes associated with chronic GVHD

ANTIMICROBIAL AGENTS FOR PROPHYLAXIS

- Acyclovir: low dose for herpes simplex virus, high dose for cytomegalovirus (see Table 230-1)
- Levofloxacin: used for prevention of bacterial infections, until fevers or infection develop
- Fluconazole: for prevention of candidiasis, starting with neutropenia
- Trimethoprim-sulfamethoxazole: agent of choice for *Pneumocystis;* also covers *Toxoplasma* and some bacteria, such as *Nocardia*. Alternatives include aerosolized pentamidine, atovaquone, and dapsone.
- Penicillin VK: prevention against *Streptococcus pneumoniae* during active chronic GVHD. Regional penicillin resistance may lead to the use of levofloxacin for this indication.
- Voriconazole or posaconazole: given in place of fluconazole to prevent mold infections
- Echinocandins (micafungin or caspofungin): intravenously administered agents that may be substituted for azoles
- Lamivudine: prevention of hepatitis B virus reactivation in anti–hepatitis B core antibody-positive, hepatitis B surface antigen–negative, and hepatitis B DNA–negative patient with hepatitis B–positive donors. Entecavir or tenofovir may be substituted for lamivudine.
- Entecavir or tenofovir: prevention of hepatitis B virus reactivation in hepatitis B surface antigen–positive patient
- Ivermectin: two doses for patients from countries with high risk for *Strongyloides* infestation

PREEMPTIVE THERAPY

- Ganciclovir, valganciclovir, or foscarnet: given to patients with cytomegalovirus reactivation based on polymerase chain reaction assay of blood or pp65 neutrophil antigen (see Table 230-1)

EMPIRICAL ANTIBACTERIAL THERAPY DURING FEVER AND NEUTROPENIA WITH NEGATIVE WORKUP

- Designated broad-spectrum agent such as ceftazidime, piperacillin-tazobactam, or cefepime
- Addition of an aminoglycoside possibly required for institutional antibiotic resistance patterns

TABLE 230-1 Suggestions for Management of Possible CMV Infection after HSCT

INDICATION	STRATEGY*	COMMENT
Prevention		
Allogeneic Transplant		
Seropositive recipient	Preemptive ganciclovir[†] induction for subclinical viremia, 5 mg/kg bid for 7-14 days, followed by 5 mg/kg daily until the end of maintenance or Ganciclovir prophylaxis[‡] at engraftment	Some cases of CMV disease may occur shortly after ganciclovir discontinuation. CMV reactivation might be delayed, occurring later after HSCT.
Seronegative recipient with seropositive donor	Preemptive ganciclovir induction for subclinical viremia, 5 mg/kg bid for 7-14 days, followed by 5 mg/kg daily until the end of maintenance and Seronegative or filtered blood products	Prophylaxis at engraftment is not recommended because of the low incidence of post-transplantation infection.
Seronegative recipient with seronegative donor	Seronegative or filtered blood products	
Autologous Transplant		
Seropositive recipient	Early ganciclovir induction of subclinical viremia, 5 mg/kg ganciclovir bid for 7 days, followed by 5 mg/kg daily for 14 days of maintenance	Because of the very low risk in some settings, monitoring is not uniformly advocated.
Seronegative recipient	Seronegative or filtered blood products	
Treatment of Disease		
CMV pneumonitis	Ganciclovir induction, 5 mg/kg bid for 14-21 days, followed by 5 mg/kg daily for at least 3-4 wk of maintenance plus IVIG every other day for the duration of induction	Extended maintenance throughout periods of severe immunosuppression (i.e., GVHD treatment) may be considered.
Gastrointestinal disease	Ganciclovir induction, 5 mg/kg bid for 14-21 days, followed by 5 mg/kg daily for at least 3-4 wk of maintenance	If deep ulcerations are present, maintenance may be required for a longer time.
Marrow failure	Foscarnet, 90 mg/kg bid for 14 days, followed by 90 mg/kg daily for 2 wk plus G-CSF	Ganciclovir plus IVIG has also been used.
Retinitis	Ganciclovir, 5 mg/kg bid for 14-21 days, followed by 5 mg/kg daily for at least 3-4 wk	Extended maintenance may be required.

CMV, cytomegalovirus; G-CSF, granulocyte colony-stimulating factor; GVHD, graft-versus-host disease; HSCT, hematopoietic stem cell transplantation; IVIG, intravenous immune globulin; PCR, polymerase chain reaction.
*Regimens should be accompanied by weekly monitoring with antigenemia or PCR-based nucleic acid testing.
[†]Oral 900-mg doses of valganciclovir produce blood levels that are similar to those for the standard intravenous dose (5 mg/kg) of ganciclovir. Foscarnet and cidofovir are acceptable alternatives. Renal dose adjustment is required for all antiviral agents.
[‡]Foscarnet, high-dose acyclovir, or valacyclovir are acceptable alternatives. Renal dose adjustment required for all antiviral agents.

- Vancomycin if any cellulitis, dysfunction with an indwelling catheter, or hemodynamic instability or colonized with methicillin-resistant *Staphylococcus aureus*.

VIRAL DISEASES IN THE TRANSPLANT RECIPIENT
- Herpes simplex virus: oral, esophageal, vaginal ulcers; autoinoculaton of other skin sites
- Varicella-zoster virus: dermatomal zoster; may disseminate; rarely severe hepatitis or visceral zoster
- Cytomegalovirus: fever, viremia, cytopenias, pneumonitis, gastrointestinal disorders (e.g., hepatitis, esophageal ulcers, mucosal changes in the duodenum or colon), retinitis

- Human herpesvirus 6: viremia, pneumonitis, encephalitis; may be associated with delayed neutrophil recovery or prolonged thrombocytopenia
- Adenovirus: hemorrhagic cystitis, pneumonitis, hepatitis
- BK polyomavirus: hemorrhagic cystitis
- Hepatitis B and C: hepatitis
- Major respiratory viruses: influenza, respiratory syncytial virus in the winter; parainfluenza virus and rhinovirus year-round.
- JC polyomavirus: progressive multifocal leukoencephalopathy
- Epstein-Barr virus: viremia or post-transplant lymphoproliferative disorder

OTHER INFECTIONS

- *Clostridium difficile* diarrhea: stool toxin polymerase chain reaction assay considered the best test
- Intravascular central catheter–related bacteremia or tunnel infection
- Typhlitis: abdominal pain and cecal edema during neutropenia
- *Pneumocystis* infection: diffuse pneumonitis among those not taking prophylaxis
- Candidiasis: candidemia originating from the gut
- Infection with *Aspergillus* and other molds: lung field abnormalities, sinusitis
- Toxoplasmosis: brain lesions

231 Infections in Solid-Organ Transplant Recipients

Nina Singh and Ajit P. Limaye

EPIDEMIOLOGY

- Infections in organ transplant recipients typically represent opportunistic infections, reactivation of latent organisms, and complications related to surgery, health care–associated infections, or both. Infections may also be donor derived.
- Advances in medical practices and preventive strategies have modified the risks and timeline of many infections in the current era.

TYPES OF INFECTIONS

- Bacterial infections are the most frequently occurring infections. Bacteremia occurs in 5% to 25% of transplant recipients.
- Fungal infections occur in 0.7% to 23% of patients. A majority of these are due to *Candida* or *Aspergillus* spp., with *Cryptococcus,* endemic mycoses, and other non-*Aspergillus* molds accounting for most of the others.
- Cytomegalovirus (CMV) is a major viral infection. In the era of routine antiviral prophylaxis, CMV disease typically occurs in the late post-transplant period. Other herpes viruses (herpes simplex virus, varicella-zoster virus, Epstein-Barr virus, human herpesvirus 6) are also seen with greater frequency and severity in transplant patients.
- Influenza and other respiratory viruses are a major cause of morbidity and mortality, especially in lung transplant recipients.
- BK virus nephropathy has emerged as an important cause of allograft dysfunction and loss in kidney transplant patients.

MANAGEMENT

- As a general principle, serologic assays, although valuable in the assessment of past exposure, are not reliable for the diagnosis of acute infections.
- Quantitative molecular assays have proved to be valuable tools for diagnosis, guiding preemptive therapy, and monitoring response to treatment for several viral pathogens (CMV, BK virus).
- Prophylaxis against *Pneumocystis* and *Toxoplasma* (heart transplant recipients) is considered standard. Preventive approaches are also routinely used for CMV, BK virus, fungal infections, and herpes simplex virus in selected transplant patients, based on risk factors.
- Evaluation should take into consideration the time elapsed since transplant, exposures, receipt of prior antimicrobial prophylactic agents, graft function, and the overall immunosuppressive state of the transplant recipient.

232 Infections in Patients with Spinal Cord Injury

Rabih O. Darouiche

DEFINITION

- Spinal cord injury (SCI) results from mechanical compression, vascular insult, or both.

PREVALENCE AND ETIOLOGY

- SCI affects almost 1 per 1000 persons.
- Causes of SCI include vehicular accidents, falls, violence, sports, and infection.
- Infection can cause or result from SCI.

URINARY TRACT INFECTION

- Urinary tract infection (UTI) is the most common infection and leading cause of rehospitalization.
- UTIs are mostly caused by usual bowel microbiota (gram-negative bacteria and enterococci).
- Intermittent catheterization is preferred to indwelling bladder catheters.
- Prevention is ineffective.
- Frequent unnecessary therapy is undertaken for failure to distinguish between clinical UTI and asymptomatic pyuria.

PNEUMONIA

- Pneumonia has the highest infection-related mortality.
- It occurs mostly in patients with tetraplegia.
- Community- and hospital-acquired microbes are comparable to those found in the general population.

INFECTION OF PRESSURE SORES AND BONE

- This diagnosis is very problematic.
- The broadest microbial etiology includes gram-positive cocci, gram-negative bacilli, and anaerobes.
- Multidisciplinary management is difficult and requires long and repeated hospital stays.

MULTIRESISTANT ORGANISMS IN SPINAL CORD INJURY UNITS

- Multiresistant organisms include methicillin-resistant *Staphylococcus aureus*, vancomycin-resistant *Enterococcus, Clostridium difficile,* and multiresistant gram-negative bacteria.
- These organisms are more prevalent in SCI units than in general hospital wards.
- Proper infection control measures reduce both colonization and infection.

233 Infections in the Elderly

Kent B. Crossley* and Phillip K. Peterson

GENERAL CONSIDERATIONS

- People living past 65 years of age are rapidly increasing in number.
- Individuals older than age 65 years have a higher incidence of most infections than do younger people.
- For nearly all infections, clinical manifestations are more subtle in the elderly.

URINARY TRACT INFECTION

- Asymptomatic bacteriuria should not be treated.
- Symptomatic infection is often caused by organisms other than *Escherichia coli.*
- Extended-duration therapy (i.e., >7 days) of symptomatic infection is not needed in either men or women.

PNEUMONIA

- Pneumonia is common and often followed by death in the year after a pneumonic illness.
- Nonbacterial causes (e.g., metapneumovirus, respiratory syncytial virus) are relatively frequent.
- Management of nursing home–associated pneumonia remains controversial.
- Immunization with influenza and pneumococcal vaccines is of significant but lesser benefit.

BACTEREMIA AND ENDOCARDITIS

- Both are more common in the elderly.
- Multidrug-resistant gram-negative organisms are commonly recovered from blood cultures of residents in long-term care facilities.

CENTRAL NERVOUS SYSTEM INFECTIONS

- Viral meningitis is uncommon in elderly individuals.
- West Nile virus infection has recently increased in frequency and is more common and more severe in the aged.

IMMUNIZATIONS

- Immunization with a serial combination of both pneumococcal vaccines is suggested for all individuals aged 65 years and older.
- A high-dose influenza vaccine is available for the elderly.
- Yellow fever vaccine is associated with prolonged viremia and delayed antibody response, with more severe adverse effects after immunization.
- Immunization against herpes zoster has been shown to reduce the incidence of disease and of postherpetic neuralgia. Recent studies have validated the safety of the vaccine.

---

*All material in this chapter is in the public domain, with the exception of any borrowed figures or tables.

234 Infections in Asplenic Patients

Janet R. Gilsdorf

EPIDEMIOLOGY

- Infection occurs in patients with congenital asplenia (rare), acquired asplenia secondary to splenectomy or sickle cell anemia, and acquired hyposplenia secondary to inflammatory or autoimmune disorders or human immunodeficiency virus–acquired immunodeficiency syndrome.
- The incidence is seven to eight severe infections per 100 person-years in postsplenectomy adults.
- Risk factors for infection include young or old age, less than 1 year after splenectomy, indication for splenectomy (immune cytopenias > trauma > incidental), lack of appropriate vaccines, and lack of prophylactic antibiotics in young children.

MICROBIOLOGY

- Encapsulated bacteria (*Streptococcus pneumoniae, Haemophilus influenzae,* and *Neisseria meningitidis*) are the classical pathogens of postsplenectomy sepsis.
- With widespread use of vaccines against encapsulated bacteria, *Staphylococcus aureus* and gram-negative enteric bacteria are seen more commonly.
- Asplenic patients are at risk for increased severity of malaria, babesiosis, and anaplasmosis.

DIAGNOSIS

- Blood culture is the most important test to identify postsplenectomy sepsis and must be obtained at the earliest sign of infection.
- White blood cell count may be elevated or depressed.
- Cerebrospinal fluid examination may be indicated in severe sepsis.
- Evidence of disseminated intravascular coagulation or vascular collapse may accompany sepsis.

TREATMENT

- Immediate empirical antibiotic therapy is key to preventing fulminant bacterial infection.
- Self-administered, oral antibiotics (amoxicillin-clavulanate, cefuroxime, or fluoroquinolone) may be used by asplenic patients at home at first sign of infection, followed by immediate visit to an emergency facility.
- Empirical systemic antibiotics (vancomycin + ceftriaxone or fluoroquinolone) must be started immediately at an emergency facility (after blood culture but before other diagnostic tests).
- Definitive antibiotic therapy will depend on the identification and antibiotic susceptibility of the infecting pathogen.

PREVENTION

- Patient education, repeatedly reinforced, is the responsibility of all health care providers.
- Avoid splenectomy if possible.

- Administer appropriate vaccines (Hib, PCV13, PPSV23, MCV4, MenB, influenza), as recommended by the Advisory Committee on Immunization Practices of the Centers for Disease Control and Prevention.
- Prophylactic antibiotics are recommended for children younger than 5 years of age, those who are immunocompromised, or patients with past history of sepsis.
- Avoid vectors that carry the parasites causing malaria, babesiosis, and anaplasmosis.

235 Infections in Injection Drug Users

Donald P. Levine and Patricia D. Brown

HOST DEFENSES

- Direct effects of opioids on the immune system include impairment of chemotaxis, phagocytosis, cytokine and chemokine production, natural killer cell activity, lymphocyte proliferation in response to mitogens, and antigen presentation by B lymphocytes. Indirect effects through the neuroendocrine system and the autonomic nervous system are also postulated.
- IgM and IgG levels are often elevated, giving rise to a high frequency of autoantibodies as well as antibodies against various microorganisms; this may cause diagnostic confusion (e.g., in interpretation of syphilis serology).
- Morphine-mediated depression of monocyte functions important to antiviral defense may contribute to the high efficiency of transmission of viruses such as hepatitis B and C viruses and human immunodeficiency virus (HIV).

SKIN AND SOFT TISSUE INFECTIONS

- Location of infection is related to the preferred location of injection; abscesses are most common, followed by cellulitis and skin ulcers.
- Infection with *Staphylococcus aureus* (particularly community-acquired methicillin-resistant *S. aureus* [MRSA]) is most common, followed by streptococci, either alone or in combination with other pathogens; infection with *Eikenella corrodens* occurs in injection drug users (IDUs) who lick their needles or contaminate their drugs with saliva; anaerobes and gram-negative bacilli are found in mixed infections.
- Incision and drainage is the mainstay of therapy for abscesses; for cellulitis, antibiotic selection and need for hospitalization must be individualized based on severity of illness; a high index of suspicion for necrotizing fasciitis should be maintained in the setting of severe pain or severe signs of systemic toxicity or both.

BONE AND JOINT INFECTIONS

- These infections are common, mainly affect the axial skeleton, and occur by the hematogenous route; contiguous spread from adjacent skin and soft tissue infection also occurs.
- Bacterial infection with *S. aureus* and group A and G streptococci are most common; infection with *Pseudomonas* is also reported; infection with *Eikenella* occurs in IDUs who lick their needles; and infection with *Candida* species is increasingly reported.
- Joint infections typically involve the extremities (most commonly the knee), although involvement of unusual sites (costochondral and sternoclavicular joints, pubic symphysis) is frequent; there is a high incidence of cervical spine involvement in persons with vertebral osteomyelitis.
- Microbiologic diagnosis should be confirmed in all cases; the use of high bioavailability oral antibiotic therapy for prolonged treatment is increasing.

INFECTIVE ENDOCARDITIS

- Incidence among IDUs appears to be increasing, perhaps owing to increased methamphetamine use (increased number of injections); IDUs with HIV are at even higher risk for infective endocarditis (IE).
- Infection with *S. aureus* is most common (the incidence of MRSA is increasing), followed by groups A, B, and G streptococci; outbreaks of gram-negative IE (caused by *Serratia* or *Pseudomonas*) are well described; and infection with *Candida* species (mainly non-*C. albicans*) have been reported.
- Tricuspid valve IE is associated with injection drug use, but the incidence of left-sided IE now exceeds that of right-sided infection in some series; multiple valves may be involved; infection of the pulmonary valve is rare.
- IDUs tend to present acutely in the first week of illness; diagnosis is usually easy to make based on the clinical signs and symptoms and supported by the results of blood cultures and cardiac imaging.
- Initial empirical therapy should be directed against *S. aureus* (with vancomycin or nafcillin in settings where MRSA is known to be rare); optimal therapy for MRSA isolates with vancomycin minimal inhibitory concentration of 2.0 µg/mL is not yet defined; many experts recommend daptomycin.
- Cefepime plus high-dose tobramycin has been used successfully in the treatment of pseudomonal IE; surgical therapy along with amphotericin plus flucytosine is the standard recommendation for candidal IE; the role of azoles and echinocandins is not yet defined; indefinite suppressive therapy with oral azoles is recommended if the patient is not a candidate for surgery.

NONCARDIAC VASCULAR INFECTIONS

- Infection with *S. aureus* most common; infection with *Pseudomonas* is also reported; polymicrobial infections are common.
- Septic thrombophlebitis presents as local pain, swelling, and fever, with bacteremia and sepsis; septic pulmonary emboli may occur; antibiotic therapy should be given for at least 4 weeks; the role of anticoagulation remains controversial—short-term anticoagulation while the patient is hospitalized may be sufficient.
- Mycotic aneurysms frequently involve the femoral veins and present as a tender, enlarging and pulsatile mass; Doppler ultrasonography, computed tomography (CT), or magnetic resonance angiography (MRA) can be used for diagnosis; surgical management is required, along with antibiotic therapy for 4 to 6 weeks.

PULMONARY INFECTIONS

- Community-acquired pneumonia caused by common respiratory pathogens is most common; patients are at risk for bacteremia, parapneumonic effusions, and empyema.
- Pulmonary tuberculosis is a major problem among IDUs, especially those infected with HIV; treatment for latent tuberculous infection is challenging; material incentives and directly observed therapy can increase adherence.

HEPATITIS

- Cocaine, methamphetamine, and buprenorphine (injected or sublingual) can be hepatotoxic; heroin is not.
- IDUs are at risk for hepatitis B virus infection and should be vaccinated if nonimmune; spontaneous reactivation of infection can occur.
- In nonendemic areas such as the United States, hepatitis D virus occurs almost exclusively in IDUs; although the overall prevalence of hepatitis D virus has decreased, the prevalence among those with chronic hepatitis B virus infection has increased.
- Superinfection of hepatitis D virus on chronic hepatitis B virus is most common; however, simultaneous infection occurs in IDUs and can result in fulminant hepatitis.
- IDUs account for the majority of hepatitis C infections in the United States, although the overall prevalence of infections in this population is decreasing; chronic infection develops

in 60% to 80% of patients; treatment is challenging and should be coupled with treatment for substance abuse.

- IDUs are at increased risk for infection with hepatitis A virus, but socioeconomic factors rather than drug use are the larger risk; nonimmune IDUs should be vaccinated.

SPLENIC ABSCESS

- Splenic abscess occurs most commonly as a complication of IE; secondary infection of a cocaine-induced splenic infarct or infection occurring after trauma also is reported; staphylococci and streptococci are the most common causative agents.
- Ultrasonography, CT, and magnetic resonance imaging can all be utilized for diagnosis; although splenectomy is generally considered the management of choice, especially in the setting of IE necessitating valve replacement, there is an increasing role for percutaneous drainage.

CENTRAL NERVOUS SYSTEM INFECTION

- Infection of the central nervous system occurs most commonly as a complication of IE (e.g., meningitis, brain abscess, mycotic aneurysms).
- Mycotic aneurysm may be diagnosed by CT, CT angiography, or MRA; optimal management is not defined; many aneurysms heal with antibiotic therapy; ruptured aneurysms require surgery or an endovascular procedure.
- The differential diagnosis of brain abscess is broad, especially in IDUs with HIV infection; microbiologic diagnosis should always be confirmed.
- Spinal epidural abscess should be suspected in IDUs who present with back pain accompanied by radicular symptoms or neurologic findings; S. aureus is the most common etiologic agent.
- IDUs are at increased risk for tetanus and wound botulism.

OCULAR INFECTIONS

- Bacterial and fungal endophthalmitis are seen, frequently as a complication of IE; Aspergillus endophthalmitis is also reported.
- Intravitreal antimicrobial agents with or without pars plana vitrectomy may be required.

HUMAN IMMUNODEFICIENCY VIRUS INFECTION

- Incidence of HIV infection among IDUs in the United States has steadily declined; however, injection drug use remains a major risk factor for HIV acquisition in other parts of the world.
- Needle exchange programs are effective at reducing HIV transmission but should ideally be coupled with access to voluntary counseling and testing, opioid substitution therapy, and combination antiretroviral therapy for those already infected.
- Injection drug use is associated with delayed entry into care and receipt of antiretroviral therapy; periods of incarceration are associated with virologic failure, but the prevalence of drug resistance is no higher than in non-IDUs.

SEXUALLY TRANSMITTED DISEASES

- Injection drug use is associated with high-risk sexual behavior, and reduction in risky sexual behavior is more difficult to achieve than reductions in risky injection behavior.
- The prevalence of common sexually transmitted infections appears to be no higher than in the general population, but because they play a role in the transmission of HIV, reducing infections in this population could reduce the transmission of HIV from IDUs to sexual partners.

236 Surgical Site Infections and Antimicrobial Prophylaxis

Thomas R. Talbot

BACKGROUND
- Surgical site infections (SSIs) are a common and unwanted outcome from most types of surgical procedures.
- The development of an SSI depends on patient-related, procedure-related, and pathogen-related factors, as well as the application of evidence-based prevention methods.
- Causative organisms of SSI are predominantly the flora present at the incision site.

RISK FACTORS FOR SURGICAL SITE INFECTIONS
(SEE TABLE 236-1)
- Patient factors include comorbid illness, colonization with pathogenic bacteria, perioperative hyperglycemia, and tobacco use.
- Procedural factors include breaks in sterile technique, operating room ventilation, and traffic.
- Proceduralist factors include surgical technique, improper application of skin antisepsis, and provider impairment.

PREVENTION OF SURGICAL SITE INFECTIONS (SEE TABLE 236-2)
- Practices to reduce bacterial inoculation into wounds include antiseptic use, sterile attire, decolonization strategies, and proper hair removal.
- Practices to improve host containment of introduced bacteria include maintenance of normothermia, minimizing tissue hypoxia, glucose control, and antimicrobial prophylaxis.

SURGICAL ANTIMICROBIAL PROPHYLAXIS
- Key principles:
  - Maintain tissue concentration of drug above minimal inhibitory concentration (MIC) of common flora (see Fig. 236-1).
  - Provide "right" drug: thus, target flora at surgical site, penetrate surgical incision site, and achieve minimal adverse events.
  - Provide "right" dose at the "right" time: provide dose in the window before incision to allow penetration into tissues (see Fig. 236-2); consider higher dose for obese patients; redose in prolonged procedures.
  - Provide "right" duration of drug: stop once incision closed or by 24 hours at the latest.
- Prophylaxis targeting resistant organisms may be warranted in select situations (e.g., known colonization with organism).
- Adherence to key principles of antimicrobial prophylaxis is used to assess overall quality of care and reimbursement from third-party payers.

SSI SURVEILLANCE
- SSI surveillance requires standardized definitions.
- Postdischarge surveillance of SSIs may lead to variability in reported outcomes and must be addressed as part of any surveillance system.

TABLE 236-1 Selected Factors Associated with an Increased Risk for Surgical Site Infection

Patient Factors

Diabetes mellitus/perioperative hyperglycemia
Concurrent tobacco use
Remote infection at time of surgery
Obesity
Low preoperative serum albumin
Malnutrition
Concurrent steroid use
Prolonged preoperative stay*
Prior site irradiation
Colonization with *Staphylococcus aureus*

Procedural Factors

Shaving of site the night before procedure
Use of razor for hair removal
Improper preoperative skin preparation/use of non–alcohol-based skin preparation
Improper antimicrobial prophylaxis (wrong drug, wrong dose, wrong time of administration)
Failure to timely redose antibiotics in prolonged procedures
Inadequate OR ventilation
Increased OR traffic
Perioperative hypothermia
Perioperative hypoxia

Proceduralist Factors

Surgical technique (poor hemostasis, tissue trauma)
Lapses in sterile technique and asepsis
Glove micropenetrations
Behavioral factors/proceduralist impairment

OR, operating room.
*Likely a surrogate marker for severity of underlying illness and comorbidities.
Modified from Mangram AJ, Horan TC, Pearson ML, et al. Guideline for prevention of surgical site infection, 1999. Hospital Infection Control Practices Advisory Committee. *Infect Control Hosp Epidemiol.* 1999;20:250-278; quiz 279-280.

TABLE 236-2 Interventional Maneuvers of Proven or Theoretical Benefit in Diminishing the Risk of Surgical Site Infection

Maneuvers to Diminish Inoculation of Bacteria into Wound

Preoperative Factors

Avoid preoperative antibiotic use (excluding surgical prophylaxis)
Minimize preoperative hospitalization
Treat remote sites of infection before surgery
Avoid shaving or razor use at operative site
Delay hair removal at operative site until time of surgery and remove hair (*only* if necessary) with electric clippers or depilatories
Ensure timely administration (including appropriate dose) of prophylactic antibiotics
Consider elimination of *Staphylococcus aureus* nasal carriage via decolonization techniques
Use standardized checklist for implementation at preprocedural time-out

Intraoperative and Postoperative Factors

Carefully prepare patient's skin with antiseptic + alcohol-based skin preparation agent (e.g., povidone-iodine-alcohol or chlorhexidine-alcohol–containing solution)
Rigorously adhere to aseptic techniques
Isolate clean from contaminated surgical fields (e.g., reglove and change instruments used to harvest saphenous vein before working in intrathoracic field)
Maintain high flow of filtered air
Redose prophylactic antibiotics in prolonged procedures
Minimize operative personnel traffic
Minimize immediate use steam sterilization of surgical instruments
Minimize use of drains
Bring drains, if used, through a separate stab wound

Continued

Part III Special Problems

TABLE 10-2   Initial Empirical Antimicrobial Regimens for Suppurative Infections of the Head and Neck—cont'd

Maneuvers to Improve Host Containment of Contaminating Bacteria

Preoperative Factors

Resolve malnutrition or obesity
Discontinue tobacco use for at least 30 days preoperatively
Maximize diabetes control

Intraoperative and Postoperative Factors

Minimize dead space, devitalized tissue, and hematomas
Consider use of supplemental oxygen therapy
Maintain perioperative normothermia (core temperature at or above 36.0° C)
Maintain adequate hydration and nutrition
Identify and minimize hyperglycemia (through 48 hours postprocedure)

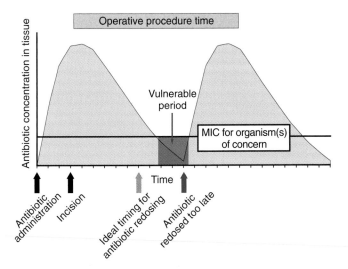

FIGURE 236-1   Tissue antibiotic concentration over time. Dynamics of tissue antibiotic concentration during the course of a surgical procedure. After an initial dose of antibiotic (noted on the far left of the x axis), tissue concentrations reach their peak rapidly, with a subsequent decline over time. As illustrated, the goal of antibiotic prophylaxis is to have tissue concentrations above the minimal inhibitory concentration (MIC) for the specific pathogens of concern at the time of the incision and throughout the procedure. Antibiotics should be redosed in prolonged procedures to prevent a period with tissue levels below the MIC *(light blue arrow)*. Failure to redose antibiotics appropriately *(dark blue arrow)* may result in a period during which the wound is vulnerable.

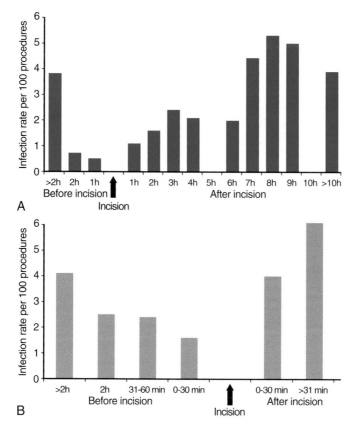

FIGURE 236-2 Timing of administration and infection rate. Relationship between timing of administration of prophylactic antibiotics and surgical site infection rate from two large studies. **A,** Data from 2847 elective surgical patients. **B,** Data from 3656 cardiac, orthopedic, and gynecologic surgical patients. (**A** from Classen DC, Evans RS, Pestotnik SL, et al. The timing of prophylactic administration of antibiotics and the risk of surgical-wound infection. *N Engl J Med.* 1992;326:281-286. **B** from Steinberg JP, Braun BI, Hellinger WC, et al. Timing of antimicrobial prophylaxis and the risk of surgical site infections: results from the Trial to Reduce Antimicrobial Prophylaxis Errors. *Ann Surg.* 2009;250:10-16.)

237 Burns

Clinton K. Murray*

DEFINITIONS

- Annually, 500,000 burn injuries receive medical treatment, and approximately 40,000 require hospitalization, of which approximately 55% are admitted to specialized burn centers.
- The primary insult from a burn is the wound itself.

EPIDEMIOLOGY

- Burn patient population: almost 70% of patients are men, with mean age 32 years, with 19% of patients younger than 5 years, and 12% age 60 years or older. The total burn size is typically less than 10% of total body surface area (TBSA) in 72% of cases.

---

*The opinions or assertions contained herein are the private views of the author and are not to be construed as official or reflecting the views of the U.S. Department of the Army, the U.S. Department of Defense, or the federal government. The author is an employee of the U.S. government, and this work was performed as part of official duties. All material in this chapter is in the public domain, with the exception of any borrowed figures or tables.

238 Bites

Ellie J. C. Goldstein and Fredrick M. Abrahamian

DEFINITION
- Bite wounds are common injuries caused by a wide variety of domestic and wild animals, as well as humans.

EPIDEMIOLOGY
- Bites occur in 4.7 million Americans yearly and account for 800,000 medical visits, including approximately 1% of all emergency department visits.

MICROBIOLOGY
- The bacteria associated with bite infections may come from the environment, the victim's skin flora, or most frequently, the oral flora of the biter, which can also be influenced by the microbiome of their ingested prey and other food.

DIAGNOSIS
- The diagnosis is made by the patient's reported history of events. Ultimately a microbiologic assessment of infected wounds is performed through aerobic and anaerobic cultures.
- Plain radiographs should be obtained if there is a high likelihood of bony injury.

THERAPY
- Irrigate wounds with copious amounts of normal saline.
- Cautiously débride devitalized or necrotic tissue.
- Primary wound closure is not usually advocated; delayed primary closure or allowing the wound to close by secondary intention is recommended.
- Loose approximation of wound edges with adhesive strips or sutures may be necessary for selected, fresh, uninfected wounds. Closure of facial wounds may be considered if coupled with copious irrigation and antimicrobial preemptive therapy.
- In most cases of terrestrial animal bites, antimicrobial therapy when indicated should include coverage for *Pasteurella* (*Eikenella* in human bites), *Streptococcus, Staphylococcus,* and anaerobes including *Fusobacterium, Porphyromonas, Prevotella,* and *Bacteroides* species.
- Oral antimicrobial choices can include the following (see Table 238-1):
  - Amoxicillin/clavulanic acid 875/125 mg one tablet by mouth twice daily
  - Clindamycin 300 mg by mouth four times daily *plus* ciprofloxacin 500 mg by mouth twice daily
  - Clindamycin 300 mg by mouth four times daily *plus* trimethoprim-sulfamethoxazole one double-strength tablet by mouth twice daily
  - Moxifloxacin 400 mg by mouth daily
  - Doxycycline 100 mg by mouth twice daily
- Intravenous antimicrobial choices can include the following:
  - Ampicillin/sulbactam 1.5 to 3 g IV every 6 hours
  - Cefoxitin 1 to 2 g IV every 6 to 8 hours

TABLE 238-1   Management of Bite Wounds

History

Animal bite: Ascertain the type of animal, whether the bite was provoked or unprovoked, and the situation/ environment in which the bite occurred. Follow rabies guidelines for details on management of bites that carry a risk of rabies.

Patient: Obtain information on antimicrobial allergies, current medications, splenectomy, mastectomy, liver disease, or immunosuppressive conditions.

Physical Examination

If possible record a diagram of the wound with the location, type, and approximate depth of injury; range of motion; possibility of joint penetration; presence of edema or crush injury; nerve and tendon function; signs of infection; and odor of exudate.

Culture

Aerobic and anaerobic cultures should be taken from infected wounds.

Irrigation

Copious amounts of normal saline should be used for irrigation.

Débridement

Devitalized or necrotic tissue should be cautiously débrided.

Radiographs

Plain radiographs should be obtained if bony penetration is possible and to provide a baseline for future evaluation of osteomyelitis.

Wound Closure

Primary wound closure is not usually advocated. Wound closure may be necessary for selected, fresh, uninfected wounds, especially large facial wounds. For larger wounds, edges may be approximated with adhesive strips in selected cases.

Antimicrobial Therapy

Early presenting (uninfected) wounds: Provide antimicrobial therapy for (1) moderate-to-severe injuries less than 8 hours old, especially if edema or significant crush injury is present; (2) bone or joint space penetration; (3) deep hand wounds; (4) immunocompromised patients (including those with mastectomy, advanced liver disease, asplenia, or chronic steroid therapy); (5) wounds adjacent to a prosthetic joint; and (6) wounds in close proximity to the genital area. In most cases, coverage should include *Pasteurella* (*Eikenella* in human bites), *Staphylococcus, Streptococcus,* and anaerobes including *Fusobacterium, Porphyromonas, Prevotella,* and *Bacteroides* species.

Infected wounds: Cover *Pasteurella* (*Eikenella* in human bites), *Staphylococcus, Streptococcus,* and anaerobes including *Fusobacterium, Porphyromonas, Prevotella,* and *Bacteroides* spp. The following antimicrobials can be considered for most terrestrial animal and human bites in adults:

- First choice: Amoxicillin/clavulanic acid 875/125 mg one tablet bid with food.
- Penicillin allergy: No alternative treatment for animal bites has been established for penicillin-allergic patients. The following regimens can be considered for adults:
  - Clindamycin 300 mg PO qid *plus* either ciprofloxacin 500 mg PO bid or levofloxacin 500 mg PO daily or trimethoprim-sulfamethoxazole one double-strength tablet PO bid
  - Doxycycline 100 mg PO bid
  - Moxifloxacin 400 mg PO daily
  - In highly penicillin-allergic pregnant patients, macrolides have been used, but because of poor antimicrobial coverage against anaerobic pathogens, the wounds must be closely followed.
- In cases where intravenous antibiotics are deemed necessary, single antimicrobial choices can include ampicillin/sulbactam, cefoxitin, ertapenem, or moxifloxacin.
- Empirical regimens for marine- and freshwater-acquired infection should also cover *Vibrio* and *Aeromonas* species, respectively, with agents such as third-generation cephalosporins (e.g., cefotaxime) and fluoroquinolones.

TABLE 238-1 Management of Bite Wounds—cont'd

Hospitalization

Indications include signs and symptoms of systemic toxicity and worsening infection.

Immunizations

Provide tetanus and rabies immunization, if indicated.

Elevation

Elevation may be required if any edema is present. Lack of elevation is a common cause of therapeutic failure.

Immobilization

For significant injuries, immobilize the extremity, especially the hands, with a splint.

Follow-up

Patients should be reminded to follow up within 48 hours or sooner for worsening or unresolved infections and continuous pain.

Reporting

Reporting the incident to a local health department may be required.

bid, two times a day; PO, orally; qid, four times a day; tid, three times a day.

- Moxifloxacin 400 mg IV daily
- Ertapenem 1 g IV daily
- Empirical regimens for marine- and freshwater-acquired infections should cover *Vibrio* and *Aeromonas* species, respectively, with agents such as third-generation cephalosporins (e.g., cefotaxime) and fluoroquinolones.

PREVENTION

- As a routine, antimicrobials are not advocated for every uninfected animal bite injury.
- In general, antimicrobial preemptive therapy is advocated for 3 to 5 days for uninfected animal bites (e.g., <24 hours after injury) in moderate-to-severe injuries, especially those to the hand or face, deep injuries penetrating bony structures, in the presence of edema, and in immunocompromised hosts.
- Provide tetanus and rabies immunization, as indicated.

239 Zoonoses

W. Ian Lipkin

DEFINITION

- A zoonosis is an infectious disease of humans that originates in animals.

EPIDEMIOLOGY

- Zoonoses account for more than half of all emerging infectious diseases and include such varied examples as human immunodeficiency virus/acquired immunodeficiency syndrome (HIV/AIDS), Ebola virus, severe acute respiratory syndrome, plague, rabies, influenza, and new-variant Creutzfeldt-Jakob disease.

DIAGNOSIS

- The majority of zoonotic diseases are diagnosed using molecular methods. Many appear in unexpected contexts; thus, a comprehensive travel and exposure history can be critical.

TREATMENT

- With the notable exception of HIV/AIDS and influenza, most viral zoonoses have not been a focus for drug development. Thus, treatment is primarily supportive. In contrast, many bacterial zoonoses can be treated with antibiotics.

PREVENTION

- Vaccines are established for only a minority of zoonotic diseases. Thus, prevention is best achieved by limiting exposure to reservoirs and vectors for transmission of infection.

240 Protection of Travelers

David O. Freedman

The pretravel office visit with an adult traveler to the developing world should follow a structured approach.

PERFORM RISK ASSESSMENT

- Exact itinerary, including regions within each country to be visited, dates of travel to assess risk of seasonal diseases, age, past vaccination history, underlying illness(es), current medications, pregnancy status, allergies, purpose of trip, risk exposures—blood, body fluids, adventure or extensive outdoor exposures, urban versus rural travel, type of accommodations, level of aversion to risk, and financial limitations that may necessitate prioritization of interventions

ADMINISTER IMMUNIZATIONS

- Routine vaccinations that are not up to date, including measles-mumps-rubella (MMR), tetanus-diphtheria–acellular pertussis (Tdap), pneumococcal, varicella, zoster
- Indicated routine travel vaccines, including hepatitis A, hepatitis B, typhoid, and influenza
- Indicated specialized vaccines, including yellow fever, rabies, polio, meningococcal, and, in certain countries, tick-borne encephalitis and cholera

PROVIDE MALARIA PREVENTION (IF INDICATED)

- Several equally effective drugs of choice may be indicated, including atovaquone/proguanil, mefloquine, and doxycycline. Ascertain which is best suited to the individual patient and itinerary.
- Educate on personal protection against arthropods.

TRAVELER'S DIARRHEA

- Recommend food and water precautions.
- Prescribe and educate on standby therapy with a quinolone antibiotic or azithromycin, and advise on use of loperamide and oral hydration if needed.

TEACH ESSENTIAL PREVENTIVE BEHAVIORS

- Most travel-related health problems, including vaccine-preventable diseases, can be avoided through simple behaviors initiated by the traveler.
- Educate on appropriate strategies in the following categories (some topics are not applicable to all destinations): blood-borne and sexually transmitted diseases, safety and crime avoidance, injury prevention, swimming safety, rabies, skin/wound care, tuberculosis, packing for healthy travel, and obtaining health care abroad.

DISCUSS OTHER APPLICABLE HEALTH ISSUES

- Advise and prescribe for altitude illness, motion sickness, or jet lag.
- Discuss prevention of specific travel-related infections that are of some risk to the traveler and have a possible preventive strategy not included in the strategies given above.
- Discuss any minimal-risk conditions (e.g., hemorrhagic fevers) that are a frequent cause of patient anxiety.

241 Infections in Returning Travelers

David O. Freedman

MAJOR SYNDROMES IN RETURNED TRAVELERS
- Fever, diarrhea (acute or persistent), skin problems, eosinophilia

TROPICAL DISEASES WITH POSITIVE PERIPHERAL BLOOD FILMS
- Malaria, babesiosis, filariasis, African trypanosomiasis, American trypanosomiasis, relapsing fever, bartonellosis

INCUBATION PERIODS OF TROPICAL DISEASES
- *Short (<10 days):* arboviral infections including dengue and yellow fever, hemorrhagic fevers, respiratory virus infections, typhoid, infection with gastrointestinal pathogens, spotted fever rickettsioses, relapsing fever, leptospirosis
- *Intermediate (10 to 20 days):* malaria, hemorrhagic fever, Q fever, typhus, typhoid, brucellosis, African trypanosomiasis, rabies, tick-borne encephalitis, Japanese encephalitis
- *Prolonged (>21 days):* viral hepatitis, malaria, rabies, tuberculosis, schistosomiasis, filariasis, amebic abscess, Q fever, Epstein-Barr virus infection

EVALUATION OF SIGNIFICANT TROPICAL FEVER
- *Any hemorrhagic manifestations?* If viral hemorrhagic fever is possible, isolate and call public health authorities; consider meningococcemia, rickettsiosis, sepsis, dengue.
- *Is malaria possible?* If there is end-organ damage, initiate empirical therapy.
- Utilize a "rule out malaria protocol," and use empirical therapy if no local expertise is available.
- Are there localizing findings? Go to syndromic approach and differential diagnosis.
- Are there no localizing findings? Consider typhoid, dengue, rickettsiosis, human immunodeficiency virus infection, leptospirosis, schistosomiasis (eosinophilia), amebic disease.
- Consult Table 241-1 for constellations of exposures and clinical presentations suggestive of particular diagnoses in returned travelers.
- Eosinophilia is caused by tissue-invasive helminths and is proportional to degree of tissue invasion.

TABLE 241-1 Constellations of Exposures and Clinical Presentations Suggestive of Particular Diagnoses in Returned Travelers*°

EXPOSURE SCENARIO	DISTINCTIVE FINDINGS	DIAGNOSIS
Any exposure in any area with documented malaria transmission	Fever with or without any other finding	Malaria
Most tropical countries	Fever and altered mental status	Malaria, meningococcal meningitis, rabies, West Nile virus
Budget travel to India, Nepal, Pakistan, or Bangladesh	Insidious-onset, high unremitting fever, toxic patient, paucity of physical findings	Enteric fever due to *Salmonella* Typhi or *Salmonella* Paratyphi
Freshwater recreational exposure in Africa	Fever, eosinophilia, hepatomegaly, negative malaria smear	Acute schistosomiasis (Katayama fever)
Bitten by *Aedes aegypti* in Central America, Southeast Asia, or the South Pacific	Fever, headache, myalgia, diffuse macular rash, mild to moderate thrombocytopenia	Dengue
Bitten by *A. aegypti* or *Aedes albopictus* in India, Malaysia, Singapore, the Caribbean, or an island in the Indian Ocean	Fever, headache, myalgia, diffuse macular rash, arthralgia, tenosynovitis often followed by chronic polyarthritis after the fever resolves	Chikungunya fever
Hunting or visiting game reserves in southern Africa	Fever, eschar, diffuse petechial rash	African tick typhus due to *Rickettsia africae*
Travel to Southeast Asia	Fever, eschar, diffuse petechial rash	Scrub typhus due to *Orientia tsutsugamushi*
Hiking, biking, swimming, rafting with exposure to fresh surface water	Fever, myalgia, conjunctival suffusion, mild to severe jaundice, variable rash	Leptospirosis
Cruise, elderly traveler	Influenza-like illness	Influenza A or B
Outdoor exposure anywhere in the Americas	Large, single furuncular lesion anywhere on body, with sense of movement inside	Myiasis due to *Dermatobia hominis* (botfly)
Clothing washed or dried out of doors in Africa	Multiple furuncular lesions around clothing contact points with skin	Myiasis due to *Cordylobia anthropophaga* (tumbu fly)
New sexual partner during travel	Fever, rash, mononucleosis-like illness	Acute human immunodeficiency virus infection
Travel to any developing country or to Western Europe	Coryza, conjunctivitis, Koplik spots, rash	Measles
Longer visit to humid areas of Africa, the Americas, or Southeast Asia	Asymptomatic eosinophilia or with periodic cough or wheezing	Strongyloidiasis
Sand fly bite in either New or Old World tropical area	Painless skin ulcer with clean, moist base in exposed area	Cutaneous leishmaniasis
Resort hotel in southern Europe, ± exposure to whirlpool spas	Pneumonia	Legionnaires' disease
Explored a cave in the Americas	Fever, cough, retrosternal chest pain, hilar adenopathy	Histoplasmosis
Ingestion of unpasteurized goat cheese	Chronic fever, fatigue	*Brucella melitensis*
Long trip to West/Central Africa	Afebrile, intensely pruritic, evanescent truncal maculopapular rash	Onchocerciasis
Long trip to West/Central Africa	Migratory localized angioedema or swellings over large joints, eosinophilia	Loiasis
Safari to game parks of East Africa	Fever, nongenital chancre, fine macular rash	East African trypanosomiasis
Travel to Australia	Fever, fatigue, polyarthritis	Ross River virus
Farming areas of India and Southeast Asia	Fever, altered mental status, paralysis	Japanese encephalitis
Forested areas of central and eastern Europe and across Russia	Fever, altered mental status, paralysis	Tick-borne encephalitis

TABLE 241-1   Constellations of Exposures and Clinical Presentations Suggestive of Particular Diagnoses in Returned Travelers*—cont'd

EXPOSURE SCENARIO	DISTINCTIVE FINDINGS	DIAGNOSIS
Rodent exposure in West Africa	Fever, sore throat, jaundice, hemorrhagic manifestations	Lassa fever
Ingestion of sushi, ceviche, or raw freshwater fish	Migratory nodules in truncal areas with overlying erythema or mild hemorrhage	Gnathostomiasis
Returning Hajj pilgrim or family contact	Fever, meningitis	Meningococcal meningitis
Ingestion of snails, fish, or shellfish in Asia or Australia	Eosinophilic meningitis	Angiostrongyliasis, gnathostomiasis
Diabetic or compromised host with exposure to moist terrain in Asia or Australia	Fever, sepsis, pneumonia or multifocal abscesses	Melioidosis
Summertime exposure to rodent droppings in Scandinavia	Fever with decreased renal function	Puumala virus
Ingestion of undercooked meat of any animal in any country	Fever, facial edema, myositis, increased creatine phosphokinase, massive eosinophilia, normal erythrocyte sedimentation rate	Trichinosis
Unvaccinated, returning from sub-Saharan Africa or forested areas of Amazonia	Fever, jaundice, proteinuria, hemorrhage	Yellow fever
Exposure to farm animals	Pneumonia, mild hepatitis	Q fever
Possible tick exposure almost anywhere	Fever, headache, rash, conjunctival injection, hepatosplenomegaly	Tick-borne relapsing fever
Poor hygienic conditions with possible body louse exposure in Ethiopia or Sudan	Fever, headache, rash, conjunctival injection, hepatosplenomegaly	Louse-borne relapsing fever

*The table includes illnesses of travelers (listed first) as well as less common diseases with presentations that should suggest the possibility of the appropriate diagnosis. Many diseases have a spectrum of presentation, and the table describes the most common presentations of these diseases. Many diseases have a spectrum of geographic origins, and the table describes the most common exposures seen in daily practice.

Index

Page numbers followed by *f* indicate figures and *t* indicate tables.